Lecture Notes: Nephrology

Welcome to the series home page for the *Lecture Notes* books for medical students and junior doctors.
- The series covers over 35 subjects providing the concise core knowledge required by medical students and junior doctors
- Each book written by an expert teacher in note form, with bullet lists, illustrations, and summary boxes
- A panel of medical students reviews each text to ensure that the coverage is exactly right for its audience
- Ideal as course textbooks or revision aids

To view the full range of other titles in the Lecture Notes series, scan this QR code:

Lecture Notes:
Nephrology
A Comprehensive Guide
to Renal Medicine

Edited by

Dr Surjit Tarafdar

General Physician and Nephrologist
Blacktown and Mt Druitt Hospital
Blacktown
New South Wales, Sydney, Australia

Conjoint Senior Lecturer
Department of Medicine
Western Sydney University
Sydney, Australia

WILEY Blackwell

This edition first published 2020

© 2020 by John Wiley & Sons Ltd

Registered Office(s)

John Wiley & Sons, Inc., 111 River Street, Hoboken, NJ 07030, USA

John Wiley & Sons Ltd, The Atrium, Southern Gate, Chichester, West Sussex, PO19 8SQ, UK

Editorial Office

9600 Garsington Road, Oxford, OX4 2DQ, UK

For details of our global editorial offices, customer services, and more information about Wiley products visit us at www.wiley.com.

Wiley also publishes its books in a variety of electronic formats and by print-on-demand. Some content that appears in standard print versions of this book may not be available in other formats.

Library of Congress Cataloging-in-Publication Data

Names: Tarafdar, Surjit, editor.

Title: Lecture notes: Nephrology : a comprehensive guide to renal medicine / edited by Dr. Surjit Tarafdar.

Other titles: Nephrology

Description: Hoboken, NJ : Wiley Blackwell, 2020. | Includes bibliographical references and index.

Identifiers: LCCN 2019035286 (print) | LCCN 2019035287 (ebook) | ISBN 9781119058045 (paperback) | ISBN 9781119058083 (adobe pdf) | ISBN 9781119058113 (epub)

Subjects: MESH: Kidney Diseases

Classification: LCC RC918.N43 (print) | LCC RC918.N43 (ebook) | NLM WJ 300 | DDC 616.6/1–dc23

LC record available at https://lccn.loc.gov/2019035286

LC ebook record available at https://lccn.loc.gov/2019035287

Cover Design: Wiley

Cover Image: © PIXOLOGICSTUDIO/Science Photo Library/Getty Images

Set in 8.5/11pt Utopia by SPi Global, Pondicherry, India

Printed and bound in Singapore by Markono Print Media Pte Ltd

10 9 8 7 6 5 4 3 2 1

To my family for their patience and support. Their belief in my ability helped me to go through those days when I was overwhelmed and exhausted.

Contents

List of Contributors

Edwin Anand
Assistant Professor
Jacobs School of Medicine & Biomedical Sciences
The State University of New York at Buffalo
Buffalo, NY, USA

Anthea Anantharajah
Clinical Immunologist / Immunopathologist
The Canberra Hospital, Garran, ACT;
Clinical Lecturer, Australian National Univeresity
Acton, Australia

Dipankar Bhattacharjee
MD(Calcutta), FRCP (Edin), FRCP (Lon), FCPS (B'Desh)
Consultant physician and Nephrologist, NHS, UK
Honorary Senior Lecturer (Ex) United Kingdom

Robert Carroll
Consultant Nephrologist, Central Northern Adelaide
Renal and Transplantation Service, Central Adelaide
LHN, SA Health, Adelaide, Australia

Philip Clayton
Consultant Nephrologist, Central Northern Adelaide
Renal and Transplantation Service, Central Adelaide
LHN, SA Health
Adelaide, Australia

Alexander Gilbert
Advances Trainee in Nephrology, Royal Prince Alfred
Hospital, Sydney, Australia

Pankaj Hari
Professor, Department of Paediatrics, All India
Institute of Medical Sciences, New Delhi, India

Yena Hye
Department of Geriatric Medicine
Nepean-Blue Mountains Hospital
Penrith, Australia

Rajini Jayaballa
MBChB, FRACP, Staff Specialist in Diabetes and
Endocrinology, Western Sydney Diabetes, Blacktown &
Mount Druitt Hospitals, Sydney, Australia

R. Jayasurya
Consultant Nephrologist, Apollo Gleneagles Hospital
Kolkata, India

Lukas Kairaitis
Head of Renal Services, Blacktown & Mount Druitt
Hospitals, Sydney; Sub-Dean, Blacktown & Mount
Druitt Clinical School, School of Medicine
Western Sydney University
Sydney, Australia

Amanda Mather
Staff Specialist Renal Physician, Royal North Shore
Hospital
Sydney, Australia

Stephen McDonald
Consultant Nephrologist, Central Northern Adelaide
Renal and Transplantation service, Central Adelaide
LHN, SA Health, Adelaide;
South Australia Executive Officer, ANZDATA Registry,
SA Health and Medical Research Institute;
Clinical Professor, Adelaide Medical School,
University of Adelaide, Adelaide, Australia

Mark McLean
Staff Specialist in Diabetes and Endocrinology,
Blacktown & Mount Druitt Hospitals, Westmead
Hospital, Sydney; Conjoint Professor of Medicine –
Western Sydney University
Sydney, Australia

Karumathil Murali
FRACP, MD Senior Staff specialist in Renal Medicine
Wollongong Hospital; Clinical Associate Professor
Graduate School of Medicine, University of
Wollongong
Wollongong, Australia

M.K. Phanish
Consultant Nephrologist, Renal Services; Lead
consultant,
Living Donor Kidney Transplantation, Epsom;
St.Helier University Hospitals NHS Trust; Lead
consultant, Diabetes-Renal Services, CUH, Epsom, UK

Priyamvada P.S.
Additional Professor, Department of Nephrology
JIPMER, Puducherry, India

Richard J. Quigg
Arthur M. Morris Professor of Medicine and
Biomedical Informatics Chief,
Division of Nephrology Jacobs School of Medicine &
Biomedical Sciences
The State University of New York, The State University
of New York, Buffalo, NY, USA

Gowri Raman
Current Palliative Care Advanced Trainee, University
of Newcastle
Australia

Wayne Rankin
Chemical Pathologist, SA Pathology and Clinical
Senior Lecturer, Discipline of Medicine, University of
Adelaide
Adelaide, Australia

Vinay Sakhuja
Emeritus Professor, Department of Nephrology, Post
Graduate Institute of Medical Education & Research
Chandigarh, India

Sarah So
Renal Advanced Trainee
Westmead and Blacktown Hospitals
Sydney, Australia

Kamal Sud
Department Head of Renal Medicine, Clinical
Associate Professor
University of Sydney - Nepean Clinical School
Nepean Hospital
Kingswood, Australia

Sanjay Swaminathan
Professor, Clinical Dean, Blacktown & Mount Druitt
Clinical School, Western Sydney University; Clinical
Immunologist, Westmead and Blacktown Hospital
Sydney, Australia

Surjit Tarafdar
Consultant Nephrologist and General Physician,
Blacktown and Mount Druitt Hospital
Blacktown, NSW, Sydney; Conjoint Senior Lecturer
Department of Medicine, Western Sydney University
Sydney, Australia

Muh Geot Wong MBBS, PhD, FRACP
Staff Specialist, Department of Renal Medicine, Royal
North Shore Hospital; Senior Clinical Lecturer
University of Sydney
Sydney, Australia

Foreword

The title 'Lecture Notes' undersells the comprehensive nature of this textbook, which fills a largely vacant niche in nephrology bookshelves, between lecture notes for medical students and junior trainees usually covering specific aspects of nephrology, and comprehensive speciality tomes targeted at those requiring specialized knowledge about any or all aspects of nephrology. *Lecture Notes: Nephrology* is aimed specifically at early-stage physician trainees who in the Australian system are preparing to undertake the basic physician trainee examination, or more senior trainees who have completed that exam, but are seeking expert knowledge as a trainee in general medicine, or are just starting specialized training in nephrology. However, its reach is much broader than that and it will appeal to anyone wanting to understand nephrology at a level greater than that found in general medical textbooks, including more advanced nephrology trainees, subspecialty nephrologists seeking knowledge beyond their subspecialty, general physicians and nephrologists wishing to brush up on all aspects of nephrology, and teachers of nephrology at any level. Whereas its reach is broad, it does not pretend to cater to those seeking highly specialized knowledge of particular aspects of nephrology. It is full of practical, contemporary information useful for day-to-day application on any aspect and at any level of renal diagnosis, investigation and management. Even the nephrologist who has been practising his or her craft for many years will find exciting new gems. In reviewing the book I found myself looking forward to reading each of the chapters at a more leisurely pace, and to applying its new knowledge for teaching and clinical practise.

The authors of *Lecture Notes: Nephrology* range from international, national and local experts on particular aspects of renal science and its clinical application, to advanced trainees in nephrology who under the supervision of senior colleagues need to have this level of expertise and knowledge for their day-to-day supervision of nephrology patients. Each chapter has been reviewed thoroughly by other authors and content experts, and achieves high standards of readability, immediacy and clinical applicability. The chapters cover all aspects of nephrology, including physiology appropriately linked to clinical disease, general nephrology, dialysis and transplantation. Of particular relevance to those preparing for nephrology examinations, and others wishing to test how well they have assimilated the book's new knowledge, is a comprehensive set of multiple choice questions, which have been written by those well placed to do so; that is, trainees preparing for or having recently completed general physician and nephrology examinations.

Surjit Tarafdar and his colleagues have produced a renal textbook of high utility, which will occupy a place of honour on nephrology bookshelves.

David CH Harris
AM, MD (USyd), BS, FRACP
Professor of Medicine,
University of Sydney
Director of Nephrology & Dialysis,
Western Sydney Renal Service
Past-President, International Society of Nephrology

Acknowledgements

I am indebted to the following groups and individuals for their contributions:

- The Histopathology Department at ICPMR, Westmead Hospital, Sydney, Australia.
- Dr Pei Dai, Advanced Trainee in Immunology at Westmead Hospital, Sydney, for the Immunofluorescence slides.
- Dr Simon Gruenewald, Consultant Nuclear Physician at Westmead Public Hospital, Sydney, and Dr Basim Alqutawneh, Consultant Radiologist at Blacktown Hospital, Sydney, for the radiographs and imaging material.
- Professor Jeremy Chapman, Associate Professor Gopala Rangan and Dr Brian Nankivell from the Department of Renal Medicine of Westmead Hospital, Sydney, and Professor Ravindra Prabhu A, Department of Nephrology at Kasturba Medical College, Manipal, India, for reviewing portions of the book.
- Dr Alexander Gilbert, renal Advanced Trainee at Prince Alfred Hospital, Sydney, for proofreading almost the entire book in addition to co-writing Chapter 14.
- Lashnika Bandaranayake and Thilan Pasanjith Subasinghe, the wonderful team of fifth-year medical students from Western Sydney University, who helped with most of the diagrams and illustrations.
- To the lovely librarians at Blacktown Hospital, Sydney, for letting me stay back in the Peter Zelas Library many a day past closing time.
- To the following junior doctors and registrars who reviewed the book and provided valuable feedback on the language and content:
  - Dr Shrikar Tummala
  - Dr Tu Hao Tran
  - Dr Hannah Jsu
  - Dr Shaun Khanna
  - Dr Sumreen Nawaz
  - Dr Ye Min Kuang
  - Dr Marlies Pinzon
  - Dr Serge Geara
- To Yogalakshmi Mohanakrishnan, the project editor from the publisher's office, for her patience, guidance and prompt responses.
- Finally, I am extremely thankful to Professor David Harris from Westmead Hospital, Sydney. Despite being the President of the International Society of Nephrology at a time when the World Congress of Nephrology was being held in Australia, Professor Harris found time to review the book and provide pearls of wisdom which added immensely to the quality of the finished work.

Clinical Implications of Renal Physiology

Surjit Tarafdar

Summary

- Besides maintaining a stable acid base, electrolyte, and fluid status of the body, kidneys also have an important endocrine role in producing and secreting 1,25-dihydroxycholecalciferol (calcitriol), renin, and erythropoietin
- More than 98% of water in the filtered urine is reabsorbed in the tubules; 90–95% of water is reabsorbed as it follows sodium (Na^+), which is avidly reabsorbed by the Na^+-deficient epithelial cells, except in the collecting duct (CD), where 5–10% of water is reabsorbed (independent of Na+) under the direct influence of vasopressin or antidiuretic hormone (ADH)
- The tubular epithelial cells constantly lose three Na^+ and gain two potassium (K^+) ions from the basolateral membrane (due to the Na+-K+-ATPase), which keeps these cells deficient in Na^+
- The countercurrent mechanism, which is dependent on the impermeability of the thick ascending limb (TAL) to water, leads to the creation of an increasing osmotic gradient from the cortex to the deeper medulla, which in turn enables ADH to reabsorb water in the CD
- Aldosterone helps in Na^+ reabsorption in the CD and also leads (directly) to K^+ and (indirectly) to hydrogen (H^+) secretion into urine
- All diuretics act by inhibiting tubular reabsorption of Na^+
- Formation of urine begins in the glomerular capillaries where the filtrate has to cross the three filtration layers: endothelium, glomerular basement membrane (GBM) and the foot processes of the podocytes; all these three layers are negatively charged and hence repel anionic proteins like albumin
- Nephrotic syndrome, which is marked by abnormally increased filtration of plasma proteins in the urine, may be due to widening of the pores in the three filtration layers, but is almost always associated with loss of negative charges in these layers
- Nephritis, which is due to glomerular inflammation, is characterized by haematuria with red blood cell (RBC) casts and dysmorphic RBCs, some degree of oliguria, hypertension, and reduction in glomerular filtration rate
- Goodpasture's disease, which is characterized by antibodies against subtype of type IV collagen, can lead to nephritis and haemoptysis, as this particular collagen is found predominantly in the GBM and alveolar membranes of the lungs
- Familial hypocalciuric hypercalcaemia, which manifests with hypercalcaemia, characteristically low urinary calcium and normal to high serum parathyroid hormone (PTH) level, is due to mutation in the calcium-sensing receptor (found in the kidney and parathyroid gland) leading to abnormally increased renal

Lecture Notes Nephrology: A Comprehensive Guide to Renal Medicine, First Edition. Edited by Surjit Tarafdar.
© 2020 John Wiley & Sons Ltd. Published 2020 by John Wiley & Sons Ltd.

reabsorption of calcium and inappropriate secretion of PTH
- Distal renal tubular acidosis (type 1 RTA) is due to an inability of the distal tubules to excrete H⁺, whilst proximal renal tubular acidosis (type 2 RTA) is due to an inability of the proximal tubules to reabsorb bicarbonate (HCO_3^-)
- Metabolic acidosis leads to hyperkalaemia and vice versa

The kidneys are paired retroperitoneal structures that are normally located between the transverse processes of the T12–L3 vertebrae, with the left kidney typically somewhat more superior in position than the right. Each kidney has an outer cortex and an inner medulla which protrudes into the pelvis. The pelvis is practically the funnel-shaped dilated upper end of the ureter.

The kidney maintains a stable acid base, electrolyte, and fluid status inside the body by selective elimination or retention of water, electrolytes, and other solutes (Table 1.1). It does so by three mechanisms:

1. Filtration of blood in the glomerulus to form an ultrafiltrate (water with low molecular weight solutes) which then enters the tubule.
2. Selective reabsorption of water, electrolytes, and solutes from the tubules into the interstitium and peritubular capillaries.
3. Selective secretion from the peritubular capillaries across the tubular epithelium into the tubular fluid.

Besides these mechanisms, the kidneys also play an active endocrine role by the production and secretion of:

- *1,25-dihydroxycholecalciferol*: cholecalciferol is derived from 7-dehydrocholesterol in the skin on exposure to the ultraviolet rays in sunlight. Cholecalciferol then undergoes two subsequent hydroxylations by 25-hydroxylase in the liver and 1-hydroxylase in the proximal tubules of the kidney to yield 1,25-dihydroxycholecalciferol

(calcitriol). Calcitriol is the active form of vitamin D, without which calcium cannot be absorbed from the intestine.
- *Renin*: discussed later under juxtaglomerular apparatus.
- *Erythropoietin (EPO)*: specialized interstitial cells in the inner cortex and outer medulla of the kidney produce and secrete EPO, which stimulates red blood cell (RBC) production in the bone marrow.

The kidney consists of nephrons with the supporting interstitium, collecting ducts (CDs), and the renal microvasculature. The nephron consists of a glomerulus and a twisted tubule which drains into the CD. The tubule consists of a proximal and a distal tubule connected by Henle's loop [1]. Each kidney has approximately one million nephrons and we cannot develop new nephrons after birth.

Cortex

This is the outer layer of the kidney and all the glomeruli are located here (Figure 1.1). The tubules of the superficial and midcortical nephrons are situated entirely within the cortex. The juxtamedullary nephrons (in the deeper regions of the cortex and nearer the medulla) have longer tubules and their loop of Henle goes down into the medulla and helps in the countercurrent mechanism, as discussed later.

Medulla

The renal medulla contains the loops of Henle of the juxtamedullary nephrons, vasa recta (peritubular capillaries surrounding the long loops of the juxtamedullary nephrons), and the CDs. The medulla consists of 7–10 conical subdivisions called pyramids, whose broad base faces the cortex, and the apical papilla points into the minor calyx. After traversing through the pyramid, the CDs open at the papilla and drain the urine into the minor calyx. Two or three minor calyces converge to form a major calyx, through

Table 1.1 Urine to plasma ratios of some physiologically important body substances

Substance	Urine to plasma ratio
Glucose	0
Sodium	0.6
Urea	60
Creatinine	150

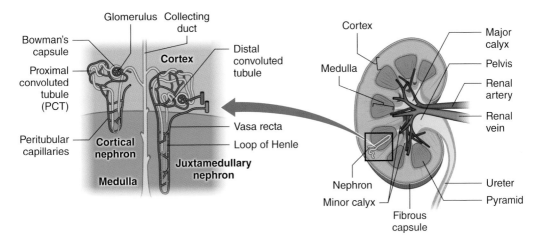

Figure 1.1 The renal cortex, medulla (with the pyramids), and minor and major calyces with their relation to the ureter and renal vasculature.

which urine continues into the renal pelvis, which is the funnel-shaped dilated proximal end of the ureter. There are usually two or three major calyces in each kidney.

Renal Vasculature

The kidneys receive 1.2–1.3l of blood per minute (about 25% of the cardiac output), making them highly vascular organs. After originating from the aorta, the renal artery enters the renal sinus and divides into the interlobar arteries, which extend towards the cortex in the spaces between the medullary pyramids. At the junction between the cortex and medulla, the interlobar arteries divide and pass over into the arcuate arteries. The arcuate arteries give rise to the interlobular arteries, which rise radially through the cortex. It is interesting to note that none of these arteries penetrates the medulla.

Afferent arterioles arise from the interlobular arteries and supply the glomerular tufts. The glomerular tufts are drained by the efferent arterioles, which then form the peritubular plexus and are of two types: cortical and juxtamedullary. The shorter cortical efferent arterioles arise from the superficial and midcortical nephrons and supply the cortex. The longer juxtamedullary efferent arterioles, which arise from the deeper nephrons, represent the sole blood supply to the medulla and are termed vasa recta. Whilst the descending vasa recta supply blood to the medulla, the ascending vasa recta drain it.

Glomerulus and Filtration across it

The glomerulus is the invagination of a tuft of capillaries into the dilated proximal end of the nephron called the Bowman's capsule (Figure 1.2). Supplied by the afferent and drained by the efferent arteriole, the glomerular capillary bunch is attached to the mesangium on the inner side and covered by the glomerular basement membrane (GBM) on the outer side. In a way, the GBM forms the skeleton of the glomeruli, with the podocytes (visceral epithelial cells with long foot processes) on the outer side and the capillaries and mesangium on the inner side. Thus, blood within the glomerular capillary is separated from the urinary space by endothelium, GBM, and podocyte.

Formation of urine begins with the filtration of blood from the glomerular capillaries. For this to happen blood must cross three layers:

- *Endothelium*: these highly fenestrated cells have 50–100nm pores with a highly electronegative luminal surface.
- *GBM*: with podocytes externally and endothelium/mesangium internally, its main constituents are collagen IV, laminin, and heparin, all of which are negatively charged.
- *Visceral epithelium (podocytes)*: a big cell body floating in the urinary space with long primary processes which affix on the glomerular capillaries by foot processes, with filtration slits sized 30–40nm

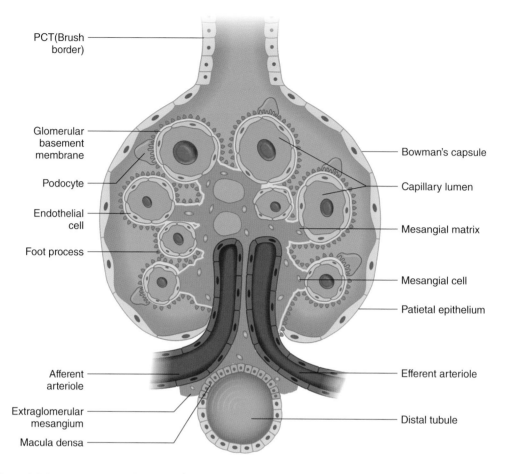

Figure 1.2 Parts of glomerulus and the juxtaglomerular apparatus (JGA). PCT, proximal convoluted tubule.

in between. These slits are bridged by the slit diaphragms, which are themselves penetrated by small pores sized about 8 nm. The luminal surfaces of both the podocyte foot processes and the slit diaphragms are rich in negatively charged proteins such as podocalyxin in the former and nephrin in the latter.

Whilst water can freely cross these three layers, the filtration of macromolecules depends on both size and charge. Molecules bigger than 8 nm are normally completely restricted by the GBM. Albumin with a diameter of 7.2 nm would have been effectively filtered were it not for its negative charge.

Clinical Notes

Common Glomerular Pathologies

- Nephrotic syndrome is characterized by proteinuria >3.5 g/24 hours, hypoalbuminaemia, generalized oedema, and hyperlipidaemia. Nephrotic syndrome is due to abnormally increased filtration of plasma proteins across the glomerular capillary. This may be due to an increase in the size of the pores mentioned earlier, but there is always an associated loss of negative charges across the filtration barrier. Proteinuria leads to hypoalbuminaemia, with a resultant decrease in plasma oncotic pressure in turn leading to oedema. In an effort to compensate for the low oncotic pressure, the liver starts to make excessive lipids, leading to hyperlipidaemia.

- Nephritis is characterized by haematuria with RBC casts and dysmorphic RBCs, some degree of oliguria, hypertension, and reduction in glomerular filtration rate (GFR). Nephritis is due to glomerular inflammation leading to leakage of RBCs across the filtration barrier. As the RBCs traverse the inflamed filtration barrier and travel down the tubules, they develop cytoplasmic blebs on their surface and are seen as dysmorphic RBCs under the microscope. Whilst travelling through the thick ascending loop of Henle, the RBCs get struck in the physiologically secreted tubular Tamm–Horsfall protein, leading to the formation of RBC casts. Thus, the presence of dysmorphic RBCs and RBC casts in a patient with haematuria helps to differentiate nephritis as the pathology rather than ureteric or bladder pathologies.
- Type IV collagen molecules are composed of three alpha chains that form triple-helical structures through specific interactions of C-terminal non-collagenous domains. GBM and alveolar capillary basement membrane collagen consist of alpha3, -4, and -5 chains, unlike other basement membranes with alpha1 (two of them) and alpha2 chains. Two disease processes pathogenetically caused by defects primarily in the GBM are:
  a. Goodpasture's disease, characterized by anti-GBM antibody against the alpha3 chain of the type IV collagen present in the GBM and alveolar membranes in the lungs [2]. Patients present with nephritis and haemoptysis.
  b. Alport syndrome, which results from mutations in genes encoding the alpha3, -4, and -5 chains of type IV collagen (80% are due to mutations in the alpha5 chain) [3]. It is the commonest inherited form of nephritis and is often associated with sensorineural deafness and ocular abnormalities due to the presence of similar alpha3, -4, and -5 chains in the type IV collagen in the basement membranes of the lens and cochlea.

Tubules

With a GFR of 125 ml/min, about 180 l of urine is formed at the glomerular level each day. Thankfully, under physiological conditions almost 98–99% of this filtered urine is reabsorbed by the tubules. More than 90% of this tubular water reabsorption is a passive process and water just follows the sodium (Na$^+$) being reabsorbed. Only in the CD is water absorbed actively and independently of Na$^+$ under the action of vasopressin or anti-diuretic hormone (ADH).

It is thus obvious that most of the water reabsorption in the tubules is dependent on the reabsorption of Na$^+$. So, what makes the tubules take up Na$^+$ so avidly?

Why do the Tubules Reabsorb Na$^+$ and Water?

The tubular epithelial cells, irrespective of which segment of the tubule they belong to, have a basolateral Na$^+$-K$^+$-ATPase that continuously pumps out three Na$^+$ ions and brings in two potassium (K$^+$) ions, thus making the cells permanently Na$^+$ deficient. Thus, the fact that the tubular epithelial cells are always deficient in Na$^+$ helps in the Na$^+$ reabsorption from the tubules. In the same vein, the fact that the tubular cells are rich in K$^+$ helps them to secrete K$^+$ into the tubular lumen.

Water is absorbed osmotically along with solutes, with Na$^+$ being the predominant solute (Table 1.2; Figure 1.3). The two exceptions are in the thick ascending limb (TAL) of the loop of Henle, which is impermeable to water, and the CD, where water is reabsorbed by the action of vasopressin, as discussed later.

Proximal Convoluted Tubule

The bulk of tubular reabsorption occurs in the proximal convoluted tubule (PCT), with 65–70% of the total Na$^+$ being reabsorbed here and about the same amount of water being reabsorbed passively. The PCT is also responsible for reabsorption of the bulk of phosphate (PO$_4^{3-}$), bicarbonate (HCO$_3$–), potassium (K$^+$), calcium (Ca$^+$) and almost all glucose, amino acids, uric acid, and low molecular weight proteins such as microglobulins and the light chain fraction of immunoglobulins.

NaHCO$_3$ is filtered in the glomeruli and dissociates in the lumen of the PCT into Na$^+$ and HCO$_3^-$. Na$^+$ is

Table 1.2 Absorption of various ions and water across different segments of the renal tubules

Ion or substance	PCT	Loop of Henle	DCT	CD
Na⁺	65–70%	30–35%	5%	1–2%
H₂O	65–70%	25%	5%	5–10%
K⁺	45–50%	40–45%		Secreted by principal cells
Ca⁺	70%	20%	10–15%	
Mg⁺	15–25%	60–70%	5–10%	
PO³⁻₄	70–80%	Insignificant	Insignificant	Insignificant
HCO₃⁻	85–90%			Secreted by beta- intercalated cells

Ca⁺: calcium; CD: collecting duct; DCT: distal convoluted tubule; HCO₃⁻: bicarbonate; H₂O: water; K⁺: potassium; Mg⁺: magnesium; Na⁺: sodium; PCT: proximal convoluted tubule; PO³⁻₄: phosphate.

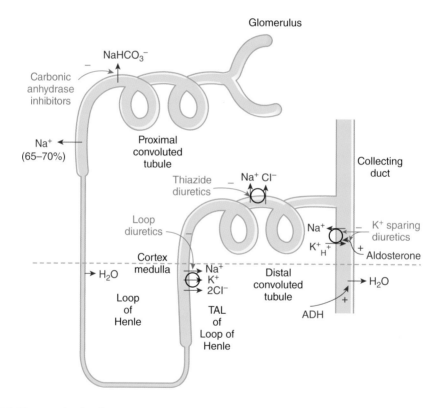

Figure 1.3 Diagram showing the movement of sodium (Na⁺), chloride (Cl⁻), potassium (K⁺), and water (H₂O) across various portions of the renal tubule, with the site of action of different diuretics highlighted. ADH: anti-diuretic hormone; NaHCO₃⁻: sodium bicarbonate; TAL: thick ascending limb.

reabsorbed by the Na⁺-hungry tubular epithelial, as already discussed. The HCO₃⁻ remaining (from the original NaHCO₃) in the lumen combines with hydrogen (H⁺) by the action of the tubular carbonic anhy-

drase (CA) to form carbonic acid (H₂CO₃), which then splits into carbon dioxide (CO₂) and water (H₂O). CO₂ enters the tubular cell and now the reaction goes in the reverse direction, with CO₂ combining with H₂O

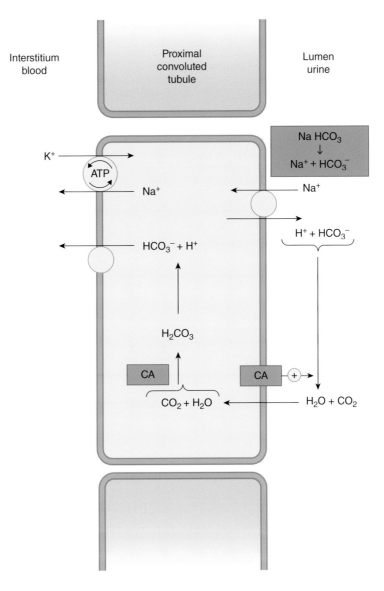

Figure 1.4 Action of carbonic anhydrase (CA) in reclaiming bicarbonate (HCO_3^-) in the proximal convoluted tubule (PCT): sodium bicarbonate ($NaHCO_3$) dissociates in the lumen of the PCT into sodium (Na^+) and HCO_3^-; Na^+ is reabsorbed by the tubular cells in exchange for hydrogen (H^+), whilst the HCO_3^- combines with the H^+ to form carbonic acid (H_2CO_3) under the influence of tubular CA. H_2CO_3 then splits into carbon dioxide (CO_2) and water (H_2O), followed by the CO_2 diffusing into the tubular cells and regenerating H_2CO_3 after combining with H_2O. Aided by the intracellular CA, this H_2CO_3 then splits to form H^+ and HCO_3^-. This H^+ is secreted into the PCT lumen in exchange for Na^+, whilst the HCO_3^- diffuses into the peritubular capillaries. ATP, adenosine triphosphate.

to form H_2CO_3, which is then split to form H^+ and HCO_3^- by the intracellular form of CA. This H^+ is then secreted into the PCT lumen in exchange for Na^+ by the Na^+-H^+ exchange transport, whilst the HCO_3^- diffuses into blood in the peritubular capillaries (Figure 1.4). Thus, for each H^+ secreted into the tubule, the body gains an HCO_3^-.

Reabsorption of Na^+ in the PCT facilitates the reabsorption of glucose, amino acids, phosphate, and uric acid.

Clinical Notes

Disorders of the Proximal Renal Tubules

- Proximal renal tubular acidosis (type 2 RTA) is due to a defect in the reabsorption of HCO_3^- leading to urinary loss of HCO_3^- and the resultant metabolic acidosis. As already explained, the reabsorption of HCO_3^- in this segment is linked to the coupled exchange of H^+ and Na^+ (Figure 1.4). As Na^+ reabsorption here is linked to the reabsorption of glucose, amino acids, phosphate, and uric acid, the patient may present with glycosuria, hypophosphataemia, and hypouricaemia (due to urinary losses), a condition that is termed Fanconi syndrome. Urine pH is usually less than 5.5 despite bicarbonaturia, as the intact distal tubules excrete excess H^+ as a compensatory mechanism for the acidosis.
- Type 2 RTA is discussed further in the clinical notes following the section on the distal convoluted tubule and collecting duct.
- Acezolamide, which is a CA inhibitor often used by ophthalmologists for the treatment of glaucoma, can also lead to a type 2 RTA-like picture, with full-blown Fanconi syndrome at times. The anti-epileptic drug topiramate and anti-HIV medication tenofovir, by their CA inhibitor activity, can also lead to proximal RTA and Fanconi syndrome [4].
- PCT is responsible for the reabsorption of the easily filtered light chain fragments of immunoglobulins. In myeloma, the excess of light chains is toxic to the PCT and may lead to proximal RTA with or without Fanconi syndrome [5].
- In prerenal AKI, serum urea increases disproportionately to creatinine due to its enhanced PCT reabsorption that follows the enhanced transport of Na^+ and water. Elevated serum urea/creatinine may also be seen in upper gastrointestinal haemorrhage, since the upper intestinal proteolytic enzymes break down haemoglobin to amino acids, which are then reabsorbed by the body and lead to the generation of urea.

Clinical Notes

Disorders of the Loop of Henle

- *Bartter syndrome*: an autosomal recessive syndrome that characteristically presents with hypokalaemia and metabolic alkalosis is described later in the chapter with Gitelman syndrome (following the section on the distal convoluted tubule and collecting duct).
- *Familial hypocalciuric hypercalcaemia (FHH)*: this benign autosomal dominant condition is caused by inactivating mutations in the gene for the CaSR.

  CaSR is predominantly found in the parathyroid gland and the kidneys. In the parathyroid gland, it decreases the secretion of PTH in response to serum Ca^+. Under normal conditions, the TAL CaSR, on being activated by Ca^+, downregulates the production of Ca^+-carrying transcellular proteins Claudrin 16 and 19 by forming Claudrin 14, which has an inhibitory effect on the two [7]. The mutated CaSR in FHH is unable to inhibit Claudrin 16 and 19, leading to uninhibited Ca^+ reabsorption and hence hypocalciuria and hypercalcaemia, and at the same time a non-suppressible serum PTH level. It is easy to confuse this condition with primary hyperparathyroidism unless one looks at the urinary Ca^+, which is characteristically low. A spot urine Ca^+/creatinine ratio of <1/100 is helpful in differentiating the hypercalcemia with inappropriately high serum PTH levels seen in FHH from primary hyperparathyroidism (where the urinary Ca+ would be high).

About 40–50% of the filtered urea is reabsorbed in the PCT. As urea is reabsorbed in this section along with Na+, in conditions of volume contraction when the PCT reabsorbs more Na^+, the net reabsorption of urea is also significantly increased. Thus, a disproportionate rise in blood urea concentration in comparison to creatinine might be a marker of a prerenal cause of acute kidney injury (AKI).

Loop of Henle

The loop of Henle consists of the thick and thin descending limbs and the thick ascending limb (TAL), with a thin ascending limb seen only in long looped nephrons.

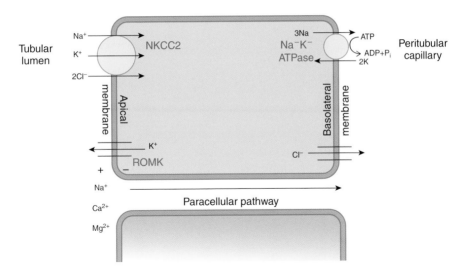

Figure 1.5 Transport mechanisms in the thick ascending limb of the loop of Henle: The basolateral (peritubular) membrane due to the action of Na+-K+-ATPase pumps three sodium (Na$^+$) out of, and two potassium (K$^+$) into, the cell. This creates a low intracellular Na$^+$ concentration, which allows the cell to absorb Na$^+$ from the urinary lumen by the electroneutral Na$^+$-K$^+$-2Cl$^-$ (NKCC2). The cell is rich in K$^+$ and so much of the reabsorbed K$^+$ recycles back into the lumen through the renal outer medullary potassium channel (ROMK) on the apical/luminal membrane. This movement of one cationic K$^+$ into the lumen plus the flux of one reabsorbed Na$^+$ (by Na-K-ATPase pump) and two chloride (Cl$^-$) out of the cell and into the peritubular capillary (via Cl$^-$ channels) causes the lumen to become more positively charged compared with the cell and peritubular capillaries/interstitium. The resultant electrical gradient promotes passive reabsorption of cations calcium (Ca$^+$) and magnesium (Mg$^+$) via the paracellular pathway. The Cl$^-$ channels require interaction with a small protein called barttin to function normally. ADP, adenosine diphosphate; ATP, adenosine triphosphate; Pi, inorganic phosphate.

The loop of Henle is responsible for the reabsorption of 30–35% of the luminal Na$^+$ but only 25% of the water, as the TAL is resistant to the movement of water across it.

The frusemide-sensitive and electroneutral Na$^+$-K$^+$-2Cl$^-$ cotransporter reabsorbs one Na$^+$ and K$^+$ each along with two Cl$^-$ ions from the TAL lumen to the tubular epithelial cell (Figure 1.5). High intracellular K$^+$ concentration (due to the basolateral Na-K-ATPase pumping out three Na$^+$ and bringing in two K$^+$ ions constantly) causes the reabsorbed K$^+$ to be secreted back into the lumen via the renal outer medullary potassium (ROMK) channel. The Cl$^-$ is absorbed into blood by the basolateral Cl$^-$ channel (ClC-Kb), which has barttin as a crucial accessory protein. Movement of one positive charge (K$^+$) into the lumen and net of one negative charge into the peritubular capillary (1 Na$^+$ and 2 Cl$^-$) causes the lumen to be more positive compared to the tubular peritubular capillary and interstitium. This electrical gradient promotes the passive reabsorption of cations Ca$^+$ and Mg$^+$ via the paracellular cleft between

the cells. Membrane proteins Claudrin 16 and 19 help in this paracellular reabsorption of Ca$^+$ and Mg$^+$ and are themselves tightly regulated by the calcium-sensing receptor (CaSR) (Figure 1.6) [6].

Countercurrent Mechanism

A major function of the loop of Henle is to create an interstitial osmotic gradient that increases from the renal cortex (290 mOsm/kg) to the tip of the medullary pyramid (1200 mOsm/kg) (Figure 1.7). This countercurrent mechanism is fundamentally dependent on the impermeability of the TAL to water. The reabsorption of Na$^+$ (and its passage to the interstitium by the basolateral Na$^+$-K$^+$-ATPase pump) in the absence of water in the ascending limb has two consequences:

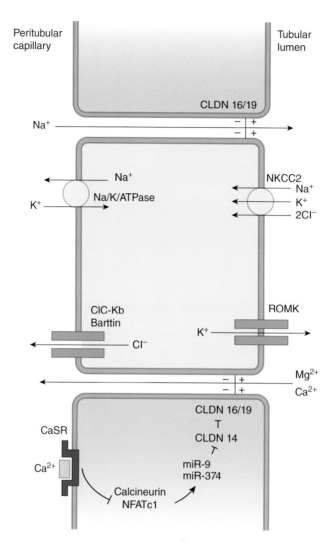

Figure 1.6 Absorption of calcium (Ca⁺) and magnesium (Mg⁺) through the paracellular pathway in the thick ascending limb of the loop of Henle. Sodium (Na⁺) is reabsorbed via the apical Na⁺-K⁺-2Cl⁻ cotransporter and pumped out basolaterally by the Na⁺-K⁺-ATPase; chloride (Cl⁻) exits via the Cl⁻ channel (ClC-Kb); and potassium (K⁺) is secreted into the tubular lumen by the renal outer medullary potassium channel (ROMK), thereby generating a lumen-positive transtubular electric potential. Ca⁺ and Mg⁺ are reabsorbed passively across the paracellular pathway because of this lumen-positive electrical potential. Claudrin 16 and 19 are the two chief transport proteins which help to carry the Ca⁺ and Mg⁺ across the paracellular cleft. Blood Ca⁺ levels regulate this process by stimulating the Ca⁺-sensing receptor (CaSR), which then upregulates Claudin-14 (CLDN14), a protein that normally binds to and inhibits Claudin 16 and -19. CaSR controls the production of Claudrin 14 by the calcineurin-NFATc1-microRNA pathway. NFAT: nuclear factor of activated T cells.

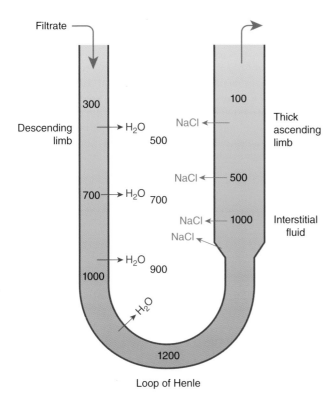

Filtrate

Descending limb

Thick ascending limb

Interstitial fluid

Loop of Henle

Figure 1.7 Countercurrent mechanism: reabsorption of sodium (Na⁺) with relative resistance to the reabsorption of water by the thick ascending limb of the loop of Henle leads to generation of the interstitial osmotic gradient; the gradient is higher for the longer loops of the juxtamedullary nephrons, which travel deeper into the medulla. H₂O, water; NaCl, sodium chloride.

1. A higher concentration of Na⁺ in the interstitium leads to higher interstitial osmotic pressure, with the highest osmotic pressure developed in tips of medullary pyramids where the longer loops of Henle reach.
2. The tubular fluid leaving the TAL is hypotonic because of excess water in comparison to Na⁺.

The creation of this gradient helps in the reabsorption of water in the medullary CD under the influence of vasopressin, with water moving from the hypoosmolar tubular environment to the hyper-osmolar medullary interstitium.

Clinical Notes

Can Frusemide Lead to Hyponatraemia?

Frusemide acts by interrupting the Na⁺ uptake in the TAL by the Na⁺-K⁺ -2Cl⁻ transporter. This interferes with the countercurrent mechanism and the generation of the medullary interstitial osmotic gradient. As discussed, without this gradient, ADH cannot reabsorb water in the medullary CD. Thus, frusemide leads to the excretion of a dilute urine which would prevent the development of hyponatraemia.

Distal Convoluted Tubule and Collecting Duct

The distal convoluted tubule (DCT) is responsible for the reabsorption of 5% of Na⁺ by the thiazide-sensitive sodium chloride (NaCl) cotransporter. Between 10% and 15% of the Ca⁺ is also reabsorbed in this segment in an active process, unlike the more passive process in the proximal parts (70% of Ca⁺ is co-transported passively with Na⁺ in the PCT). Ca⁺ enters tubular cells via the transient receptor potential vanilloid 5 (TRPV5) channel, and 5–10% of the total Mg⁺ reabsorption also occurs in this segment by the transient receptor potential melastatin 6 (TRPM6) and TRPM7 channels.

The CD is responsible for reabsorption of up to 2% of the Na⁺ and water, but this can vary depending on the needs of the body. The two chief types of cells found in the CD are:

- Principal cells, which are responsible for Na⁺ reabsorption and K⁺ secretion (under the influence of aldosterone) and water reabsorption (under the influence of ADH).

- Intercalated cells, which are responsible for the secretion of H⁺ (by alpha-intercalated cell) or HCO₃⁻ (by beta-intercalated cell).

ADH

ADH is synthesized in the supraoptic and paraventricular nuclei of the hypothalamus and travels down the pituitary stalk to be stored in the posterior pituitary. Secreted in response to decreased intravascular volume or increased plasma osmotic pressure as in dehydration, the main physiological effects of ADH are retention of water by the kidneys and vasoconstriction.

There are three types of ADH receptors: V1A, V1B, and V2. V1A receptors cause vasoconstriction by increasing vascular smooth muscle intracellular Ca⁺ concentration, whilst V1B receptors lead to adrenocorticotropic hormone (ACTH) release by the pituitary gland. V2 receptors are found on the principal cells in the CD and via the cyclic adenosine monophosphate (cAMP) pathway lead to movement and fusion of the aquaporin 2 (AQP2) water channels to the luminal membrane (Figure 1.8). The medullary osmotic gradient established due to the selective reabsorption of Na⁺ in the TAL helps in the water being reabsorbed in the CD.

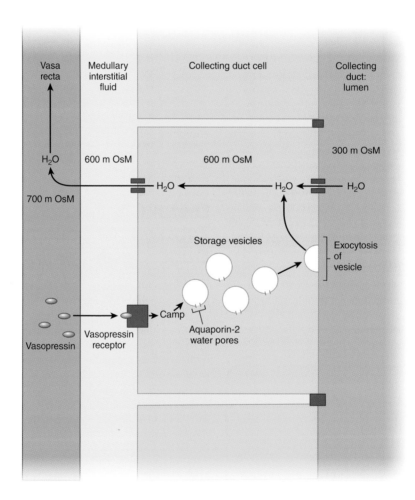

Figure 1.8 Anti-diuretic hormone (vasopressin), acting through cyclic adenosine monophosphate (cAMP), increases the total number of aquaporin-2 molecules in the principal cells of the collecting duct; aquaporin-2 aids in water reabsorption in this part of the renal tubule. H₂O: water.

Aldosterone

Aldosterone is secreted by the zona glomerulosa of adrenal cortex and helps in Na^+ reabsorption and K^+ and H^+ excretion by the distal portions of the tubules. On binding to the mineralocorticoid receptor, aldosterone upregulates and activates the basolateral Na^+-K^+-ATPase in the principal cells, causing lower intracellular Na^+, and at the same time upregulates epithelial sodium channels (ENaC), increasing apical membrane permeability for Na^+. The resultant intracellular movement of Na^+ causes luminal negativity, leading in turn to secretion of the positively charged K^+. The Na^+ and K^+ movement is not a strict one-to-one exchange and more Na^+ is reabsorbed than K^+ is lost. So, the same luminal negativity leads to H^+ secretion by the neighbouring alpha-intercalated cells. The potassium-sparing diuretics (amiloride and triamterene) act by directly inhibiting ENaC channels; spironolactone acts by competing with aldosterone for binding to the mineralocorticoid receptor (Figure 1.9).

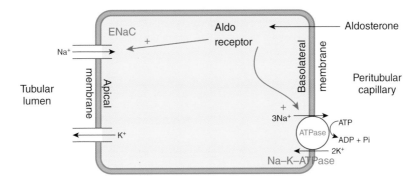

Figure 1.9 Ion transport in collecting tubule principal cells. Aldosterone, after combining with the cytosolic mineralocorticoid receptor (aldo-receptor), leads to enhanced sodium (Na^+) reabsorption and potassium (K^+) secretion by increasing both the number of open Na^+ channels and the number of Na^+-K^+-ATPase pumps. Whilst spironolactone competes with aldosterone for the aldosterone receptor, amiloride and triamterene act by directly inhibiting the epithelial Na^+ channel. ENaC: epithelial sodium channel.

Clinical Notes

Diuretics, the Distal Tubules, Vasopressin and Aldosterone
- The unifying mechanistic principle of action of all diuretics is to prevent tubular Na^+ reabsorption. Both thiazide and loop diuretics can lead to hypokalaemia and metabolic alkalosis by the following mechanisms:
  a. With more Na^+ flowing to the distal parts of the nephron, the tubular cells try to reclaim the excess Na^+, resulting in loss of positive charges from the lumen. The tubular cells try to compensate by secretion of the positively charged K^+ (by principal cells) and H^+ (by alpha-intercalated cell) into the lumen.
  b. Intravascular volume contraction because of diuretics causes activation of the renin-angiotensin-aldosterone (RAS), which contributes to the urinary K^+ and H^+ losses due to the effect of aldosterone.
- Potassium-sparing diuretics can lead to hyperkalaemia and metabolic acidosis. Spironolactone competes with aldosterone for binding to the mineralocorticoid receptor, whilst amiloride and triamterene act by directly inhibiting the ENaC. The resultant effect is inhibition of K^+ and H^+ secretion.
- Effects of diuretics on Ca^+: Let us recapitulate that the paracellular reabsorption of Ca^+ in the loop of Henle is dependent on the positive electrical gradient in the lumen (Figures 1.6). Loop diuretics by inhibiting the Na^+-K^+-$2Cl^-$ transporter inhibit generation of this gradient and hence prevent reabsorption of Ca^+ in this segment of the tubule. On the other hand, thiazide diuretics increase proximal Na^+ and water reabsorption due to volume depletion, leading in turn to increased passive proximal calcium reabsorption. Thus, whilst frusemide helps to excrete Ca^+ in the urine, thiazide diuretics decrease urinary Ca^+ excretion and lead to hypercalcaemia.

- Lithium causes nephrogenic diabetes insipidus by causing decreased expression of AQP 2 genes.
- Primary hyperaldosteronism should always be suspected in a patient with hypokalaemia, metabolic alkalosis, and hypertension (more than half of patients are normokalaemic). This is discussed in more detail in Chapter 3.
- Bartter and Gitelman syndromes, both autosomal recessive disorders, are characterized by hypokalaemia, metabolic alkalosis, and low to normal blood pressure, with hypomagnesaemia being an additional distinctive feature of Gitelman syndrome, which tends to present in adults and is generally the milder of the two. The tubular defects in sodium chloride reabsorption in Bartter and Gitelman syndromes are almost identical to those seen with chronic ingestion of loop and thiazide diuretics, respectively [8, 9, 10]. Additional down-regulation of the Mg^+-reabsorbing TRPM6 channel in Gitelman syndrome causes Mg^+ wasting and the resultant characteristic hypomagnesaemia. These disorders are discussed in more detail in Chapter 3.
- Distal renal tubular acidosis (type 1 RTA) is due to an inability of the distal tubules to excrete H^+, leading to metabolic acidosis. The kidney characteristically cannot lower the urinary pH to less than 5.5 due to a deficiency of H in the urine, in contrast to type 2 RTA where the urinary pH is usually greater than 5.5 (Table 1.3) [11].

Table 1.3 Differences between types 1 and 2 renal tubular acidosis (RTA)

RTA1 (distal RTA)	RTA2 (proximal RTA)
Inability to secrete H^+	Inability to reabsorb HCO_3^-
Urine pH >5.5 (absence of H^+ in urine)	Urine pH <5.5 (compensatory rise in DCT secretion of excess H^+)
Associations: Sjögren's syndrome, systemic lupus erythematosus, primary biliary cirrhosis, autoimmune hepatitis	Associations: myeloma, Wilson's disease, tenofovir, acetazolamide, gentamicin
No Fanconi syndrome	Fanconi syndrome may be seen: glycosuria, phosphaturia, uric aciduria, and aminoaciduria (low serum phosphate and urate concentrations)
Proximal tubules reabsorb all alkali including citrate, which normally keeps Ca^+ in urine soluble, leading to increased predisposition to nephrolithiasis and nephrocalcinosis	No renal stones
Treat with alkali and K^+ replacement	Same treatment, but needs bigger doses of alkali as glomeruli lose the administered alkali and tubules cannot reabsorb it due to the nature of the defect

DCT: distal convoluted tubule; H^+: hydrogen; HCO_3^-: bicarbonate; K^+: potassium.

Glomeruli and Tubule Balance each other

An increase or decrease in glomerular filtration is balanced by increased or decreased tubular reabsorption. Similarly, an increase in tubular flow leads to a decrease in glomerular filtration and vice versa.

Glomerulotubular Balance

Increased filtration of protein-free fluid across the glomeruli leads to the blood flowing to efferent and peritubular arterioles being more concentrated. The resultant increased oncotic pressure in the peritubular capillaries aids in enhanced reabsorption of water across the tubular epithelium.

Tubuloglomerular Feedback

As more urine flows though tubules it causes decreased glomerular filtration and vice versa via macula densa constricting or dilating the afferent arterioles. The mechanism is explained in the next section.

Juxtaglomerular Apparatus

The juxtaglomerular apparatus (JGA) comprises the modified tubular epithelial cells called macula densa, the terminal portion of afferent arteriole with its renin-producing modified smooth muscle cells (granular or juxtaglomerular cells) and the extraglomerular mesangial cells.

At the point where the afferent arterioles enter the glomerulus and the efferent arteriole leaves it, the tubule touches the arterioles of the glomerulus from which it arose. At this location, which marks the ending of the TAL and the beginning of the DCT, the tubular epithelium is modified into narrowly packed cells with large nuclei called the macula densa. Macula densa sense the Na^+ and Cl^- levels in the tubular fluid and in the case of low flow, as seen in hypovolaemia or renal artery stenosis, relay this information via the extraglomerular mesangial cells to the granular cells. Granular cells are modified smooth muscle cells in the terminal portion of the afferent arterioles that contain and secrete renin when stimulated by the macula densa.

Renin splits the 32-amino acid polypeptide angiotensinogen formed in liver to yield the physiologically inactive decapeptide angiotensin1. As this angiotensin1 circulates through the lungs, angiotensin-converting enzyme (ACE) splits two more amino acids off it to form the octapeptide angiotensin II. Apart from being a potent vasoconstrictor, angiotensin also leads to aldosterone release (Figure 1.10).

Note that angiotensin II constricts efferent more than afferent arterioles in the kidney, thus effectively increasing filtration pressure and glomerular filtration.

In the case of high tubular flow and raised luminal Na^+ and Cl^-, the macula densa cells secrete adenosine triphosphate (ATP) into their surroundings. This ATP is converted into adenosine, which binds to the surrounding extraglomerular mesangial cells and raises their intracellular Ca^+ levels. This Ca^+ signal is then propagated via gap junctions to adjacent cells, including the granular cells of the JGA and the vascular smooth muscle cells of the afferent arteriole, resulting in a decrease in renin

---

Clinical Notes

Angiotensin-Converting Enzyme Inhibitors (ACE-I) and Angiotensin Receptor Blockers (ARB)

In renal artery stenosis, diabetic nephropathy or chronic kidney disease, the intrarenal perfusion pressure is already reduced and GFR is maintained in part by an angiotensin II-induced increase in resistance at the efferent arteriole [13, 14]. Blocking this response with an ACE-I or ARB will sequentially relax the efferent arteriole, lower intraglomerular pressure and reduce the GFR (and as a result decrease proteinuria). Renal function should be checked at five to seven days when an ACE-I or ARB is begun and the drug should be discontinued if serum creatinine concentration increases more than 30% above the baseline value.

---

release and vasoconstriction. Both these changes decrease the GFR [12].

Hydrogen Ion and the Kidney

As discussed previously, in the PCT H^+ is secreted in exchange for Na^+ and an HCO_3^- is regenerated with the aid of CA. In the more distal tubule and CD, H^+ is secreted by the type A intercalated cell via the luminal H^+-ATPase. Aldosterone indirectly helps this H^+ secretion by enhancing Na^+ reabsorption in neighbouring principal cells. Na^+ absorption generates a lumen-negative potential that drives both K^+ secretion by principal cells as well as H^+ by the alpha-intercalated cells [15]. H^+-K^+-ATPase pumps, which secrete H^+ and reabsorb K^+, are also present in the luminal membrane of alpha-intercalated cells. Whilst they are not normally a major player in K^+ homeostasis, the number and activity of these pumps are increased by K^+ depletion (Figure 1.11).

H^+ in the urine needs buffers, otherwise urine would quickly become saturated with it. The chief buffer that helps to carry the secreted H^+ in urine is ammonia, which becomes converted to ammonium after accepting the H^+:

$$NH_3 + H^+ \leftrightarrow NH_4^+$$

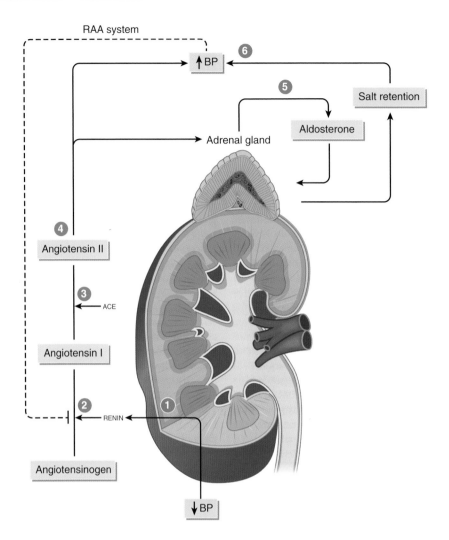

Figure 1.10 Relation between blood pressure and renin–angiotensin–aldosterone (RAA) system. Low tubular flow due to hypovolaemia/hypotension leads to renin secretion (1), which breaks angiotensinogen produced by the liver to yield angiotensin-1 (2); angiotensin-1 is cleaved by angiotensin-converting enzyme (ACE) in the lungs to yield angiotensin-2 (3, 4); angiotensin-2 causes vasoconstriction as well as aldosterone secretion by the adrenal gland (5); the combined effects of the vasoconstriction and salt retention by aldosterone help to raise the blood pressure (6).

Two ammonia are derived from the breakdown of glutamine in the PCT cells by the enzyme glutaminase. This ammonia is secreted and subsequently reabsorbed by the TAL cells by the Na^+ K^+2Cl^- channels as the K^+ is substituted by ammonia. The ammonia then enters the medullary interstitium and is secreted into the CD, where it helps to buffer H^+. Hypokalaemia induces renal ammonia production by increasing the cellular uptake of glutamine and increasing the activity of glutaminase (this facilitates the excretion of H^+ by making more ammonia available for buffering it in the tubular lumen).

Potassium and Acid Base Balance

In metabolic acidosis, excess H^+ enters cells to be buffered and the intracellular electroneutrality is maintained by intracellular K^+ moving out, leading to a raised plasma K^+ concentration while the reverse happens in metabolic alkalosis (refer figure 7.2 in chapter 7 - Chronic Kidney Disease). We need to remember that metabolic acidosis and hyperkalemia

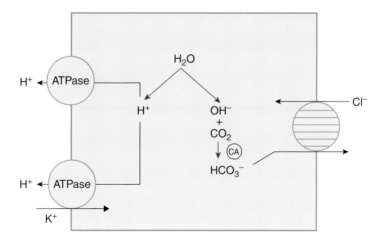

Figure 1.11 Mechanism of hydrogen (H^+) secretion and bicarbonate (HCO_3^-) and potassium (K^+) reabsorption in the type A intercalated cell. Water within the cell dissociates into hydrogen (H^+) and hydroxide (OH^-) ions. Whilst H^+ is secreted into the lumen by the $H+$-ATPase pumps, the OH^- ions in the cell combine with carbon dioxide (CO_2) to form HCO_3^- in a reaction catalysed by carbonic anhydrase (CA). The cellular HCO_3^- enters the peritubular capillaries in exchange for extracellular chloride (Cl^-) via Cl^--HCO_3 exchangers. In addition, H^+-K^+-ATPase pumps, which secrete H^+ and reabsorb K^+, are also present in the luminal membrane of the type A intercalated cell. The number and activity of these pumps are increased by K^+ depletion.

often go together while metabolic alkalosis is often associated with hypokalemia.

Hyperkalaemia potentiates metabolic acidosis by three mechanisms:

- Excess K^+ enters the cell and in exchange H^+ comes out of the cell.
- K^+ competes with H^+ for secretion by the CD.
- Hyperkalaemia, by decreasing renal ammonia production, inhibits H^+ excretion in urine (ammonia is the chief buffer for urinary H^+).

References

1. Kriz, W., Bankir, L., Bulger, R.E. et al. (1988). A standard nomenclature for structure of the Kidney. The Renal Commission of the International Union of Physiological Sciences (IUPS). *Pflugers Arch.* 411: 113–120.
2. Kotur, G., Kotur, G., Horvatić, I. et al. (eds.) (2015 May-Jun). Goodpasture's syndrome – case reports. *Lijec. Vjesn.* 137 (5–6): 171–176.
3. Truong, J., Deschênes, G., Callard, P. et al. (2017 Feb). Macroscopic hematuria with normal renal biopsy – following the chain to the diagnosis: questions. *Pediatr. Nephrol.* 32 (2): 277–278. https://doi.org/10.1007/s00467-015-3266-4.
4. Mirza, N., Marson, A.G., and Pirmohamed, M. (eds.) (2009). Effect of topiramate on acid-base balance: extent, mechanism and effects. *Br. J. Clin. Pharmacol.* 68 (5): 655.
5. Batuman, V. (2007). Proximal tubular injury in myeloma. *Contrib. Nephrol.* 153: 87–104.
6. Yu, A.S. (2015). Claudins and the kidney. *J. Am. Soc. Nephrol.* 26 (1): 11.
7. Gong, Y., Renigunta, V., Himmerkus, N. et al. (2012 Apr). Claudin-14 regulates renal Ca^{++} transport in response to CaSR signalling via a novel microRNA pathway. *EMBO J.* 31 (8): 1999–2012.
8. Simon, D.B., Bindra, R.S., Mansfield, T.A. et al. (1997). Mutations in the chloride channel gene, CLCNKB, cause Bartter;s Syndrome type III. *Nat. Genet.* 17 (2): 171–178.
9. Simon, D.B., Bindra, R.S., Mansfield, T.A. et al. (1997). Mutations in the chloride channel gene, CLCNKB, cause Bartter's syndrome type III. *Nat. Genet.* 17 (2): 171.
10. Konrad, M., Vollmer, M., Lemmink, H.H. et al. (eds.) (2000). Mutations in the chloride channel gene CLCNKB as a cause of classic Bartter syndrome. *J. Am. Soc. Nephrol.* 11 (8): 1449–1459.
11. De Jong, J.C., Van Der Vliet, W.A., Van Den Heuvel, L.P. et al. (2000). Functional expression of mutations in the human NaCl cotransporter: evidence for impaired routing mechanisms in Gitelman's syndrome. *J. Am. Soc. Nephrol.* 11 (8): 1449.
12. De Jong, J.C., Van Der Vliet, W.A., Van Den Heuvel, L.P. et al. (2002). Functional expression of mutations in the human NaCl cotransporter: evidence

for impaired routing mechanisms in Gitelman's syndrome. *Am. Soc. Nephrol.* 13 (6): 1442.

13. Vallon, V. (2003). Tubuloglomerular feedback and the control of glomerular filtration rate. *News Physiol. Sci.* 18 (4): 169–174. https://doi.org/10.1097/01.ASN.0000023430.92674.E5.

14. Toto, R.D., Mitchell, H.C., Lee, H.C. et al. (1991). Reversible renal insufficiency due to angiotensin converting enzyme inhibitors in hypertensive nephrosclerosis. *Ann. Intern. Med.* 115 (7): 513.

15. Bakris, G.L. and Weir, M.R. (2000). Angiotensin-converting enzyme inhibitor-associated elevations in serum creatinine: is this a cause for concern? *Arch. Intern. Med.* 160 (5): 685.

Questions and Answers

Questions

1. In the proximal convoluted tubule, sodium is reabsorbed in exchange for:
   a. Hydrogen
   b. Magnesium
   c. Calcium
   d. Glucose, amino acids, and phosphate
   e. Potassium and chloride

2. Fanconi syndrome should be suspected in:
   a. Hyperuricaemia
   b. Hyperphosphataemia
   c. Hypophosphataemia
   d. Hyperkalaemia
   e. Alkalosis

3. Which part of the renal tubule is impermeable to water?
   a. Proximal convoluted tubule
   b. Distal convoluted tubule
   c. Cortical duct
   d. Descending limb of loop of Henle
   e. Ascending limb of loop of Henle

4. The following electrolyte profile may be associated with both thiazide and loop diuretics
   a. Hyperkalaemia with metabolic alkalosis
   b. Hypokalaemia with metabolic alkalosis
   c. Hyperkalaemia with metabolic acidosis
   d. Hypokalaemia with metabolic acidosis
   e. Hyperkalaemia

5. The correct statement regarding macula densa is
   a. The macula densa senses the total amount of NaCl in tubular urine
   b. If the delivery of NaCl is lower than normal, then macula densa signals special cells in the afferent arteriole to release renin
   c. Renin release has no effect on aldosterone production
   d. a and b are correct
   e. All of them are correct

6. The effect of aldosterone on renal H^+ secretion is:
   a. It has no effect
   b. Increases secretion
   c. Decreases secretion
   d. Can do both at different parts of the tubule
   e. Reabsorb H^+

7. Primary hyperaldosteronism is characterized by:
   a. Hypokalaemia
   b. Hyperkalaemia
   c. Metabolic alkalosis
   d. Metabolic acidosis
   e. a and c

Answers

1. a. In the PCT, the reabsorption of Na$^+$ is coupled to the secretion of H$^+$. Glucose, amino acids, phosphate, and uric acid are co-transported with the Na$^+$. Ca$^+$ and Mg$^+$ are also reabsorbed here though the bulk of Mg$^+$ reabsorption occurs in the TAL.

2. c. Type 2 RTA is due to a proximal tubular defect in the reabsorption of HCO$_3^-$ leading to urinary loss of HCO$_3^-$ and metabolic acidosis with hypokalaemia. The absorption of HCO$_3^-$ in this segment is linked to the coupled exchange of H$^+$ and Na$^+$. As this reabsorption of Na$^+$ is linked to the reabsorption of glucose, amino acids, phosphate, and uric acid, the patient may present with glycosuria, hypophosphataemia, and hypouricaemia (due to urinary losses) and this condition is termed as Fanconi syndrome.

3. e. The countercurrent mechanism is fundamentally dependent on the impermeability of the ascending limb of loop of Henle to water. The reabsorption of Na$^+$ by the Na$^+$-K$^+$-2Cl$^-$ transporter in the absence of water reabsorption in longer loops of the juxtamedullary nephrons leads to establishment of the medullary osmotic gradient. It is worth remembering that without this gradient water reabsorption in the medullary collecting duct under the influence of ADH would not be possible.

4. b. All diuretics act by inhibiting the tubular reabsorption of Na$^+$. In case of loop and thiazide diuretics, with more Na$^+$ flowing to the distal nephron, the tubular cells reclaim some of the excess Na$^+$ leading to decrease in luminal positivity. The tubular cells try to compensate for this by secretion of the positively charged K$^+$ and H$^+$ into the lumen. Also, intravascular volume contraction because of diuretics cause activation of the renin-angiotensin-aldosterone system (RAAS), which in turn leads to urinary K$^+$ and H$^+$ losses under the influence of aldosterone.

5. d. Macula densa (modified tubular epithelial cells at the ending of TAL and beginning of DCT) senses Na$^+$ and Cl$^-$ level in the tubular fluid and in case of low levels, stimulates granular cells, which are modified smooth muscle cells in the afferent arteriole to secrete renin. Renin breaks down hepatic angiotensinogen to yield angiotensin I, which is then cleaved further by the angiotensin-converting enzyme in the lung to yield angiotensin II. Angiotensin II apart from being a very potent vasoconstrictor also stimulates aldosterone release by the adrenal gland.

6. b. Aldosterone aids in the reabsorption of Na$^+$ and secretion of K$^+$ and H$^+$ in the collecting duct. Aldosterone upregulates the basolateral Na$^+$-K$^+$-ATPase (in principal cell) causing lower intracellular Na$^+$ and at the same time upregulates epithelial sodium channels (ENaC), thus increasing apical membrane permeability for Na$^+$. The movement of Na$^+$ from the lumen to the epithelial cells leads to luminal negativity which triggers K$^+$ secretion by the epithelial cells to correct the potential difference. However, the Na$^+$ to K$^+$ exchange is not strictly a one-to-one phenomenon and more Na$^+$ is reabsorbed than K$^+$ is secreted. H$^+$ gets secreted by the neighbouring alpha-intercalated cells to make up for this difference.

7. e. Primary hyperaldosteronism should always be suspected in the hypertensive patient with hypokalaemia and metabolic alkalosis (although more than half the patients are normokalemic) who is not on thiazide or loop diuretics. Aldosterone leads to reabsorption of Na$^+$ in the CD and the resulting tubular negativity aids in the excretion of K$^+$ and H$^+$.

2

Investigation of Renal Diseases

Karumathil Murali and Wayne Rankin

Summary

- Evaluation of renal disease involves multiple modalities including urine dipstick test and microscopy, imaging, laboratory analysis of urine and blood, and at times renal biopsy
- Non-contrast computed tomography (CT) scan is highly sensitive for the detection of urinary calculi including uric acid stones, which may be radiolucent in plain X-ray
- Ultrasound is highly reliable to exclude urinary obstruction
- Whilst nuclear scans are not used as the initial imaging modality of choice for the evaluation of renal diseases, they are often used to derive functional information to supplement structural details obtained from ultrasound or CT scans
- Normally 10% of urinary creatinine is derived from secretion by the proximal tubule: during acute kidney injury, tubular secretion of creatinine can increase up to 40% of the total urinary creatinine, due to a decrease in filtered creatinine and an increase in tubular creatinine secretion, primarily driven by the rise in serum creatinine levels. Therefore overall creatinine excretion may not decrease until late in renal failure
- The Chronic Kidney Disease Epidemiology Collaboration (CKD-EPI) equation for estimation of the glomerular filtration rate is currently recommended by most experts for the classification and staging of chronic kidney disease
- Renal biopsy is often undertaken to establish diagnosis in patients with nephrotic syndrome, unexplained renal failure, glomerular haematuria, and/or proteinuria >1 g/day

Multiple investigative modalities are available for the evaluation of renal disease. The judicial combination of bedside examination, urine dipstick testing, imaging, laboratory analysis of urine and blood and at times renal biopsy helps to establish diagnosis, selection of appropriate treatment options, and prediction of prognosis.

Radiological Investigation of Kidney Disease

The choice of radiological investigation depends on the clinical indication and a combination of

Lecture Notes Nephrology: A Comprehensive Guide to Renal Medicine, First Edition. Edited by Surjit Tarafdar.
© 2020 John Wiley & Sons Ltd. Published 2020 by John Wiley & Sons Ltd.

tests is often required to establish an accurate diagnosis.

Plain X-ray

Plain X-rays are rarely used to investigate kidney disease in modern practice. The renal outlines in plain films are frequently obscured by bowel gas shadows. Calculi in the kidneys or along the urinary tract may be visible, but phleboliths and faecoliths can cause confusion. Although a plain X-ray of the abdomen can identify calcium-containing, struvite, and cystine stones, it may fail to delineate radiolucent uric acid and xanthine stones [1]. A plain X-ray may also miss small radiopaque stones or stones overlying bony structures.

Ultrasound

Ultrasound is a frequently used non-invasive imaging modality and has the advantage of not exposing the patient to ionizing radiation or nephrotoxic contrast agents. It is relatively inexpensive, but has the disadvantage of being operator dependent. Ultrasound is highly reliable to exclude urinary obstruction and also distinguish whether a lesion in the renal parenchyma is cystic or solid. Doppler ultrasound scanning in experienced hands provides valuable information regarding blood flow to and from the kidneys (Figures 2.1 and 2.2).

Renal size varies between 9 and 12 cm and shrinkage usually indicates chronic renal parenchymal disease. Mild renal enlargement may be seen in diabetes, amyloidosis, and myeloma. In these conditions, renal size may be preserved even when the patient reaches end-stage renal disease (ESRD).

The renal cortical outline is usually smooth and regular. Mild cortical lobularity, known as foetal lobulation, is a normal variant. Marked cortical irregularity however indicates renal scarring. Generalized scarring is non-specific and may result from a variety of chronic renal diseases. In reflux nephropathy, scars

(a)

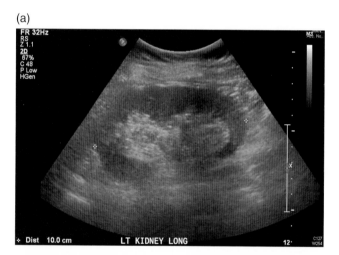

(b)

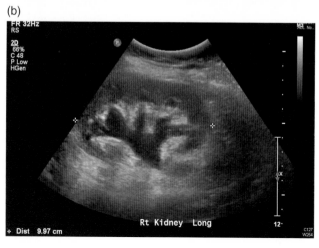

Figure 2.1 Ultrasound images of normal kidney and in hydronephrosis. (a) Normal kidney shows a smooth and regular outline with adequate cortical thickness. The central echo complex is predominantly echogenic due to an abundance of renal sinus fat. The pelvi-calyceal system is normally not identifiable except when dilated (b), as in hydronephrosis.

(a)

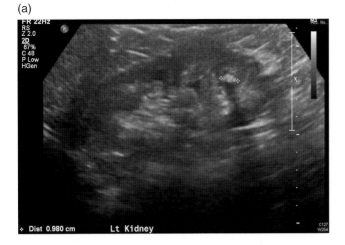

(b)

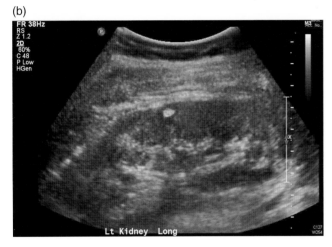

Figure 2.2 Ultrasound images of renal echogenic lesions. Ultrasound is sensitive to detect renal calculi, which are identified as echogenic foci with an acoustic shadowing (a). Similarly, echogenic lesions may be due to angiomyolipoma (b), which are dense due to the fat content, but lack acoustic shadowing and are seen as hypodense lesions in computed tomography scan.

are most prominent in the upper and lower poles. Focal scars may result from renal infarcts or severe pyelonephritis.

Cortical thickness is measured from the surface to the base of the medullary pyramids, which are less echogenic than the parenchyma. Diffuse cortical thinning is suggestive of chronic kidney disease (CKD), whilst localized cortical thinning is often associated with a cortical scar.

The commonest abnormality seen in the renal parenchyma is renal cysts (Figure 2.3). Simple cysts are characterized by a thin wall, and the absence of septa or solid components. They can be multiple and bilateral.

Bosniak Classification of Renal Cysts

The Bosniak classification was developed to risk-stratify cysts based on findings in urinary tract imaging to estimate the probability of cancer [2]. This classification helps in the evaluation and follow-up of renal cysts, which are very common and seen in over 25% of patients above the age of 50 years (Figure 2.4).

- *Bosniak I*: hairline-thin wall without internal septa, calcifications or solid areas; clear contents without contrast enhancement. Very low risk of cancer.
- *Bosniak II*: may contain thin septa, some calcification in the wall or septa, includes uniformly high-attenuation lesions <3 cm, but no contrast enhancement. Low risk of cancer.
- *Bosniak IIF*: may have multiple septa, mildly thickened septum or wall with areas of nodular calcification, uniformly attenuating lesions >3 cm are also included, but again without significant contrast enhancement. These are diagnosed as complicated cysts and require radiological follow-up after three to six months to ensure stability.
- *Bosniak III*: includes indeterminate cysts with thickened or irregular walls or septa, which may or

(a)

(b)

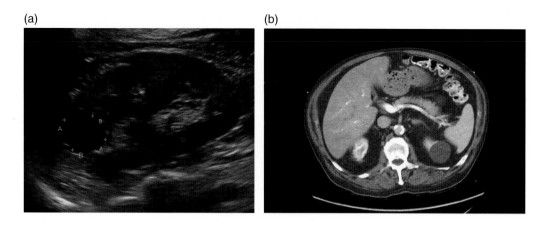

Figure 2.3 Simple renal cyst seen on (a) ultrasound and (b) computed tomography scan.

(a)

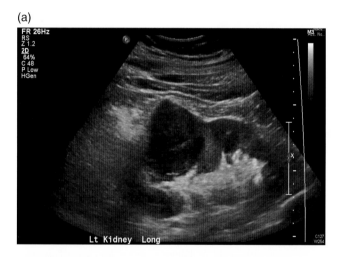

(b)

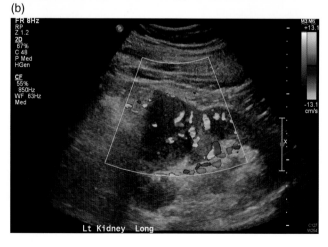

Figure 2.4 Ultrasound images of Bosniak IV category renal cyst. Solid areas (a) in a cyst with increased vascularity (b) classify a complex cyst to Bosniak IV category with 80–100% risk of renal cell cancer.

may not show contrast enhancement. Up to 40–60% of these lesions represent renal cell cancer.

- *Bosniak IV*: have enhancing soft tissue densities in addition to the features of Bosniak III cysts. Up to 80–100% of these lesions are neoplastic.

Markedly enlarged kidneys with multiple bilateral cysts suggest autosomal dominant polycystic kidney disease. Renal calculi are visualized as bright or echogenic foci, and the presence of acoustic shadowing is diagnostic. Shadowing is absent in angiomyolipomas, which are also bright due to the abundance of fat. Renal masses can be identified by ultrasound, but a computed tomography (CT) scan provides better delineation.

The ureters are visible in ultrasound only when dilated. The urinary bladder should be adequately distended for optimal evaluation, otherwise there is a risk of over-diagnosing trabeculations and mucosal lesions. Measurement of residual urine is important, especially in patients with prostatomegaly, lower urinary tract symptoms or recurrent urinary infections.

Renal Artery Doppler Scans

These scans evaluate vascular flow in both renal arteries and veins. They are usually used for evaluation of renal artery stenosis, renal vein thrombosis, and renal infarction.

Markedly increased peak systolic velocity in the renal artery, especially when compared to aortic peak systolic velocity (renal/aortic ratio), is suggestive of renal artery stenosis. Prolonged acceleration time (the time from start of flow to peak flow) with a slow rising pulse (tardus–parvus isoform) also indicates resistance to systolic flow due to luminal stenosis.

Renal artery Doppler should preferably be done in the fasting state, as image quality can be compromised by bowel gas. The test is highly operator dependent and often needs a long examination time.

Resistive Index

The resistive index (RI) is measured as:

Peak systolic velocity – end diastolic velocity / peak systolic velocity

A normal RI is <0.70.

Although there has been a decrease in the initial enthusiasm for the use of the RI in renal transplant patients, it is still commonly used to monitor the transplant in early post-transplant days. Causes for a raised RI in the transplant kidney include:

- Acute tubular necrosis (ATN)
- Acute or chronic transplant rejection

- Immunosuppression toxicity
- Renal vein thrombosis
- Renal artery stenosis
- Perinephric fluid collection

A prospective study of 321 renal transplant recipients found that an RI >0.8 was associated with an increased risk for a composite endpoint of a 50% decrease in graft function, need for dialysis or recipient death [3]. RI is considered a poor marker of renal parenchymal disorders and is rarely used in the evaluation of native kidneys.

Computed Tomography

CT often provides complementary information to that obtained with renal ultrasonography, and has the advantage of allowing simultaneous evaluation of adrenal lesions and abnormalities in other abdominal organs. Non-contrast CT is highly sensitive for the detection of urinary calculi, including uric acid stones, which may be radiolucent in plain X-ray. It is superior to ultrasound in the detection of ureteric calculi and identifying the level of ureteric obstruction. It is less sensitive than ultrasound in differentiating between solid and cystic lesions in the kidneys; however, solid lesions with high fat content, such as angiomyolipomas, have a distinct hypodense appearance in CT scan. Non-contrast CT has largely replaced intravenous pyelography in urological evaluation for suspected nephrolithiasis.

Enhancement of a lesion after administration of intravenous contrast may suggest increased vascularity, a hallmark of malignant renal tumours. Vascular lesions such as arteriovenous malformations are also highlighted by contrast enhancement, whilst renal infarcts classically appear as wedge-shaped non-enhancing hypodensities.

Magnetic Resonance Imaging

Whilst not recommended as a first-line urinary tract imaging modality, magnetic resonance imaging (MRI) is useful to evaluate renal lesions which are inconclusive on CT or when contrast-enhanced CT scan is not advisable, for example in a patient with contrast allergy. MRI provides better delineation of wall thickening and nodularity of renal lesions compared to CT or ultrasound. It can also provide useful information about the contents of cysts, such as hyperdensity seen in cyst haemorrhage. Diffusion-weighted MRI may be helpful to distinguish between inflammatory and neoplastic masses when evaluating indeterminate renal lesions. There are no diagnostic features in MRI that will confidently distinguish between benign and malignant renal lesions, therefore clinical and imaging follow-up may be necessary for equivocal lesions. Gadolinium enhancement is the most prominent feature of malignant renal tumours.

CT Angiography

CT angiography (CTA) is often used to evaluate suspected renal artery stenosis. It easily identifies atherosclerotic renal artery stenosis and demonstrates the calcification burden in the aorta and renal ostium.

Radiocontrast used for CT imaging has the potential to cause nephrotoxicity [4]. Vulnerability is greater in patients with underlying CKD, diabetes, heart failure, and multiple myeloma. Strategies to mitigate the risk of contrast nephrotoxicity include using the lowest possible dose of contrast agent and choosing a low-osmolality non-ionic agent. Prehydration with intravenous fluids, either saline or sodium bicarbonate, has been shown to be effective in reducing the incidence of contrast nephrotoxicity. The use of oral N-acetylcysteine is no longer advised for prevention of contrast nephrotoxicity.

Magnetic Resonance Angiography

Magnetic resonance angiography (MRA) of the renal arteries with gadolinium enhancement is used to diagnose renal artery stenosis with greater accuracy compared to Doppler ultrasound imaging. When MRA is performed without gadolinium, the test is less reliable. Although gadolinium-enhanced MRA gives image resolution comparable to CTA, it is not very sensitive for calcification, which is better delineated by CT imaging. MRA can also miss mid and distal vessel lesions seen in fibromuscular dysplasia (FMD) and the renal artery aneurysms seen in polyarteritis nodosa (PAN).

In patients with advanced kidney disease, use of gadolinium has been implicated in the systemic disease nephrogenic systemic fibrosis (NSF) [5]. Most reported cases of NSF have occurred in patients on dialysis, but gadolinium should be avoided in patients with estimated glomerular filtration rate (eGFR) <30 ml/min/1.73 m^2. Gadolinium is safe in patients with eGFR >60 ml/min/1.73 m^2, but its safety in patients with eGFR between 30 and 60 ml/min/1.73 m^2 is unclear. The benefits should be weighed against the potential risks in such patients. NSF runs a variable course and can be progressive. Although ESRD patients with NSF have shown improvement in symptoms with restoration of normal kidney function following kidney transplantation, there is no definitive cure for this condition; therefore, prevention is the key. Apart from avoiding gadolinium altogether, prompt post-MRI institution of haemodialysis can reduce the load of the agent in patients with advanced renal failure or those on established dialysis. Peritoneal dialysis (PD) is not very effective in the removal of gadolinium and therefore patients on PD are offered urgent haemodialysis if they are exposed.

Renal Digital Subtraction Angiography/Arteriography

Digital subtraction angiography (DSA) is rarely needed as a diagnostic test, because less invasive tests such as CTA and MRA provide similar information. However, the image resolution of DSA is far superior. It has higher sensitivity and specificity for subtle abnormalities as in mild cases of FMD and PAN (Figure 2.5). Renal artery interventions such as revascularization (angioplasty/stenting), renal sympathetic denervation or selective branch occlusion, such as coil embolization to control post-procedure bleeding, require arteriography. In addition to the risk of contrast toxicity, arteriography also entails the risk of cholesterol embolization due to dislodgement of atherosclerotic plaques and arterial injury, including intimal dissection.

Micturating Cystourethrography

Micturating cystourethrography (MCU) involves filling the urinary bladder with radiocontrast using a urethral catheter and taking serial X-rays when the patient is voiding to detect vesicoureteric reflux. This is most commonly performed in children. Vesicoureteric reflux can also be diagnosed using indirect radionuclide cystography, which does not require urethral catheterization, but does not provide the same detailed anatomical information as obtained with MCU.

Retrograde/Antegrade Pyelography

Retrograde/antegrade pyelography is usually done during invasive investigation or treatment of suspected urinary obstruction. The former requires cystoscopic ureteric cannulation and the latter requires percutaneous transrenal puncture of the collecting system under radiological guidance. The resolution of the images is higher than CT urography or intravenous urography and the test can detect mucosal filling defects, which can occur due to transitional cell cancers involving the ureter or renal pelvis.

(a)

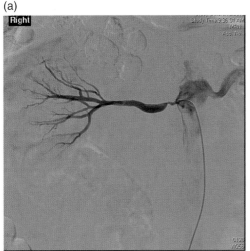

(b)

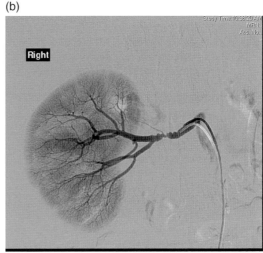

Figure 2.5 Digital subtraction angiography distinguishes between atherosclerotic renal artery stenosis (a) where the narrowing is in the proximal portion of artery near its origin from aorta with post-stenotic dilatation, and fibromuscular dysplasia (b) which is characterized by more distally located multiple narrowing and dilatation leading to a 'beaded' appearance.

Retrograde studies can be useful in localizing the obstruction when there is insufficient renal function to excrete intravenous contrast.

Antegrade pyelography is resorted to when retrograde pyelography is less feasible. Ureteral pressures can be measured, and the examination is often performed as a prelude to nephrostomy placement.

Nuclear Imaging

Nuclear imaging of the kidney is never employed as primary renal imaging, but is often used to derive functional information to supplement structural details obtained from ultrasound or CT scans. Nuclear scans can evaluate renal perfusion, excretion, and obstruction, with the option of refining functional information using pharmacological agents. The radionuclide agents commonly used include ^{99m}Tc diethylene triamine pentaacetic acid (DTPA), ^{99m}Tc mercapto acethyl triglycine (MAG3), and ^{99m}Tc dimercapto succinic acid (DMSA). DTPA is cleared by glomerular filtration and is ideal for dynamic imaging and studies to assess function. MAG3 is secreted in the proximal tubule, but is rapidly cleared and is suited for dynamic imaging, similar to DTPA. Because of its lesser dependence on glomerular filtration for clearance, the more expensive MAG3 is superior in patients with reduced GFR. DMSA is taken up by proximal tubular cells and accumulates there for several hours before clearing. DMSA is therefore suitable for static renal imaging, for example for detection of scars in reflux nephropathy.

A radionuclide renal scan (renogram) provides information about blood flow as well as renal uptake and excretion (Figure 2.6). The initial phase of the study shows blood flow through both kidneys and the aorta. The images are taken every few seconds up to a minute after bolus injection of the radiotracer. This part of the test therefore helps to evaluate perfusion of the kidneys.

The second phase of the renogram evaluates renal function by measuring radiotracer uptake and excretion by the individual kidneys. Pictures are taken every 2 minutes for up to 30 minutes, with peak renal cortical concentration normally occurring between 3 and 5 minutes after injection of the tracer. Delayed transit of the tracer can be due to renal dysfunction (e.g. rejection or ATN) or obstructive uropathy.

In cases of suspected obstructive uropathy based on delay in clearance of the tracer from the pelvicalyceal system, a diuretic renogram can be helpful (Figure 2.7). A loop diuretic is injected intravenously whilst radiotracer activity is still present in the renal pelvis and serial images are obtained to assess tracer clearance. A computer-generated washout curve is then obtained. In patients with true obstruction, the radiotracer activity will remain in the collecting system despite the administration of the loop diuretic, whilst it will quickly wash out in the absence of true obstruction.

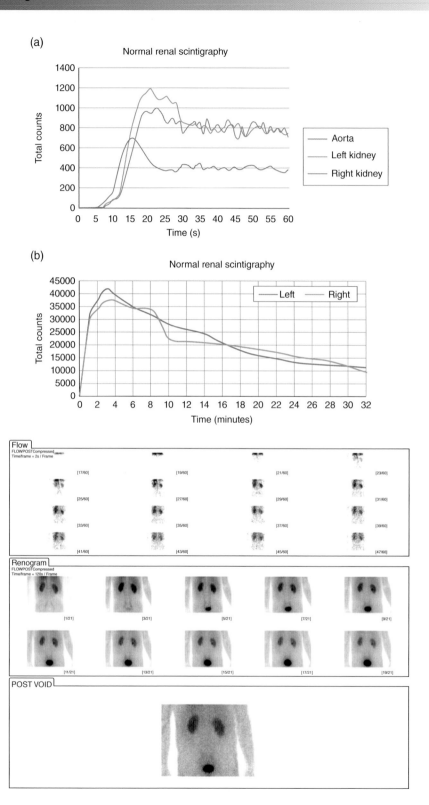

Figure 2.6 Normal renal scintigraphy: (top) renal blood flow in 0–60 seconds; (bottom) renal uptake and excretion of tracer over 0–30 minutes.

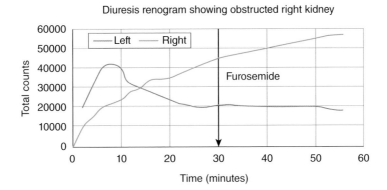

Figure 2.7 Diuresis renogram showing obstructed right kidney causing tracer to continue accumulating in the right kidney despite intravenous administration of frusemide.

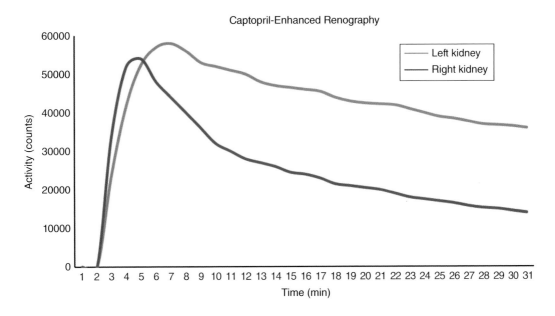

Figure 2.8 Captopril renogram showing delayed peak activity and excretion of tracer in the left kidney with renal artery stenosis.

Captopril Renogram

A captopril renogram is useful as a screening test for unilateral renal artery stenosis (Figure 2.8) [6]. The test is based on the principle that patients with renal artery stenosis maintain their parenchymal perfusion by compensatory angiotensin II-mediated efferent arteriolar constriction to increase the intra-glomerular pressure and thereby preserve glomerular filtration. After a baseline DTPA/MAG3 scan to assess perfusion and initial excretion, captopril, a short-acting angiotensin-converting enzyme inhibitor, is administered to counter the angiotensin II-mediated increase in filtration pressure. This lowers excretion on the affected side, as detected by a second set of scans, and suggests functionally significant renal artery stenosis. The test detects the differential reduction in GFR and therefore is not reliable in the diagnosis of bilateral renal artery stenosis.

Laboratory Evaluation of Renal Function

A variety of tests which assess glomerular filtration as well as immunological and microbiological tests to evaluate the aetio-pathogenesis of renal disease are undertaken in the routine evaluation of patients with kidney disease.

Glomerular Filtration Rate

The GFR provides an overall measure of filtration occurring at all functioning nephrons and reflects the total number of functioning nephrons. However, the relationship between GFR and nephron number is not a simple linear relationship, being complicated by factors such as compensatory hyperfiltration, muscle mass, diet, tubular secretion of creatinine, and extra-renal clearance of creatinine:

- An increase in single-nephron GFR due to a compensatory increase in glomerular capillary pressure and glomerular hypertrophy can compensate for the decrease in nephron number, and therefore the GFR may not reflect the nephron loss.
- Creatinine is derived from the metabolism of phosphocreatine in muscle, as well as excessive dietary creatine from high meat intake or creatine supplements sometimes used by body builders. Increased muscle mass and excess intake of meat therefore can lead to raised plasma creatinine without alteration in GFR. For the same reason, creatinine may be low in vegetarians and those with amputation.
- Creatinine is freely filtered across the glomerulus and is neither reabsorbed nor metabolized by the kidney. Under normal conditions, approximately 10% of urinary creatinine is derived from secretion by the proximal tubule. As the GFR falls, tubular secretion of creatinine is enhanced to up to 40% of the total urinary creatinine, thus causing the plasma creatinine to remain unchanged. Thus, a relatively stable plasma creatinine in the normal or near normal range does not exclude renal impairment. Also, drugs like cimetidine and trimethoprim interfere with the proximal tubular secretion of creatinine and thus increase the plasma creatinine levels without any change in the actual GFR.
- Creatinine is contained in intestinal secretions and degraded by bacteria. When GFR is reduced, the amount of creatinine eliminated through this extra-renal route is increased due to intestinal bacterial overgrowth and increased bacterial creatininase activity. On the other hand, antibiotics can raise plasma creatinine by destroying intestinal bacteria and thus inhibiting this extra-renal pathway of creatinine secretion.

Clearance Studies

Laboratory techniques do not allow for direct measurement of GFR; however, GFR can be approximated via measurement of the clearance of a filtration marker. Ideally, this marker should be freely filtered at the glomerulus, not secreted or reabsorbed by the tubules, and not synthesized or catabolized during its excretion. For any filtration marker, the clearance can be calculated from the concentration of the marker in urine (U) and plasma (P) and the urine formation rate (volume/time; V/t) according to the general equation:

$$Clearance = (U \times V/t)/P$$

For an ideal filtration marker, the filtered load is equal to the rate of urinary excretion and, theoretically, the clearance is equal to the GFR.

Inulin Clearance

The polysaccharide inulin has been used as an ideal exogenous filtration marker since it meets the criteria discussed. However, inulin clearance determination is of historical interest only, as it never became a routine investigation because testing was expensive, invasive – requiring venous cannulation and bladder catheterization – and there were technical difficulties associated with inulin assays.

Because of the limitations of inulin clearance estimation, the focus turned to the clearance of endogenous markers. Although no endogenous marker meets the criteria for an ideal marker, knowledge of the limitations of a given marker means that resultant clearance values can be interpreted accordingly.

Creatinine Clearance

Creatinine clearance is determined from the concentrations of creatinine in plasma and a timed urine sample, usually a 24-hour collection. Creatinine is freely filtered at the glomerulus and is not reabsorbed or metabolized by the kidney. However, with worsening renal function up to 40% of the creatinine in urine arises from secretion in the proximal tubule, leading to overestimation of the GFR.

Additional errors are introduced in the collection of the required timed urine sample, usually over 24 hours, particularly in the outpatient setting, because of patient difficulties in both timing the collection and capturing the full collection volume.

Estimated Glomerular Filtration Rate

As the inverse relation between plasma creatinine and creatinine clearance/GFR is not linear, regression equations have been derived to estimate GFR from a single plasma creatinine measurement. These formulae take into consideration the well-established relationship between creatinine production, muscle mass, and age. The three best-characterized equations are the Cockcroft–Gault, Modification of Diet in Renal Disease (MDRD), and Chronic Kidney Disease Epidemiology Collaboration (CKD-EPI) formulae. It should be noted that these formulae are not applicable in all populations. They are only useful when renal function (and thus creatinine concentration) is stable and are not recommended for use in pregnant women, acutely unwell and hospitalized patients, or in cases of acute kidney injury. Care should also be taken in applying these equations to people with extremes in muscle mass, including amputees, paraplegics, body builders, the obese, and those with muscle-wasting and neuromuscular disease. Dietary extremes should also be considered, and care taken in people with malnutrition, vegetarians, and those taking creatine dietary supplements. These formulae are not applicable in people under the age of 18 years.

Cockcroft–Gault Formula

This estimates GFR based on plasma creatinine and patient age, weight, and sex:

$$Estimated\,GFR(ml\,/\,min) = \{(140 - Age) \times weight(kg) \times F\} /$$
$$(plasma\,creatinine[\mu mol\,/\,l] \times 0.815)$$

where F = 1 if male and 0.85 if female.

This formula was derived from a small study of predominantly male subjects and, despite its validation in subsequent studies, questions remain as to its applicability across multiple population groups. Being the only creatinine estimation formula that includes weight in the equation, this formula overestimates GFR in the obese and oedematous patients. Although the Cockcroft–Gault formula is still used in some drug dosing applications, its use has been predominantly supplanted by the more rigorously derived MDRD and CKD-EPI formulae, both of which were developed and validated against I^{125}-iothalamate clearance, considered a gold standard measure of GFR in clinical practice.

MDRD Formula

This was developed in a study involving over 1600 predominantly male subjects, most with renal disease, and is based on plasma creatinine, age, and gender:

$$eGFR(ml\,/\,min\,/\,1.73m^2) = 175 \times$$
$$(plasma\,creatinine[\mu mol\,/\,l] \times 0.0113)^{-1.154} \times age^{-0.203}$$

$$(\times 0.742\,if\,female) - (1.210\,if\,African\,American)$$

This formula can lead to systematic underestimation of GFR at values above 60 ml/min/1.73 m^2.

CKD-EPI Equation

The CKD-EPI equation should be used when Scr is reported in mg/dL:

$$GFR = 141 \times min\,(Scr/\kappa,1)^{\alpha} \times max\,(Scr/\kappa,1)^{-1.209} \times 0.993^{Age}$$
$$\times 1.018\,[if\,female] \times 1.159\,[if\,black]$$

where Scr is serum creatinine in mg/dL, κ is 0.7 for females and 0.9 for males, α is –0.329 for females and –0.411 for males, min indicates the minimum of Scr/κ or 1, and max indicates the maximum of Scr/κ or 1.

The CKD-EPI equation is as accurate as the MDRD study equation amongst individuals with an estimated GFR less than 60 ml/min per 1.73 m^2, and somewhat more accurate in those with higher GFRs [7, 8].

Current international guidelines addressing the classification and staging of CKD generally recommend use of the CKD-EPI formula, but do allow for other formulae to be used if considered appropriate to the patient population.

Of note is that tubular secretion of creatinine is disproportionally high in patients with nephrotic syndrome and sickle cell disease, and therefore these patients may have a GFR that is substantially lower than is estimated from the serum creatinine.

Cystatin C is a cysteine protease inhibitor present on the surface of all nucleated cells. It has a molecular weight of approximately 13.4 kDa and, after being shed into the plasma, is cleared by glomerular filtration. As its production is independent of diet, muscle mass, age, and sex, measurement of cystatin C has been suggested to provide a better indicator of GFR than creatinine [9]. Uptake of this test has been limited primarily by expense and availability. It should also be noted that cystatin C concentrations are increased by corticosteroid treatment in a dose-dependent manner, which can lead to underestimation of the GFR; caution is therefore advised in the use of cystatin C in assessing GFR in renal transplant patients receiving steroid as part of anti-rejection treatment.

Calcium, Phosphate, and Parathyroid Hormone

Calcium, phosphate, and parathyroid hormone (PTH) levels are frequently measured in patients with CKD. Plasma calcium is approximately 50% bound to albumin, whilst 5% is bound to anions such as bicarbonate and citrate. The remaining calcium that exists in a free ionized form represents the biologically active component of the total plasma calcium. Approximate corrections for decreased albumin concentrations can be made using simple formulae, the most commonly used being:

$$Calcium_{Corrected} (mmol/l) = Calcium_{Measured} (mmol/l) + 0.02 \times (40 - serum\ albumin[g/L])$$

Measurement of total calcium and albumin and application of this equation are adequate in most circumstances; however, if more precise assessment of calcium homeostasis is required, the ionized fraction of calcium should be measured.

Phosphate is commonly measured in the plasma of patients with CKD. Though most of the body content of phosphate is intracellular and organic, nearly all the phosphate in the extracellular fluid is inorganic and easily measurable.

A marked increase in phosphate levels, whether acute or chronic, can lead to a reciprocal reduction in calcium levels due to extravascular calcium phosphate precipitation [10]. Specific combination patterns of abnormalities in calcium, phosphate, and PTH levels can provide valuable clues to the underlying clinical problem (Table 2.1).

Additional Tests

In addition to the traditional renal function tests, other routine tests can provide insight into renal pathology and its prognosis. Derangement in liver function tests can provide an impetus to assess for hepatitis-associated renal disease or, in the setting of ischaemic ATN, may point to ischaemic liver injury. Increased alkaline phosphatase activity in the absence of obstructive liver disease may be an indicator of renal bone disease [11]. If doubt exists as to the

origin of the alkaline phosphatase, isoenzyme fractionation could be considered.

Decreased albumin can be indicative of nephrotic syndrome. The lipid profile is also markedly altered in nephrotic syndrome, leading to both hypercholesterolaemia and hypertriglyceridaemia.

Measurement of uric acid is important in both nephrolithiasis and suspected urate nephropathy. Acute urate nephropathy occurs with intratubular precipitation of uric acid crystals following the production and excretion of large amounts of uric acid in conditions such as tumour-lysis syndrome and can lead to renal failure. In contrast, chronic urate nephropathy is the consequence of chronic inflammation in response to uric acid precipitation within the renal medulla leading to tubulointerstitial fibrosis and atrophy, with resultant CKD.

Haematological tests are important in renal disease and may provide indications about the nature or severity of the underlying disease. Erythropoietin is synthesized by the renal interstitial cells and stimulates erythrocyte production by the bone marrow. As CKD progresses, erythropoietin production is compromised and results in anaemia. This can be complicated by the possible presence of iron deficiency as well as the chronic inflammatory environment associated with CKD that can lead to functional iron deficiency and associated anaemia of chronic disease. Renal anaemia is typically normocytic normochromic; however, with overt iron deficiency it may be microcytic hypochromic. Iron studies performed to assess the nature of the anaemia should be interpreted with the CKD in mind, with ferritin values increased in response to inflammation, and values as high as 100 μg/l might still represent iron deficiency. Ferritin levels above 200 μg/l and transferrin saturation above 20% are desirable in patients who are receiving recombinant erythropoietin for renal anaemia.

In the setting of acute kidney injury (AKI), new anaemia in the absence of overt blood loss may indicate a haemolytic process. Intravascular haemol-

Table 2.1 Calcium, phosphate, and parathyroid hormone levels in different types of hyperparathyroidism

Calcium	Phosphate	Parathyroid hormone (PTH)	Probable clinical condition
High	Low	High (or not appropriately suppressed)	Primary hyperparathyroidism
Low or normal	High	High	Secondary hyperparathyroidism
High	High	High	Tertiary hyperparathyroidism

ysis due to a variety of causes can cause haemoglobi-nuria and AKI, whilst microangiopathic haemolytic processes cause kidney injury due to microvascular thrombosis. The latter is characterized by new onset of thrombocytopenia. Whilst thrombocytopenia may be due to a number of aetiologies, the presence of fragmented red cells (schistocytes) in the peripheral blood film and biochemical markers of haemolysis like elevated reticulocyte count and decreased serum haptoglobin point to thrombotic microangiopathy as the cause of thrombocytopenia. Leukocytosis is non-specific but may indicate an infectious process, whilst leukopaenia may be related to a number of aetiologies, including drug-related side effects or systemic lupus erythematosus (SLE).

Autoantibodies

Autoantibody screening is common practice in the evaluation of renal disease. The kidneys alone may be affected or the renal disease may be part of a systemic autoimmune disease like SLE.

Anti-nuclear antibodies (ANA) represent a family of autoantibodies that bind to components of the cell nucleus and can be detected by indirect immunofluo-rescence (IIF) or enzyme-linked immunosorbent assay (ELISA). ANAs can be subtyped to extractable nuclear antigens (e.g. anti Ro/anti La linked to Sjögren's syndrome; anti-Scl-70 linked to scleroderma) or other nuclear antigens can be spe-cifically identified (e.g. anti-double-stranded DNA linked to SLE; anti-histone antibody indicative of drug-induced lupus).

Autoantibodies are crucial in the diagnosis of rapidly progressive glomerulonephritis. Antibody against glomerular basement membrane points to Goodpasture's disease in the appropriate setting [12]. Anti-neutrophil cytoplasmic antibody (ANCA) is a marker of small vessel vasculitis [13]. Diffuse cyto-plasmic staining (c-ANCA), corresponding to anti-bodies against neutrophil proteinase-3, is associated with granulomatosis with polyangiitis (previously known as Wegener's granulomatosis), whilst perinu-clear staining (p-ANCA), corresponding to antibodies against neutrophil myeloperoxidase, is associated with microscopic polyangitis.

Serum Complement Levels

Measurement of complement components C3 and C4 is useful in the evaluation of glomerulonephritis (GN). Low C3 and C4, indicating classical complement path-way activation, are typically seen in SLE, whilst iso-lated reduction of C3, indicating alternate complement pathway activation, is seen in C3 GN, including dense deposit disease, or in the acute phase of post-strepto-coccal GN and other infection related GNs.

Several infections are associated with renal disease and the serological markers present evi-dence of relevant infections. Hepatitis B, hepatitis C, and HIV are associated with several glomeru-lar diseases. For example hepatitis B and C are linked to secondary membranous nephropathy and mesangiocapillary/membranoproliferative GN respectively while HIV is linked to secondary focal segmental glomerulosclerosis. Viral markers are therefore critical in the evaluation of suspected glo-merular disease. Hepatitis C-related membranopro-liferative GN can be associated with cryoglobulins, which can be detected in the serum. Antibodies to streptolysin O and anti-DNAse B provide clues to recent streptococcal infection.

Paraproteins and Immunoglobulins

Multiple myeloma and related monoclonal plasma cell dyscrasias, which produce abnormal immunoglobulins (paraproteins) and immunoglobulin components such as free light chains, have long been recognized as a cause of kidney injury. The classical pathogenesis of renal failure in myeloma involves the tubular deposi-tion of free light chains to produce light chain cast nephropathy (myeloma kidney) [14]. Myeloma can also cause renal disease through deposition of monoclonal immunoglobulin and immunoglobulin light chains, leading to amyloid light chain (AL) amyloidosis, light and/or heavy chain deposition disease, and prolifera-tive GN due to monoclonal immunoglobulin G depo-sition. Renal injury may also occur through direct interstitial plasma cell infiltration or hypercalcaemia.

Serum and urine protein electrophoresis are used to identify monoclonal proteins in the serum and the spillover of excess light chains into the urine. Free light chains can be quantitated in the serum and abnormal ratios of κ to λ light chains may indi-cate the presence of unidentified myeloma or light chains disease, which has recently been shown to be important in the identification of monoclonal gammopathy of renal significance [15]. This entity represents cases in which the diagnostic criteria for overt myeloma are not met, but in which renal injury can be linked to the presence of paraprotein. Measurement of serum free light chains should therefore be considered in all patients with kidney disease of undetermined aetiology. Serial quantita-tion of paraprotein and serum free light chain con-centrations is also used in monitoring of disease treatment and progression.

Urinalysis

Simple bedside examination of a freshly passed urine sample using dipstick-based testing and microscopy can provide a great deal of information regarding the underlying pathology in renal disease. Minimal equipment is required and these simple tests can guide further sophisticated analyses.

Appearance

Normal urine is typically clear and yellow in colour, due to the presence of urobilin (urochrome). Changes in urine colour can result from the presence of pigments such as haemoglobin and myoglobin, crystals or chyle, or from other endogenous or exogenous pigmented molecules.

Turbid urine might indicate the presence of infection, crystals, or chyle and should prompt further examination by microscopy. Specimens that have been stored and/or cooled before examination might artefactually contain large amounts of crystals but with little significance.

Urine Dipstick Analysis

The presence of leukocytes and nitrite may indicate the presence of urinary tract infection.

Protein

Measurement by dipstick provides gross assessment of the presence of proteinuria. The standard dipsticks detect albumin only; although they can provide a semi-quantitative indication of the degree of albuminuria, they have poor sensitivity and may not detect microalbuminuria (urine albumin 3–30 mg/mmol creatinine). When quantitation of albumin excretion is required, formal laboratory testing as either 24 hours urinary albumin or spot urine albumin/creatinine ratio is useful.

Haemoglobin

Haemoglobin is detected by urine dipstick based on chemical reaction catalysed by pseudoperoxidase activity of the haem moiety of haemoglobin [16]. A positive test result can be seen in the absence of haematuria due to:

- Haemoglobinuria due to intravascular haemolysis
- Myoglobinuria due to rhabdomyolysis
- High concentration of bacteria with pseudoperoxidase activity, e.g. enterobacteriaceae, staphylococci, and streptococci

False negative results may occur in the presence of high concentrations of vitamin C [17].

Urine pH

This provides an indicator of tubular capacity to appropriately acidify urine and thus excrete protons: normal urine pH is acidic. Urine pH assessment is useful in the investigation of renal calculus formation and the evaluation of suspected renal tubular acidosis. Urinary tract infection with urease-producing organisms can cause high urine pH due to the liberation of ammonia from urea.

In the presence of a normal anion gap, metabolic acidosis, and suspicion of renal tubular acidosis (RTA), the urinary pH allows differentiation between distal (type I) and proximal (type II) RTA. In the context of metabolic acidosis one would expect a highly acidic urine, as the kidney will try to compensate by secreting extra hydrogen ions; however, in distal RTA where the pathophysiology involves inability of the distal tubules to secrete hydrogen, the urine pH does not drop below 5.3 [18].

Urine Microscopy

Urine microscopy is used to demonstrate the presence of cells, bacteria, casts, and crystals in urine. Care must be taken in obtaining samples: $>10 \times 10^6$ squamous epithelial cells indicates perineal contamination and thus unsatisfactory collection. Examination of centrifuged sediment by an experienced morphologist helps to identify cell morphology as well as casts and crystals.

Pyuria

Three or more white cells per high-power field in the centrifuged sediment, or $>8 \times 10^6$ white cells/l, generally indicates infection, but can be seen in inflammatory conditions like interstitial nephritis. Similarly, the presence of corresponding numbers of red cells indicates microhaematuria, which may be due to a variety of causes, but the presence of dysmorphic red blood cells (RBCs) in a freshly voided specimen indicates glomerular haematuria.

Urine Casts

Cylindrical structures formed in the distal renal tubules are known as casts. Their matrix is formed of Tamm–Horsfall protein (uromodulin), which is secreted by the thick ascending limb of loop of Henle tubular cells. Whilst the physiological significance of this protein is not known, trapping of cells such as RBCs, white cells, and degenerating tubular cells in the matrix causes the formation of different types of casts.

Hyaline casts are innocuous, whilst granular casts are formed from degenerate tubular cells and may indicate tubular injury. RBC casts consist of RBCs trapped in a protein matrix and are diagnostic of GN, whilst white cell casts imply pyelonephritis or interstitial nephritis.

Crystals in the urine may be normal or pathological. The shape and abundance of the crystals are important in identification of their nature and significance and are discussed in Chapter 4.

Proteinuria

In the healthy adult, less than 100 mg of protein appears in the urine over 24 hours, despite the glomerular membrane being exposed to 65–70 kg of protein across that period. The glomerular membrane restricts the passage of larger molecular weight proteins by molecular sieving based on molecular diameter and shape, whilst the membrane's net negative charge repels negatively charged small plasma proteins such as albumin and thus prevents their filtration. Small peptides such as insulin and low molecular weight proteins such as β2-microglobulin pass into the proximal tubular fluid, from which they are almost completely reabsorbed and catabolized by tubular cells.

Isolated proteinuria is defined as proteinuria without haematuria or reduction in GFR. The patient is usually asymptomatic and the proteinuria is discovered incidentally on dipstick examination of urine. The urine sediment is unremarkable (fewer than 3 erythrocytes per high-power field and no casts), protein excretion is less than 3.5 g/day (usually less than 1 g/day), serological markers of systemic disease are absent, and there is no hypertension, diabetes, oedema, or hypoalbuminaemia.

Proteinuria may be:

- *Glomerular*: due to increased passage of proteins such as albumin across the glomerular membrane, a sensitive marker of glomerular diseases such as diabetic nephropathy. Nephrotic range proteinuria (>3.5 g/day/1.73 m^2) is diagnostic of glomerular disease. Low-level glomerular proteinuria can occur in benign situations such as orthostatic or exercise-induced proteinuria.
- *Tubular*: compromised proximal tubular reabsorption of filtered proteins. Low molecular weight proteins such as beta-2-microglobulin and retinol-binding protein are seen on urine protein electrophoresis.
- *Overflow*: passage of low molecular weight proteins into the glomerular filtrate in amounts that exceed

proximal tubular resorptive capacity is seen with immunoglobulin light chains (Bence Jones protein) in multiple myeloma, myoglobin in rhabdomyolysis, and haemoglobin in intravascular haemolysis [19].
- *Post-renal*: can occur with urinary tract infection, nephrolithiasis or urinary tract malignancy.

Urine protein quantitation methods may detect total protein or albumin alone, and samples may be timed (24 hours) or single void specimens. Timed urine collections avoid variations in urine flow rate and protein excretion and results are expressed as mass of protein per unit time. However, timed urine collections can be incomplete and inconvenient. Timed 24-hour collections have a role in the initial assessment of proteinuria, and allow for the diagnosis of nephrotic syndrome. Measurement of protein in a single void early morning sample and reported as protein or albumin expressed as a ratio to creatinine concentration is reproducible and reliable.

Urine Electrolytes

Urine sodium can be used for categorization of AKI, with calculation of the fractional excretion of sodium (FE_{Na}):

$$FE_{Na}(\%) = 100 \times (Urine[Na^+] \times Plasma[Creatinine]) / (Plasma[Na^+] \times Urine[Creatinine])$$

FE_{Na} <1% indicates prerenal uraemia, but can also be seen in acute GN, heart failure and hepatorenal syndrome, whilst FE_{Na} >2% is consistent with ATN but can also be seen with diuretic therapy, obstructive neuropathy, CKD, and osmotic diuresis. Urine sodium >20 mmol/l, associated with a high urine osmolality in a patient with hyponatraemia, may indicate failure to dilute urine and point to a diagnosis of syndrome of inappropriate anti-diuretic hormone secretion (SIADH).

Measurement of urinary potassium is important in assessing hypokalaemia, with values <25–30 mEq/day on a 24-hour urine collection indicating extra-renal loss.

Urinary chloride <20 mmol/l in a patient with metabolic alkalosis indicates volume contraction and implies saline responsiveness. Urine sodium is not reliable to assess volume depletion in the setting of metabolic alkalosis.

Urine Microbiology

Urine microscopy (see earlier discussion) and culture of freshly voided mid-stream samples are important in the identification and management of urinary tract infections. In patients with pyuria without bacteriuria, infective agents such as tuberculosis should be considered.

Identification of viruses, yeasts and fungi, and parasites can also be performed using basic techniques such as microscopy, along with sophisticated techniques such as DNA analysis using the polymerase chain reaction.

Urine Cytology

Urine cytology aids in the identification of urinary tract malignancy (usually bladder cancer) and is an important adjunct to cystoscopy in the investigation of haematuria. Though diagnostic yields are low for upper urinary tract malignancy, cells from high-grade urothelial malignancies may be seen.

In addition, urine cytology can be used to identify infection with human polyomaviruses in renal transplant recipients; however, the morphological changes seen are non-specific and require follow-up with DNA-based or other techniques to confirm the infectious agent.

Renal Biopsy

Histological examination of a core biopsy sample of the renal cortex is often undertaken to establish accurate diagnosis in patients with nephrotic syndrome, unexplained renal failure, glomerular haematuria, and/or proteinuria >1 g/day. The evaluation of the biopsied specimen involves examination by light microscopy, electron microscopy, and immunofluorescence.

In many patients with significant kidney disease, a presumptive diagnosis may be possible with non-invasive evaluation and renal biopsy may not be indicated. For example, in a long-standing diabetic patient with diabetic retinopathy, renal dysfunction, proteinuria, and benign urine sediment, a presumptive diagnosis of diabetic nephropathy can be made. Even when glomerular disease is suspected, a biopsy may not be warranted when renal histology will not alter management decisions. For example, renal biopsy might not be necessary in a patient with stable isolated microhaematuria, who does not have proteinuria or renal dysfunction. On the other hand, in patients with severe renal failure with bilateral shrunken kidneys, renal biopsy is often futile, because the most likely finding will be severe scarring and the disease is usually irreversible.

When indicated, percutaneous biopsy of both native and transplant kidneys can be safely undertaken using ultrasound or CT guidance. Protocol biopsies are taken at predetermined intervals after kidney transplantation to assess presymptomatic histological changes.

Indications for Kidney Biopsy

- Nephrotic syndrome, with or without renal insufficiency in adults. In children, the first presentation of nephrotic syndrome is empirically treated as minimal change disease, and biopsy is done only in treatment-resistant cases or when non-minimal change disease is suspected.
- Rapidly progressive renal failure.
- AKI of unknown aetiology, when obstruction, prerenal uraemia and ATN appear unlikely and especially when renal impairment is progressive.
- Acute nephritic syndrome in adults often requires biopsy to guide treatment, whether it is primary or secondary to a systemic disease. When presentation is classical, as in post-infectious GN or Henoch–Schönlein purpura (immunoglobulin A nephritis), biopsy may not be necessary if renal function is stable or improves promptly on follow-up.
- In non-nephrotic proteinuria, biopsy may be indicated when proteinuria is >1 g/day.
- In isolated microscopic haematuria after structural lesions have been ruled out and there is new onset of hypertension, proteinuria >1 g/day, or renal failure.
- Systemic disease with renal involvement warrants characterization of renal histology to guide treatment, e.g. patients with SLE and acute nephritic syndrome, or multiple myeloma with suspected light chain cast nephropathy.
- Renal transplant biopsy is commonly performed to evaluate allograft dysfunction. It is also indicated when transplant patients develop features of renal parenchymal disease, raising suspicion of a recurrence of the original disease or de novo glomerular disease.

Complications and Contraindications of Kidney Biopsy

Bleeding is the commonest complication of both native and transplant kidney biopsy, but the absolute risk is <1.5%. Generally, post-biopsy bleeding is self-limiting, but rarely it may be severe enough to require transfusion or endovascular procedures to control bleeding, or very rarely it can end up in nephrectomy or death.

Contraindications for kidney biopsy include a solitary functioning native kidney, bleeding disorders, uncorrected coagulopathies or current treatment with anti-coagulants or anti-platelet agents, uncontrolled hypertension, active urinary tract infections, or skin and soft tissue infections along the biopsy track. The presence of multiple cysts and anatomical abnormalities can make the biopsy more challenging. CT guidance for the procedure may be beneficial in these circumstances.

References

1. Richmond, J. (2007). Radiological diagnosis of kidney stones. *Nephrology* 12: S34–S36. https://doi.org/10.1111/j.1440-1797.2007.00780.x.
2. Bosniak, M.A. (2012). The Bosniak renal cyst classification: 25 years later. *Radiology* 262 (3): 781–785. https://doi.org/10.1148/radiol.11111595.
3. Naesens, M., Heylen, L., Lerut, E. et al. (2013). Intrarenal resistive index after renal transplantation. *N. Engl. J. Med.* 369 (19): 1797–1806.
4. Detrenis, S., Meschi, M., Musini, S., and Savazzi, G. (2005). Lights and shadows on the pathogenesis of contrast-induced nephropathy: state of the art. *Nephrol. Dial. Transplant.* 20 (8): 1542.
5. Braverman, I.M. and Cowper, S. (2010). Nephrogenic systemic fibrosis. *F1000 Med. Rep.* 2: 84. https://doi.org/10.3410/M2-84.
6. Sultana, N., Begum, S.M.F., Parveen, R. et al. (2015). DTPA captopril renogram: still an invaluable tool for probability assessment in suspected cases of renovascular hypertension. *Bangladesh J. Nucl. Med.* 18 (2): 131–134.
7. Levey, A.S. and Stevens, L.A. (2010). Estimating GFR using the CKD epidemiology collaboration (CKD-EPI) creatinine equation: more accurate GFR estimates, lower CKD prevalence estimates, and better risk predictions. *Am. J. Kidney Dis.* 55 (4): 622–627. https://doi.org/10.1053/j.ajkd.2010.02.337.
8. White, S.L., Polkinghorne, K.R., Atkins, R.C., and Chadban, S.J. (2010). Comparison of the prevalence and mortality risk of CKD in Australia using the CKD epidemiology collaboration (CKD-EPI) and Modification of Diet in Renal Disease (MDRD) study GFR estimating equations: the AusDiab (Australian diabetes, obesity and lifestyle) study. *Am. J. Kidney Dis.* 55 (4): 660–670.
9. Hoek, F.J., Kemperman, F.A.W., and Krediet, R.T. (2003). A comparison between cystatin C, plasma creatinine and the Cockcroft and Gault formula for the estimation of glomerular filtration rate. *Nephrol. Dial. Transplant.* 18 (10): 2024–2031. https://doi.org/10.1093/ndt/gfg349.
10. Larsson, T., Nisbeth, U.L.F., Ljunggren, Ö. et al. (2003). Circulating concentration of FGF-23 increases as renal function declines in patients with chronic kidney disease, but does not change in response to variation in phosphate intake in healthy volunteers. *Kidney Int.* 64 (6): 2272–2279.
11. Kovesdy, C.P., Ureche, V., Lu, J.L., and Kalantar-Zadeh, K. (2010). Outcome predictability of serum alkaline phosphatase in men with pre-dialysis CKD. *Nephrol. Dial. Transplant.* 25 (9): 3003–3011. https://doi.org/10.1093/ndt/gfq144.
12. Hirayama, K., Yamagata, K., Kobayashi, M., and Koyama, A. (2008). Anti-glomerular basement membrane antibody disease in Japan: part of the nationwide rapidly progressive glomerulonephritis survey in Japan. *Clin. Exp. Nephrol.* 12 (5): 339–347.
13. Berden, A., Göçeroğlu, A., Jayne, D. et al. (2012). Diagnosis and management of ANCA associated vasculitis. *BMJ* 344: e26. https://doi.org/10.1136/bmj.e26.
14. Finkel, K.W., Cohen, E.P., Shirali, A., and Abudayyeh, A. (2016). Paraprotein–related kidney disease: evaluation and treatment of myeloma cast nephropathy. *Clin. J. Am. Soc. Nephrol.* 11 (12): 2273–2279. https://doi.org/10.2215/CJN.01640216.
15. Steiner, N., Göbel, G., Suchecki, P. et al. (2018). Monoclonal gammopathy of renal significance (MGRS) increases the risk for progression to multiple myeloma: an observational study of 2935 MGUS patients. *Oncotarget* 9 (2): 2344–2356. https://doi.org/10.18632/oncotarget.23412.
16. Fogazzi, G.B., Verdesca, S., and Garigali, G. (2008). Urinalysis: core curriculum 2008. *Am. J. Kidney Dis.* 51 (6): 1052–1067.
17. Nagel, D., Seiler, D., Hohenberger, E.F., and Ziegler, M. (2006). Investigations of ascorbic acid interference in urine test strips. *Clin. Lab.* 52 (3–4): 149.
18. Strife, C.F., Clardy, C.W., Varade, W.S. et al. (1993). Urine-to-blood carbon dioxide tension gradient and maximal depression of urinary pH to distinguish rate-dependent from classic distal renal tubular acidosis in children. *J. Pediatr.* 122 (1): 60.
19. Barratt, J. and Topham, P. (2007). Urine proteomics: the present and future of measuring urinary protein components in disease. *CMAJ* 177 (4): 361.

Further Reading

Agarwal, S.K., Sethi, S., and Dinda, A.K. (2013). Basics of kidney biopsy: a nephrologist's perspective. *Indian J. Nephrol.* 23 (4): 243–252.

Amann, K. and Haas, C.S. (2006). What you should know about the work-up of a renal biopsy. *Nephrol. Dial. Transplant.* 21 (5): 1157–1161.

Durand, E., Chaumet-Riffaud, P., and Grenier, N. (2011). Functional renal imaging: new trends in radiology and nuclear medicine. *Semin. Nucl. Med.* 41 (1): 61–72.

Faubel, S. (2014). Moving points in nephrology: renal relevant radiology. *Clin. J. Am. Soc. Nephrol.* 9 (2): 371–429.

Grenier, N., Quaia, E., Prasad, P.V., and Juillard, L. (2011). Radiology imaging of renal structure and function by computed tomography, magnetic resonance imaging, and ultrasound. *Semin. Nucl. Med.* 41 (1): 45–60.

Questions and Answers

Questions

1. A 35-year-old male presents with acute onset of right loin pain radiating to groin with vomiting. He is afebrile and hemodynamically stable. Urine dipstick shows blood and leukocytes. Which of the following imaging test is most reliable in confirming or excluding ureteric colic due to suspected calculus obstruction?
   a. Plain X-ray abdomen AP and Right lateral views
   b. Ultrasound KUB
   c. Non-contrast CT scan KUB
   d. Gadolinium enhanced MRI scan of KUB

2. A 56-year-old female is referred for evaluation of a single cyst in the left kidney, which has grown in size over the last six months and the cyst has some solid-looking areas in ultrasound. Which of the following findings would raise most concerns about a renal cell carcinoma?
   a. Increase in size of the cyst of >3 cm in six months
   b. Calcification of the cyst wall noted in non-contrast CT scan
   c. Hyperdense contents of the cyst noted in MRI scan
   d. Enhancement of solid areas in the cyst wall noted in contrast CT scan

3. A 25-year-old male is noted to have marked left hydronephrosis and dilatation of renal pelvis without ureteric dilatation, when evaluated for flank pain noticed after an alcoholic binge. His renal function is normal and urine examination does not show protein or blood. Which of the following statements about further assessment is true?
   a. CT urography will provide confirmatory diagnosis
   b. DTPA scan with diuretic administration will confirm or exclude complete obstruction
   c. DMSA is superior to DTPA scan in further evaluation
   d. Obstruction cannot be confidently diagnosed without an antegrade pyelography

4. Renal biopsy is urgently indicated in the evaluation of the following patients except:
   a. 58-year-old hypertensive male with microhaematuria, 1 g/day proteinuria and creatinine rise from 120 to 350 µmol/l in four weeks.
   b. 40-year-old type 1 diabetic female with retinopathy who has 4 g/day of proteinuria, benign urine sediment, and creatinine 150 µmol/l
   c. 28-year-old female with SLE, who has 1 g/day of proteinuria, microhaematuria, and creatinine 110 µmol/l
   d. 70-year-old male with multiple myeloma who has 3 g/day of proteinuria, benign urine sediment, and creatinine 600 µmol/l

5. Haemoglobin is detected by urine dipstick based on chemical reaction catalyzed by pseudoperoxidase activity of the heme moiety of haemoglobin. Which of the following conditions is NOT associated with a positive result?
   a. Glomerulonephritis
   b. Heavy Vitamin C intake
   c. Intravascular haemolytic anaemia
   d. Rhabdomyolysis

Answers

1. c. Non-contrast CT scan is highly sensitive to detect stones including uric acid stones which are radiolucent in plain X-ray. CT scan also has the advantage of being able to accurately locate the level of obstruction. While ultrasound is excellent to diagnose obstruction and identify renal calculi, it is less reliable in detecting ureteric stones.

2. d. Contrast enhancement in the solid areas of the cyst, which imply increased vascularity, will classify the complicated cyst to Bosniak IV category, which carries 80–100% risk to be a renal cell cancer. In some cases the increased vascularity may be detected in a colour Doppler examination, though the sensitivity is poor. Hyperdense contents in a cyst in MRI scan may indicate bleeding into the cyst. Gadolinium enhancement is the most compelling MRI feature that raises suspicion of renal cancer. While calcification of walls, internal septation, nodularity of the cyst wall, and rapid increase in size are all features that raise concerns, none of them is as specific for cancer as contrast enhancement.

3. b. Dilated pelvicalyceal system without ureteric dilatation and worsening symptoms precipitated by alcohol-related increase in urine flow rate in a young patient is highly suspicious of congenital pelvi-ureteric junction obstruction. Ultrasound is very sensitive to diagnose dilatation of the collecting system and CT urography will not provide any additional information. In patients with dilated collecting system, urinary obstruction can be confirmed by DTPA scan, by the failure to clear the radionuclide tracer pooled in the collecting system, spontaneously and following administration of a diuretic. DMSA concentrates in the kidney and takes a long time to clear under normal conditions, which make it an ideal agent for static renal imaging, e.g. for the detection of renal cortical scars. It is not suitable for excluding urinary obstruction. Antegrade pyelography is an invasive test, usually done in the context of procedures to treat obstruction, when a retrograde pyelography is not feasible (e.g. inability to cannulate the ureter or negotiate the ureteric obstruction with a guide wire).

4. b. Renal biopsy provides accurate information about the nature of renal injury which is important in establishing the aetiology of renal disease and guiding treatment. It is essential in the evaluation of a patient with rapidly progressive renal failure to diagnose crescentic nephritis (a) and systemic disease like SLE with renal involvement (c), where treatment decision will depend on severity of histological abnormalities. Establishing a diagnosis of myeloma cast nephropathy will modify therapeutic options in a patient with myeloma and acute kidney injury, and biopsy is essential to guide therapy (d). In a diabetic with established microvascular disease like retinopathy and proteinuric renal impairment associated with benign urine sediment (b), a presumptive diagnosis of diabetic nephropathy can be made with reasonable certainty.

5. b. Apart from glomerular haematuria seen with glomerulonephritis, positive result for urine dipstick haemoglobin can be seen due to:

   - Haemoglobinuria due to intravascular haemolysis
   - Myoglobinuria due to rhabdomyolysis
   - High concentration of bacteria with pseudoperoxidase activity, e.g. enterobacteriaceae, staphylococci, and streptococci

   False negative results may occur in the presence of high concentrations of vitamin C.

3

Disorders of the Renal Tubules Leading to Disturbances of Acid–Base and Potassium

Surjit Tarafdar

Summary

- Disorders of the renal tubules can lead to either metabolic acidosis or alkalosis as well as hypokalaemia or hyperkalaemia
- Metabolic alkalosis with hypokalaemia when associated with hypertension may be a manifestation of primary aldosteronism
- Primary aldosteronism is a common cause of secondary hypertension
- Metabolic alkalosis with hypokalaemia when associated with low to normal blood pressure can be a manifestation of Bartter or Gitelman syndromes
- Renal tubular acidosis (RTA) can be described as a group of disorders characterized by normal anion gap (hyperchloraemic) metabolic acidosis with either hypokalaemia or hyperkalaemia
- Both types 1 and 2 RTA are associated with hypokalaemia and result from tubular inability to excrete hydrogen or reabsorb bicarbonate, respectively
- Type 4 RTA is associated with hyperkalaemia and is due to diminished production or reduced tubular effectiveness to aldosterone

Defects in the ability of the renal tubules to perform the normal functions required to maintain acid–base balance and reabsorb sodium (Na^+) can lead to various disorders. These disorders can be broadly classified into:

- *Conditions associated with metabolic alkalosis and/or hypokalaemia*: Further sub-divided into two groups depending on the blood pressure (BP):

Low–normal BP

  o Bartter syndrome
  o Gitelman syndrome

High BP

  o Primary aldosteronism (commonest cause in this group)

Lecture Notes Nephrology: A Comprehensive Guide to Renal Medicine, First Edition. Edited by Surjit Tarafdar.
© 2020 John Wiley & Sons Ltd. Published 2020 by John Wiley & Sons Ltd.

- Liddle syndrome
- Chronic liquorice ingestion
- Apparent mineralocorticoid excess (AME)
- Familial hyperaldosteronism (FH; including glucocorticoid-remediable aldosteronism)

- *Conditions associated with metabolic acidosis*: Include renal tubular acidosis (RTA) types 1, 2, and 4. The metabolic acidosis is characteristically associated with a normal anion gap and hypokalaemia in the first two conditions and hyperkalaemia in the latter.

It must be remembered that increased gastrointestinal losses can lead to hypokalaemia due to the associated hypovolaemia causing activation of the renin–angiotensin–aldosterone system (RAAS).

Whilst upper gastrointestinal losses are usually associated with metabolic alkalosis due to loss of gastric hydrochloric acid, lower gastrointestinal losses tend to lead to metabolic acidosis due to the loss of bicarbonate-rich pancreatic secretions.

Disturbance of Na$^+$ Reabsorption: Metabolic Alkalosis and Hypokalaemia

In all the tubular epithelial cells, the basolateral Na$^+$-K$^+$-ATPase pumps out three Na$^+$ and pumps in two potassium (K$^+$) ions from the interstitium/surrounding peritubular capillaries, creating a state of intracellular Na$^+$ deficiency and K$^+$ excess. This intracellular Na$^+$ deficiency in turn allows passive reabsorption of Na$^+$ by the tubular cells from the urinary lumen.

In the proximal tubules, the apical Na$^+$ –H$^+$ exchange protein facilitates the reabsorption of Na$^+$ whilst secreting hydrogen (H$^+$) (Figure 1.4). This exchange protein is inhibited by the carbonic anhydrase inhibitor acetazolamide.

In the thick ascending limb (TAL) of the loop of Henle, the electro-neutral Na$^+$-K$^+$-2Cl$^-$ co-transporter (NKCC2) reabsorbs one Na$^+$ and K$^+$ each along with two chloride (2Cl$^-$) ions (Figure 1.5). The higher intracellular K$^+$ concentration causes the reabsorbed K$^+$ to be promptly secreted back into the lumen by the adenosine triphosphate (ATP)-sensitive renal medullary K channel (ROMK). The two Cl$^-$ ions are absorbed into peritubular capillary blood by the basolateral Cl channel (ClC-Kb), which has barttin as a crucial accessory protein while the basolateral Na+-K+-ATPase pumps the Na+ into the peritubular capillary or interstitium. The movement of one positively charged K$^+$ back into the tubular lumen and two negatively charged 2Cl$^-$ and one positively charged Na+ (net gain of one electronegative charge) into the peritubular capillaries creates an electrical gradient with more positive charge in the tubular lumen. This leads to a compensatory paracellular reabsorption of positively charged calcium (Ca$^+$) and magnesium (Mg$^+$). Loop diuretics act by inhibiting the NKCC2 co-transporter and as a result, also lead to decreased reabsorption of Ca$^+$ and Mg$^+$. This is why loop diuretics are used for the treatment of hypercalcaemia. Defects in the reabsorption of Na$^+$ in the ascending limb can result in Bartter syndrome.

In the distal tubules, Na$^+$ is reabsorbed by the apical sodium chloride (NaCl) co-transporter (NCCT) (Figure 3.1). Inhibition of NCCT by thiazide diuretic leads to volume contraction, leading in turn to an increased reabsorption of Na$^+$ in the proximal tubule and loop of Henle. As already discussed, increased Na$^+$ reabsorption in the TAL of the loop of Henle leads to increased Ca$^+$ reabsorption, which explains the hypercalcaemia associated with thiazide diuretics. Defect in the NCCT can lead to Gitelman syndrome.

In the collecting duct, Na$^+$ reabsorption is mediated by the apical epithelial Na$^+$ channel (ENAC) in the principal cells (sensitive to triamterene and amiloride).

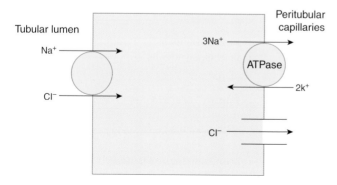

Tubular lumen

Na$^+$

Cl$^-$

Peritubular capillaries

3Na$^+$

ATPase

2k$^+$

Cl$^-$

Figure 3.1 Ion transport mechanisms in the distal convoluted tubule. The Na$^+$-K$^+$-ATPase pump in the basolateral membrane pumps three sodium (Na$^+$) ions out of and two potassium (K$^+$) ions into the cell. The resultant low intracellular Na$^+$ concentration leads to reabsorption of Na$^+$ from the tubular lumen; chloride (Cl$^-$) is co-transported with Na$^+$.

This Na$^+$ reabsorption is coupled with the tubular secretion of K$^+$ and is under the control of aldosterone (Figure 1.9). However, as more positively charged Na$^+$ is reabsorbed then K$^+$ is secreted, the urinary lumen still needs more positive charges. To compensate, H$^+$ is secreted by the neighbouring intercalated cells in the collecting duct. Thus aldosterone directly leads to absorption of Na$^+$ with secretion of K$^+$ by the principal cells, whilst it causes indirect secretion of H$^+$ by the intercalated cells. Excessive activity of the ENAC channel can lead to Liddle syndrome.

Both loop and thiazide diuretics can lead to hypokalaemia and metabolic alkalosis by the following mechanisms:

- Diuretics act by decreasing tubular Na$^+$ reabsorption, leading to increased luminal concentration of Na$^+$. As the Na$^+$-rich urine flows to the distal parts of the tubule, the tubular cells try to reabsorb some of the Na$^+$ and in exchange secrete positively charged K$^+$ and hydrogen (H$^+$) into the lumen.
- Diuretics lead to an element of volume contraction, which leads to activation of the RAAS; aldosterone leads to increased urinary loss of K$^+$ directly and H$^+$ indirectly, as explained earlier.

The key factors to consider in a patient (not known to be on thiazide or loop diuretics) who presents with hypokalaemia and metabolic alkalosis are:

- Is the patient hypertensive or normotensive?
- Is there any suspicion of surreptitious vomiting or diuretic abuse?

If there is no suspicion of surreptitious vomiting or diuretic use, then patients with low to normal BP are likely to have Bartter or Gitelman syndromes. Those with hypertension are likely to have primary aldosteronism or the rarer Liddle syndrome, have high chronic intake of liquorice, AME or one of the FH subtypes, including glucocorticoid-remediable aldosteronism (GRA).

Loss of hydrochloric acid-rich gastric secretion in patients with surreptitious vomiting leads to metabolic alkalosis. The resultant hypovolaemia-induced RAAS activation leads to aldosterone-induced increased urinary K$^+$ loss and the resultant hypokalaemia.

Conditions with Hypokalaemia, Metabolic Alkalosis, and Normal or Low Blood Pressure

Bartter and Gitelman Syndromes

Bartter and Gitelman syndromes are autosomal recessive disorders characterized by hypokalaemia, metabolic alkalosis, and low to normal BP [1]. Bartter syndrome is usually seen in the perinatal period or childhood, whilst Gitelman syndrome is mostly a disorder of adulthood, with hypomagnesaemia being a striking feature. The prevalence of Gitelman syndrome is 1 in 40 000 compared with 1 in 1 000 000 for Bartter syndrome [2].

The tubular defects of Na reabsorption in Bartter and Gitelman syndromes are almost identical to those seen with chronic ingestion of loop and thiazide diuretics respectively. Impaired Na$^+$ reabsorption in both conditions leads to mild volume contraction and activation of the RAAS. The combination of secondary hyperaldosteronism and increased distal delivery of Na$^+$ causes increased secretion of K$^+$ and H$^+$, leading to the characteristic hypokalaemia and metabolic alkalosis. BP is on the lower side in both the conditions due to Na$^+$ loss and resultant volume contraction. In addition, Bartter syndrome is characterized by increased renal release of vasodilator prostaglandins due to decreased NaCl uptake into the macula densa cells at the end of the TAL of the loop of Henle, contributing to the low BP.

Bartter syndrome is due to a defect in Na$^+$ reabsorption in the TAL and may be classified into four types depending on the mutation in the protein involved (NKCC2 type 1, ROMK type 2, ClC-Kb type 3, and barttin type 4; see Figure 3.2) [3, 4]. Types 1, 2, and 4 are collectively called antenatal Bartter syndrome and lead to presentation in the perinatal life or polyhydramnios and premature delivery. Infants may present with vomiting and failure to thrive with polyuria, hypercalciuria, and characteristically raised urinary chloride. In contrast, type 3 is less severe and usually presents in the first two to five years of life.

Gitelman syndrome is due to mutations in the gene coding for the thiazide-sensitive Na$^+$-Cl$^-$ co-transporter in the distal tubule [5]. As discussed, the resultant volume contraction in Gitelman syndrome leads to increased NKCC2 activity in the TAL, which in turn leads to increased Ca$^+$ reabsorption and subsequent low urinary Ca$^+$. However, whilst one would have expected the urinary Mg$^+$ to be low due to the same mechanism, downregulation of the distal tubule epithelial Mg$^+$ channel (TRPM6) in Gitelman syndrome causes Mg$^+$ wasting and the resultant characteristic hypomagnesaemia [6]. Patients often present in adult life with cramps, polyuria, and nocturia.

Both the conditions are characterized by high urinary Cl$^-$, which is essentially because Cl$^-$ binds to the excess urinary Na$^+$. Urinary Ca$^+$ is high in Bartter syndrome and low in Gitelman syndrome, findings which mimic the use of loop and thiazides diuretics respectively.

Patients who abuse diuretics will show variable urinary Cl$^-$ levels depending on the timing of diuretic

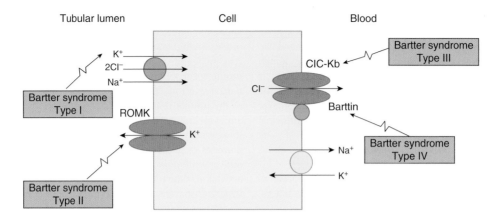

Figure 3.2 Points of mutation in the four types of Bartter syndrome. Chloride channel Kb (ClC-Kb) is the Cl⁻ channel, whilst barttin is its subunit. Type 1 is due to defective function of the Na⁺-K⁺-2Cl⁻ (NKCC2) cotransporter in the luminal membrane; type 2 is due to a defective renal outer medullary potassium channel (ROMK); type 3 is due to a defective ClC-Kb; type 4 is due to defect in the barttin subunit of the ClC-Kb.

abuse, and in cases of doubt a urine diuretic screen may be helpful [7].

Those who chronically induce vomiting often develop characteristic physical findings such as scarring on the dorsum of the hand (from insertion into the mouth), dental erosions from exposure to acidic gastric secretions, and parotitis. The urinary Cl⁻ is characteristically low, as hypovolaemia leads to increased Na⁺ reabsorption in the tubules, with the accompanying Cl⁻ reabsorption.

Initial therapy in patients with Bartter syndrome is often a combination of non-steroidal anti-inflammatory drug (NSAID) and potassium-sparing diuretic such as spironolactone or amiloride [8]. Patients will often need potassium supplementation.

Gitelman syndrome is not characterized by raised vasodilatory prostaglandin and hence there is no role for NSAIDs. Initial therapy consists of a potassium-sparing diuretic, but magnesium and potassium supplementation are often needed.

Treatment is lifelong for both conditions.

Conditions with Hypokalaemia, Metabolic Alkalosis, and High Blood Pressure

Primary Aldosteronism

Primary aldosteronism (which is also known as Conn's syndrome) should always be suspected in a patient with metabolic alkalosis and/or hypokalaemia with hypertension (more than half of patients are normokalaemic). The condition could arise because of aldosterone producing adenoma (35%)

or bilateral idiopathic hyperplasia (>60%). An elevated plasma aldosterone to renin ratio (PAC/PRA) is suggestive of the diagnosis of primary aldosteronism. Using this criterion, it is estimated that 5–13% of all patients with hypertension have primary hyperaldosteronism [9].

Confirmatory tests include demonstration of the non-suppressibility of aldosterone production after intravenous saline infusion or heavy oral salt loading. This is followed with computed tomography (CT) or magnetic resonance imaging (MRI) scan of the adrenal gland, but one must be aware of the potential of an incidental non-secretory benign adrenal mass (incidentaloma). In equivocal cases, adrenal vein sampling is the gold standard [10]. Adenoma is associated with a marked (usually fourfold greater than contralateral adrenal) increase in aldosterone concentration on the side of the tumour.

Treatment consists of surgery for unilateral adenomas and aldosterone receptor blockade with spironolactone or eplerenone for bilateral adrenal hyperplasia.

Liddle Syndrome (Pseudohyperaldosteronism)

Liddle syndrome is a rare autosomal-dominant condition which usually presents in teenagers with hypokalaemic metabolic alkalosis and hypertension. A mutation in the ENAC channel (the Na⁺-reabsorbing channel in the collecting duct under the control of aldosterone) renders it resistant to normal degradation [11]. The resultant persistence of the ENAC channel leads to enhanced Na⁺ reabsorption (with compensatory K+ and H+ secretion by the tubular cells) and the resultant hypertension with hypokalaemic metabolic alkalosis. Liddle syndrome is characteristically associated with low plasma renin and aldosterone and hence can be easily differentiated from primary aldosteronism.

Therapy consists of Na$^+$ restriction and K$^+$ supplementation. Triamterene and amiloride, which block the ENAC channels, are useful. A direct aldosterone receptor antagonist like spironolactone is obviously not helpful. Lifelong therapy is needed.

Apparent Mineralocorticoid Excess and Chronic Liquorice Ingestion

AME is a rare form of severe juvenile hypertension that is usually transmitted as an autosomal recessive trait and is accompanied by hypokalaemic metabolic alkalosis.

Cortisol binds as avidly as aldosterone to the mineralocorticoid receptor and the plasma cortisol concentration is approximately 100-fold higher than the PAC. In the kidney, 11-beta-hydroxysteroid dehydrogenase enzyme type 2 isoform (11-beta-HSD2) converts cortisol into the inactive cortisone. The syndrome of AME is due to deficiency in this enzyme, leading to an elevated level of cortisol in the kidneys; the renal cortisol stimulates the mineralocorticoid receptor, which simulates hyperaldosteronism both clinically and biochemically [12]. Whilst primary hyperaldosteronism is characterized by raised plasma aldosterone to plasma renin activity, in AME both plasma aldosterone levels and plasma renin activity are characteristically low. A 24-hour urine collection reveals abnormally high urine cortisol to cortisone levels, supporting the diagnosis.

Treatment consists of K$^+$ supplementation and mineralocorticoid blockade with drugs like spironolactone or amiloride. If mineralocorticoid antagonism is not effective or not tolerated, then oral dexamethasone to suppress adrenocorticotropic hormone (ACTH) and thus reduce endogenous cortisol secretion is suggested.

Liquorice contains glycyrrhetinic acid, which inhibits 11-beta-HSD2, the same enzyme that is deficient in AME. Chronic liquorice ingestion can therefore lead to a clinical presentation similar to AME.

Familial Hyperaldosteronism

FH is an uncommon subset of primary aldosteronism. There are four recognized types:

- *FH type I* or glucocorticoid-remediable aldosteronism (GRA): due to a *CYP11B1/CYP11B2* chimeric gene (discussed in the next section).

- *FH type II*: this is the largest group amongst the four known types of FH. Characterized by autosomal-dominant inheritance, this condition is clinically indistinguishable from sporadic primary aldosteronism. Whilst the exact mutation is not known, it is suspected to have a linkage to chromosome 7p22.
- *FH type III*: caused by germline mutations in the potassium channel subunit KCNJ5, patients usually present early with massive adrenal hyperplasia.
- *FH type IV*: caused by germline mutations in the *CACNA1H* gene, which encodes the alpha subunit of an L-type voltage-gated calcium channel (Cav3.2). Whilst CT may show cortical adenoma, bilateral hyperplasia or normal-appearing adrenal glands, adrenal venous sampling shows bilateral aldosterone hypersecretion.

FH Type 1 or Glucocorticoid-Remediable Aldosteronism

Both cortisol and aldosterone are synthesized and secreted from the adrenal cortex. Whilst cortisol production is under the control of ACTH secreted by the anterior pituitary gland, aldosterone production is under the control of angiotensin II and serum K$^+$ levels. One of the enzymes involved in the biosynthetic pathways of both cortisol and aldosterone, termed 11B-hydroxylase (isoenzymes B-1 in cortisol synthesis and B-2 in aldosterone synthesis) has 95% homology between the two isoenzymes. The genes for both the isoenzymes are located close to each other on chromosome 8. Unequal meiotic crossovers may produce a hybrid enzyme which is involved in both cortisol and aldosterone synthesis and as a result, both cortisol and aldosterone production are controlled by ACTH [13]. Administration of exogenous corticosteroids will lead to suppression of endogenous ACTH and hence aldosterone, leading to reversal of the hypertension and the hypokalaemic metabolic alkalosis.

Positive family history and typical onset of hypertension before age 21 with metabolic alkalosis should lead to suspicion. Hypokalaemia is typically mild or absent, but becomes pronounced if diuretics are given. There is a high prevalence of haemorrhagic stroke secondary to ruptured intracranial aneurysms.

The plasma aldosterone is elevated and plasma renin activity is suppressed, though the aldosterone/renin ratio is typically not as high as with primary aldosteronism. Administration of dexamethasone 0.5 mg 6-hourly for 48 hours leads to suppression of aldosterone to undetectable levels. Genetic testing to detect the hybrid gene is the preferred mode of diagnosis.

Treatment with low-dose corticosteroids is effective. Mineralocorticoid receptor antagonists such as spironolactone or ENAC antagonists such as amiloride and triamterene are also useful.

Renal Tubular Acidosis

RTA can be described as a group of disorders characterized by normal anion gap (hyperchloraemic) metabolic acidosis with either hypokalaemia or hyperkalaemia and a relatively well-preserved glomerular filtration rate. Defects in H$^+$ secretion in the distal tubules lead to RTA type 1 (also called distal RTA), whilst inability to reabsorb bicarbonate (HCO3) in the proximal tubules leads to RTA type 2 (proximal RTA). Both conditions are associated with hypokalaemia. Type 4 RTA is due to either aldosterone deficiency or tubular resistance to the action of aldosterone and is associated with hyperkalaemia.

Normal anion gap (hyperchloraemic) metabolic acidosis may also be due to extra-renal causes such as chronic diarrhoea with faecal loss of bicarbonate-rich pancreatic secretions. The urine anion gap (UAG) calculation helps to differentiate between renal and extra-renal causes of normal anion gap acidosis, being positive in the former and negative in the latter [14].

$$UAG(\text{in meq/l or mmol/l}) = Urine(Na^+ + K^+ - Cl^-)$$

The UAG is positive (between 20 and 90) in healthy individuals because the dietary and hence urinary Na$^+$ and K$^+$ are normally more than Cl$^-$. With non-renal causes of metabolic acidosis, the kidney will appropriately respond by excreting a heavy load of H$^+$, which will also need increased ammonia to buffer it. Since ammonia in the urine exists as ammonium chloride (NH$_4$Cl), this leads to increased urinary Cl$^-$, with the result that the UAG becomes negative. In distal RTA, since the defect is in the secretion of H$^+$ and hence NH$_4$Cl would be low, the UAG remains positive.

Types 1 and 2 Renal Tubular Acidosis

Type 1 RTA is caused by the inability of the distal tubules to secrete H$^+$. The kidney characteristically cannot lower the urinary pH to less than 5.5 due to a deficiency of H$^+$ in the urine [15].

Although type 1 RTA may be inherited, acquired causes are not uncommon in adults and include Sjögren's syndrome, systemic lupus erythematosus, hypergammaglobulinaemic states, primary biliary cirrhosis, autoimmune hepatitis, hypercalciuria, obstructive uropathy, and renal transplantation. The drug amphotericin can lead to type 1 RTA by causing an excessive back leak of H$^+$ in the distal tubules.

In type 2 RTA the proximal tubule has a reduced capacity to reabsorb HCO$_3$ [16]. As the kidneys lose HCO$_3$ and plasma HCO$_3$ concentration falls, the filtered load of HCO$_3$ decreases, reaching a level that can be reabsorbed and a new steady-state serum HCO$_3$ concentration is reached. Because of this ability of the kidney to decrease HCO$_3$ excretion as well as the compensatory increase in H$^+$ secretion by the distal tubules, urinary pH will usually be less than 5.5. Reabsorption of Na$^+$ (linked to the reclaiming of HCO$_3$) in the proximal tubules helps to co-transport amino acid, glucose, uric acid, and phosphate. Type 2 RTA can occur as an isolated defect in HCO$_3$ reabsorption or as a generalized defect in proximal tubular reabsorption, with amino aciduria, phosphaturia, glycosuria, and uric aciduria, when the condition is termed Fanconi syndrome.

Although type 2 RTA may be familial, it can be secondary to myeloma, where the filtered immunoglobulin light chains cause proximal tubular toxicity [17]. It can be seen with the use of carbonic anhydrase inhibitors such as acetazolamide and topiramate. Other causes include Wilson's disease, cystinosis, Lowe syndrome, outdated tetracycline, and lead or mercury poisoning.

The metabolic acidosis in both types 1 and 2 RTA causes bones to release calcium salts to act as a buffer. This can over time lead to progressive osteomalacia and osteopenia. This also leads to increased urinary calcium excretion. Under normal circumstances urinary citrate binds with calcium and makes it soluble. However, citrate is an effective alkaline buffer and hence in type 1 RTA, the proximal tubules tend to reabsorb increased amounts of citrate in an effort to combat the acidosis. The resultant deficiency of citrate in urine in type 1 RTA tends to make the urinary calcium insoluble. In addition, the alkaline urine markedly diminishes the urinary calcium solubility. The end result is increased incidence of nephrocalcinosis and nephrolithiasis in type 1 RTA. Expectedly, in type 2 RTA the defect in proximal tubular reabsorption limits the ability to reabsorb citrate, which in turn helps to excrete the excess calcium by making it more soluble. The low urinary pH also aids in calcium excretion.

Table 3.1 Differentiating features between types 1 and 2 renal tubular acidosis (RTA)

Type 1 RTA (distal RTA)	Type 2 RTA (proximal RTA)
Inability to secrete H^+	Inability to reabsorb HCO3
Urine pH >5.5 (low H^+ in urine)	Urine pH <5.5 (compensatory increase in distal tubular H^+ secretion)
Nephrolithiasis and nephrocalcinosis	No renal stones
No Fanconi syndrome	May have Fanconi syndrome: glycosuria, phosphaturia, uric aciduria, and aminoaciduria
Treat with alkali and K^+ replacement	Same treatment, but often need bigger doses of alkali

H^+: hydrogen; HCO_3: bicarbonate; K^+: potassium.

Type 1 or 2 RTA should be considered in patients with normal anion gap (hyperchloraemic) metabolic acidosis and hypokalaemia. Type 1 RTA is characteristically associated with urinary pH more than 5.5. In contrast, the urinary pH is usually lower than 5.5 in type 2 RTA, except when the patient is being treated with massive doses of alkali. Hypophosphataemia, hypouricaemia, and glycosuria in the absence of raised blood glucose can point towards Fanconi syndrome.

A similar biochemical picture may be seen in chronic diarrhoeal states, as discussed earlier, but the UAG will be negative in diarrhoea and positive in type 1 RTA.

Treatment of both types 1 and 2 RTA consists of potassium replacement and alkali therapy. One should be careful when administering sodium bicarbonate, because the resultant Na^+ loss in urine may increase K^+ secretion and thus exacerbate hypokalaemia. In this setting, it is advisable to replace K^+ before the acidosis is corrected.

Type 2 RTA often needs much bigger doses of alkali because of the tendency of the kidneys to excrete more HCO_3 as the serum HCO_3 concentration increases (Table 3.1).

Type 4 RTA

Type 4 RTA (hyperkalaemic distal tubular acidosis) is the commonest amongst the RTAs and should always be suspected in patients presenting with normal anion gap metabolic acidosis and hyperkalaemia [18]. The pathophysiology involves either decreased production of aldosterone or diminished responsiveness of the cortical duct to aldosterone. Under normal circumstances, secretion of H^+ and K^+ in the collecting duct is dependent on the intraluminal negativity generated as a consequence of aldosterone-induced reabsorption of Na^+. With hypoaldosteronism or tubular unresponsiveness to aldosterone, less Na^+ is reabsorbed and hence less H^+ and K^+ are secreted into the tubules.

Many of the patients have mild to moderate impairment in renal function, but the magnitude of hyperkalaemia and acidosis is disproportionate to the degree of renal failure. Most commonly associated with diabetes mellitus, type 4 RTA may also be seen with use of NSAIDs, angiotensin-converting enzyme inhibitors (ACE-Is), angiotensin II receptor blockers, calcineurin inhibitors (cyclosporine and tacrolimus), and chronic heparin therapy, as all of these lead to diminished aldosterone production. Impaired responsiveness of the collecting duct to aldosterone can be seen with structural damage to the kidney, as in sickle cell nephropathy; it may also result from use of K^+-sparing diuretics, such as spironolactone, amiloride or triamterene. Mostly patients are asymptomatic, but sometimes there may be dangerous elevation of K^+ needing urgent treatment.

In patients who are not hypertensive or volume overloaded, administration of a synthetic mineralocorticoid such as fludrocortisone may be effective. In patients with hypertension or fluid overload, a thiazide or loop diuretic may help by increasing distal delivery of Na^+ and consequently increasing the secretion of H^+ and K^+ [19].

References

1. Kurtz, I. (1998). Molecular pathogenesis of Bartter's and Gitelman syndromes. *Kidney Int.* 54 (4): 1396.

2. Ji, W., Foo, J.N., O'Roak, B.J. et al. (2008). Rare independent mutations in renal salt handling genes contribute to blood pressure variation. *Nat. Genet.* 40 (5): 592.

3. Simon, D.B., Bindra, R.S., Mansfield, T.A. et al. (1997). Mutations in the chloride channel gene, CLCNKB, cause Bartter's syndrome type III. *Nat. Genet.* 17 (2): 171.

4. Konrad, M., Vollmer, M., Lemmink, H.H. et al. (2000). Mutations in the chloride channel gene CLCNKB as a cause of classic Bartter syndrome. *J. Am. Soc. Nephrol.* 11 (8): 1449.

5. De Jong, J.C., Van Der Vliet, W.A., Van Den Heuvel, L.P. et al. (2002). Functional expression of mutations in the human NaCl cotransporter: evidence for impaired routing mechanisms in Gitelman's syndrome. *J. Am. Soc. Nephrol.* 13 (6): 1442.

6. Gross, P. and Heduschka, P. (2010). Inherited disorders of sodium and water handling. In: *Comprehensive Clinical Nephrology*, 4e (eds. J. Floege, R.J. Johnson and J. Feehally), 573–583. Mosby.

7. Sasaki, H., Kawasaki, T., Yamamoto, T. et al. (1986). Pseudo-Bartter's syndrome induced by surreptitious ingestion of furosemide to lose weight: a case report and possible pathophysiology. *Nihon Naibunpi Gakkai Zasshi* 62 (8): 867.

8. Dillon, M.J., Shah, V., and Mitchell, M.D. (1979). Bartter's syndrome: 10 cases in childhood. Results of long-term indomethacin therapy. *Q. J. Med.* 48 (191): 429–446.

9. Young, W.F. (2007). Primary aldosteronism: renaissance of a syndrome. *Clin. Endocrinol.* 66 (5): 607.

10. Young, W.F., Stanson, A.W., Thompson, G.B. et al. (2004). Role for adrenal venous sampling in primary aldosteronism. *Surgery* 136 (6): 1227.

11. Botero-Velez, M., Curtis, J.J., and Warnock, D.G. (1994). Liddle's syndrome revisited – a disorder of sodium reabsorption in the distal tubule. *N. Engl. J. Med.* 330: 178–181.

12. Dave-Sharma, S., Wilson, R.C., Harbison, M.D. et al. (1998). Examination of genotype and phenotype relationships in 14 patients with apparent mineralocorticoid excess. *J. Clin. Endocrinol. Metab.* 83 (7): 2244.

13. Lifton, R.P., Dluhy, R.G., Powers, M. et al. (1992). A chimaeric 11-beta-hydroxylase/aldosterone synthase gene causes glucocorticoid-remediable aldosteronism and human hypertension. *Nature* 355: 262–265.

14. Palmer, B.F. and Alpern, R.J. (2010). Metabolic acidosis. In: *Comprehensive Clinical Nephrology*, 4e (eds. J. Floege, R.J. Johnson and J. Feehally), 155–166. Mosby.

15. Soriano, J.R. Renal tubular acidosis: the clinical entity. *J. Am. Soc. Nephrol* 13 (8): 2160–2170. https://doi.org/10.1097/01.ASN.0000023430.92674.E5.

16. Rodríguez Soriano, J., Boichis, H., Stark, H., and Edelmann, C.M. Jr. (1967). Proximal renal tubular acidosis. A defect in bicarbonate reabsorption with normal urinary acidification. *Pediatr. Res.* 1: 81–98.

17. Lazar, G.S. and Feinstein, D.I. (1981). Distal tubular acidosis in multiple myeloma. *Arch. Intern. Med.* 141 (5): 655–656.

18. DeFronzo, R.A. (1980). Hyperkalemia and hyporeninemic hypoaldosteronism. *Kidney Int.* 17 (1): –118.

19. Sebastian, A., Schambelan, M., and Sutton, J.M. (1984). Amelioration of hyperchloremic acidosis with furosemide therapy in patients with chronic renal insufficiency and type 4 renal tubular acidosis. *Am. J. Nephrol.* 4 (5): 287.

Questions and Answers

Questions

1. A 52 year-old woman presents to ED feeling generally unwell. Blood tests reveal metabolic acidosis with a normal anion gap and hypokalaemia. Her urinary pH is 5.7. The rest of the blood tests including phosphate and uric acid are normal. What could have led to this condition?
   a. Myeloma
   b. Sjögren's syndrome
   c. Wilson's disease
   d. Diabetes mellitus

2. What is the diagnosis in the above case?
   a. RTA type 4
   b. RTA type 1
   c. RTA type 2
   d. RTA type 3

3. Which of the following is true?
   a. Nephrocalcinosis is commonly seen in RTA type 1
   b. Nephrocalcinosis is commonly seen in RTA type 2
   c. Nephrocalcinosis is commonly seen in RTA type 4
   d. Nephrocalcinosis is equally seen in RTA types 1 and 2

4. Which of the following can lead to normal anion gap acidosis?
   a. CRF
   b. Acetazolamide
   c. Lactic acidosis
   d. Starvation

5. Fanconi syndrome should be suspected in:
   a. Hyperuricaemia
   b. Hyperphosphataemia
   c. Hypophosphataemia
   d. Hyperkalaemia

6. Bartter syndrome is due to a defect in:
   a. Na^+ reabsorption in the distal convoluted tubule
   b. Na^+ reabsorption in the collecting duct
   c. K^+ reabsorption in the collecting duct
   d. Na^+ reabsorption in the ascending limb of loop of Henle

7. Which of the following is true about thiazide diuretics?
   a. Can lead to hypercalciuria
   b. Can lead to hyperkalaemia
   c. Can lead to hypocalciuria
   d. Can lead to mild metabolic acidosis

8. A 23 year-old thin-looking female presents feeling unwell and investigations reveal a hypokalaemic metabolic alkalosis with variable urinary chloride levels on repeat testing. Rest of the bloods including creatinine, calcium, and magnesium are normal. Her blood pressure is 98/68 mmHg. What is the likely diagnosis?
   a. Bartter syndrome
   b. Gitelman syndrome
   c. Diuretic abuse
   d. Chronic vomiting

9. A 17 year-old male is found to have persistent hypertension. He has a strong family history of early onset hypertension and blood tests reveal a hypokalaemic metabolic alkalosis. Further investigations reveal both plasma aldosterone levels and plasma renin activity are severely low. What is the likely diagnosis?
   a. Conn's syndrome
   b. Primary hyperaldosteronism
   c. Liddle syndrome
   d. Glucocorticoid-remediable aldosteronism (GRA)

10. Chronic liquorice ingestion can lead to:
   a. Hyperkalaemic metabolic acidosis
   b. Hypokalaemic metabolic alkalosis
   c. Hypokalaemic metabolic acidosis
   d. Hyperkalaemic metabolic alkalosis

Answers

1 and 2. Answer to both the questions is b. The normal anion gap acidosis with hypokalaemia points towards either RTA 1 or 2 but the urinary pH > 5.5 is suggestive of RTA 1 which may be associated with Sjögren's syndrome. Myeloma has a strong association with type 2 RTA.

3. a. Nephrocalcinosis is seen in type 1 RTA due to the following reasons:

I. Metabolic acidosis from any cause including the various RTAs causes bones to release calcium salts to act as a buffer, which in turn leads to high urinary concentration of calcium. Under normal circumstances urinary citrate binds with calcium and makes it soluble. However, in type 1 RTA, the proximal tubules tend to reabsorb increased amounts of citrate as it is a buffer (in an effort to combat the acidosis). The resultant deficiency of citrate in urine in type 1 RTA tends to make the urinary calcium insoluble.

II. Alkaline urine markedly diminishes the urinary calcium phosphate solubility and RTA 1 is characterized by urinary pH > 5.5 despite the metabolic acidosis.

4. b. Acetazolamide causes reversible inhibition of carbonic anhydrase which leads to decreased bicarbonate reabsorption in the proximal tubules. The presentation is essentially that of type 2 RTA. All the remaining choices are associated with high anion gap metabolic acidosis.

5. c. Reabsorption of Na^+ (linked to reclaiming of HCO_3) in the proximal tubules helps to co-transport bicarbonate, amino acid, glucose, uric acid, phosphate, and uric acid. A defect in this mechanism leading to impaired reabsorption of bicarbonate causes type 2 RTA and when associated with defective reabsorption of the co-transported amino acid, glucose, uric acid, phosphate, and uric acid as well is known as Fanconi syndrome. The diagnosis may be suspected by hypophosphataemia, hypouricaemia, or glycosuria in the absence of diabetes mellitus.

6. d. Bartter syndrome is due to defect in Na^+ reabsorption in the ascending limb of loop of Henle, while defect in Na^+ reabsorption in the distal convoluted tubule leads to Gitelman syndrome. A reminder – Bartter and Gitelman syndromes resemble the effects of chronic use of loop and thiazide diuretics, respectively.

7. c. Inhibition of Na^+ uptake in the distal convoluted tubule by thiazide diuretic leads to volume contraction, which in turn leads to increased reabsorption of Na^+ in other parts of the tubule. As discussed above, reabsorption of Na^+ by the Na^+-K^+-$2Cl^-$ co-transporter in the ascending limb of loop of Henle is followed by the back diffusion of the K^+ into the tubular lumen, while the Na^+ and the $2Cl^-$ ions diffuse into the peritubular capillary blood. This creates an electrical gradient with more positivity in the tubular lumen and to neutralize that, Ca^+ and Mg^+ are reabsorbed via the paracellular cleft. With increased activity of the Na^+-K^+-$2Cl^-$ co-transporter in response to the volume contraction induced by thiazide diuretic, increased amount of Ca^+ is reabsorbed.

8. c. The variable urinary chloride is the hint here. Both Gitelman and Bartter syndromes are characterized by decreased Na^+ reabsorption. The Na^+ which is lost in urine is mostly bound to Cl^- and hence urinary Cl^- concentration will be consistently high. In chronic vomiting urinary Cl^- is low as hypovolaemia leads to increased Na^+ reabsorption in the tubules with the accompanying Cl reabsorption. Urinary Cl^- levels will be variable in cases of diuretic abuse depending on the timing of urine collection in relation to diuretic use. In equivocal cases, urine diuretic screen is helpful.

9. c. Primary hyperaldosteronism is characteristically associated with raised plasma aldosterone to renin ratio (PAC/PRA). In GRA, the plasma aldosterone is elevated and plasma renin activity is suppressed, though the aldosterone–renin ratio is typically not as high as with primary aldosteronism. In Liddle syndrome, the apical epithelial Na^+ channel (ENAC) which is normally under the control of aldosterone is mutated and reabsorbs Na^+ independent of the aldosterone levels. As a feedback, both the plasma renin activity and aldosterone concentration are low.

10. b. In the kidney, 11-beta-hydroxysteroid dehydrogenase enzyme type 2 isoform (11-beta-HSD2) converts cortisol to the inactive cortisone, thus preventing cortisol from its natural tendency of binding to the mineralocorticoid receptor. Cortisol has a potent mineralocorticoid action and the plasma levels of cortisol are significantly higher than that of aldosterone. Liquorice contains glycyrrhetinic acid, which inhibits 11-beta-HSD2, the same enzyme that is deficient in the syndrome of apparent mineralocorticoid excess (AME). Therefore, chronic use of liquorice leads to elevated level of cortisol in the kidneys, which in turn leads to exaggerated stimulation of the mineralocorticoid receptor and hypertension with hypokalaemic metabolic alkalosis.

4

Renal Stones

Yena Hye and Surjit Tarafdar

Summary

- Calcium stones are the commonest type of renal stones (75%), whilst struvite (10–15%), uric acid (8%), and cystine (less than 1%) stones make up the remainder
- Stones less than 5 mm in diameter have a high chance of spontaneous clearance, whilst stones over 10 mm usually need urological intervention
- Low fluid intake or high fluid losses, e.g. from sweating or gastrointestinal losses, are major risk factors for renal stones
- Uric acid stones are more common in acidic urine, whilst struvite and calcium phosphate stones are commoner in alkaline urine
- Both non-contrast computed tomography of the abdomen and pelvis and ultrasonography are considered initial diagnostic studies of choice for renal stones
- Medical expulsive therapy for renal stones consists of calcium-channel blockers (usually nifedipine) and alpha-blockers (usually tamsulosin)

Renal stones include nephrolithiasis, which refers to stone formation within the renal tubule or collecting duct, nephrocalcinosis, which refers to diffuse renal parenchymal calcification, and ureterolithiasis, which refers to stones within the ureter.

Whilst patients with renal stones may present with classic symptoms of renal colic and haematuria, others may be asymptomatic or may experience atypical symptoms, such as vague abdominal pain with nausea or urinary urgency.

There are various types of kidney stones and it is clinically important to identify the stone type, since it often guides selection of the optimal preventive regimen and prognosis. Calcium stones (calcium oxalate or the less common calcium phosphate) are seen most commonly (75%), whilst struvite (10–15%), uric acid (8%), and cystine (less than 1%) stones make up the rest. Some stones are a mixture of crystal types (e.g. calcium oxalate and calcium phosphate) and also contain protein in the stone matrix. On the other hand, the same patient may have different types of stones concurrently (e.g. calcium oxalate and uric acid). Rarely, stones are composed of medications, such as acyclovir, indinavir, and triamterene [1]. In Mediterranean and Middle Eastern countries, up to 75% of renal stones are composed of uric acid, presumably because of the hot weather conditions leading to concentrated and acidic urine.

Kidney stones less than 5 mm in diameter have a high chance of being passed out spontaneously with urine, whilst those that are 5–7 mm have only a 50% chance. Stones over 10 mm in diameter almost always require urological intervention [2].

The calcifications in nephrocalcinosis are usually calcium phosphate or calcium oxalate and may be deposited in the cortex or medulla.

Lecture Notes Nephrology: A Comprehensive Guide to Renal Medicine, First Edition. Edited by Surjit Tarafdar.
© 2020 John Wiley & Sons Ltd. Published 2020 by John Wiley & Sons Ltd.

Epidemiology

Nephrolithiasis is a global disease and data suggest that the prevalence is increasing, likely due to dietary changes with sedentary lifestyles leading to increasing body mass index (BMI) and incidence of type 2 diabetes mellitus. There are data to suggest that up to 1 in 5 men and 1 in 10 women will develop at least one stone during their lifetime. The prevalence and incidence of nephrolithiasis vary by age, sex, and race. The peak incidence occurs between the ages of 40 and 49 years and it is more common in men than women, with a ratio of 2.5 : 1. The prevalence and incidence rates are highest for Caucasians, followed by Hispanics, then people of African origin and Asians, in that order [3].

Cystinuria is a genetic cause of kidney stones with an average prevalence of 1 in 7000 births. Although cysteine stones are found in about 1% of stone formers, they represent a higher percentage of stones in children (about 5%).

In addition to the costs associated with treatment of renal stones, this condition has a substantial economic impact since the individuals affected are often of working age. Once an individual has been diagnosed with nephrolithiasis, preventing a recurrence is essential.

Aetiology and Pathogenesis

There are two theories regarding calcium stone formation. The first states that when urine has calcium and oxalate in a concentration more than that in which they can stay dissolved – that is, the urine is supersaturated with these elements – they combine to form a more stable and solid phase, a process called nucleation. In homogenous nucleation, similar ions join into crystals, whilst the more common heterogeneous nucleation results when crystals grow around dissimilar crystals or other substances in the urine, examples being calcium oxalate crystals nucleating around uric acid crystals or sloughed epithelial cells. The second theory argues that rather than intraluminal nucleation, crystals in the urine become attached to exposed crystalline deposits of calcium phosphate (termed Randall's plaques) on renal papilla [1]. Calcium phosphate precipitates in the basement membrane of the thin loops of Henle, erodes into the interstitium and then accumulates in the subepithelial space of the renal papilla. These Randall's plaques eventually erode through the papillary urothelium. Urinary calcium phosphate and calcium oxalate gradually deposit on the plaques to create urinary calculus.

Struvite stones, which are composed of magnesium ammonium phosphate, form only when urinary ammonia production is increased and the urine pH is persistently alkaline (>7.0). In humans, this situation only arises with upper urinary tract infection (UTI) with urease-producing organisms such as *Proteus*, *Pseudomonas* or *Klebsiella*.

Urease breaks down urinary urea into ammonia (NH_3) and carbon dioxide (CO_2):

$$Urea \longrightarrow^{(urease)} 2NH_3 + CO_2$$

The ammonia produced by this reaction then combines with water to form ammonium (NH_4^+) and hydroxide (OH^-), which raises the urinary pH:

$$NH_3 + H_2O \longrightarrow NH_4^+ + OH^-$$

Women are more prone to pure struvite stones, as they are more likely to develop upper UTIs because of their shorter urethra. Patients with an increased susceptibility to urinary infection, such as those with neurogenic bladder or urinary diversion, also form pure struvite stones [1, 3].

In patients with mixed calcium and struvite stones, it is presumed that the primary event is calcium oxalate stone formation, with secondary infection and struvite deposition. A comprehensive medical evaluation should be performed to uncover the underlying metabolic defect(s) responsible for calcium stone formation [2]. On the other hand, patients with pure struvite stones will not benefit from a metabolic evaluation, but would rather benefit from determining the cause of the recurrent upper UTIs.

Cystinuria is an inherited autosomal-recessive disease that is characterized by high concentrations of the amino acid cystine in urine, leading to the formation of cystine stones. The condition is characterized by decreased proximal tubular reabsorption of filtered cystine, resulting in increased urinary cystine excretion and cystine nephrolithiasis.

Different Types of Renal Stones and Risk Factors

Certain diseases and dietary habits can affect urine composition, which in turn influences the risk of nephrolithiasis. The universal risk factor is low urine output, due to either low fluid intake or high fluid losses, for example from sweating or gastrointestinal

Table 4.1 Risk factors for renal calcium stones

Urinary factors	Higher calcium
	Higher oxalate (calcium oxalate stones)
	Lower citrate
	Higher pH (calcium phosphate stones)
	Lower volume
Underlying conditions	Primary hyperparathyroidism
	Medullary sponge kidney
	Distal renal tubular acidosis
	Pancreatic insufficiency
	Inflammatory bowel disease
	Bowel resection
	Bariatric surgery
	Jejunoileal or gastric bypass surgeries
	Primary hyperoxaluria
Dietary factors	High animal protein diet
	High salt and sugar intakes
	Increased intake of high oxalate-containing foods
	Low calcium intake
	Excessive vitamin C and D supplementation
Medications	Loop diuretics
	Corticosteroids
	Vitamin D/calcium supplements
	Theophylline
	Acetazolamide
	Amphotericin B

losses [4]. Tables 4.1 and 4.2 list the major risk factors for developing calcium and non-calcium renal stones.

Calcium Stones

Stones composed of calcium oxalate can occur in various disorders. In general, calcium phosphate stones are associated with the same risk factors as calcium oxalate stones (other than alkaline urine for the former and hyperoxaluria for the latter). Risk factors for developing calcium stones can be grouped under urinary factors, underlying medical conditions, dietary factors, and medications [5].

Urinary risk factors for developing renal calcium stones include:

- Higher urine calcium excretion, with or without hypercalcaemia.
- Higher urine oxalate excretion, which may be present in up to 40% of male and 15% of female stone formers and is a major risk factor for calcium oxalate stone formation. Marked hyperoxaluria may be

Table 4.2 Risk factors for non-calcium renal stones

Stone types	Risk factors
Uric acid	Urine pH <5.5 (e.g. chronic diarrhoea, chronic metabolic acidosis)
	Overproduction and excretion of uric acid (e.g. gout)
	Medications (e.g. salicylates, probenecid or allopurinol)
Struvite	Upper urinary tract infection with a urease-producing organism (e.g. Proteus, Pseudomonas or Klebsiella)
Cysteine	Cystinuria

secondary to the increased intestinal absorption of oxalate (enteric oxaluria) or inherited enzymatic defects causing overproduction of oxalate (primary oxaluria).

○ *Enteric oxaluria:* fat malabsorption is the commonest cause of increased intestinal oxalate absorption. In patients with fat malabsorption, intestinal calcium binds to unabsorbed fatty acids, leaving oxalate free to be absorbed and then filtered by the kidney. Fat malabsorption leading to hyperoxaluria and renal stones may be seen in pancreatic insufficiency, inflammatory bowel disease, bowel resection, bariatric surgery, jejunoileal or gastric bypass surgeries.

○ *Primary hyperoxaluria*: this is a rare autosomal-recessive disorder that is characterized by enzymatic defects in glyoxylate metabolism, causing enhanced oxalate production with consequent calcium oxalate stone formation. End-stage renal disease (ESRD) occurs in about half of patients by young adulthood. As the glomerular filtration rate falls below 30–40 ml/min per 1.73 m², the combination of oxalate overproduction and reduced urinary oxalate excretion leads to calcium oxalate deposition in the heart, blood vessels, joints, bone, and retina. Patients may present with unexplained cardiomyopathy or cardiac conduction defects, poor peripheral circulation and gangrene, joint pain, bone pain, spontaneous fractures, and diminished visual acuity. Liver transplantation is the only definitive therapy known, as that helps to replace the defective hepatic enzymes. In case of ESRD, as oxalate is not removed by dialysis, renal transplantation is the preferred therapy.

- Low urinary citrate, which may be seen in chronic metabolic acidosis predisposes to urinary calcium stones. Under normal conditions, citrate inhibits urinary calcium stone formation by binding with calcium to form a soluble complex, which is excreted in urine. Chronic metabolic acidosis leads to enhanced citrate reabsorption by the proximal tubules because of citrate's alkaline nature, except in proximal renal tubular acidosis (RTA), where the defect is in the proximal tubule and therefore citrate cannot be reabsorbed. The resultant low urinary citrate concentration can predispose to urinary calcium stone formation.
- Hyperuricosuria contributes to nephrolithiasis in 10–15% of calcium stones, as calcium oxalate crystals nucleate around uric acid crystals.
- A persistently alkaline urine pH, as seen with type I (distal) RTA due to an inability to excrete hydrogen (H⁺) ion, is associated with calcium phosphate stone formation (as mentioned, calcium phosphate stones are more common in alkaline urine).
- Low urine volume, which increases the concentrations of the lithogenic factors.

Underlying medical conditions that predispose to calcium stone formation include:

- Primary hyperparathyroidism, which is suspected because of the presence of hypercalcaemia that is often mild and intermittent [6]. Affected patients are more prone to have calcium phosphate stones.
- Medullary sponge kidney (MSK), a congenital disorder characterized by dilatation of the terminal collecting ducts in the renal pyramids, which is often associated with hypercalciuria and hypocitraturia. It is estimated that this disorder is present in 12–20% of recurrent calcium stone formers [7]. Diagnosis of MSK does not change the evaluation or the treatment recommendations, as the condition has an excellent long-term prognosis.

The dietary risk factors for calcium stone formation include:

- A high animal protein diet, which can lead to increased urinary excretion of calcium and uric acid as well as decreased excretion of citrate.
- High salt and sugar intakes, which increase urinary calcium excretion.
- Increased intake of high oxalate-containing foods, particularly spinach and nuts. The exact contribution of dietary oxalate to urinary oxalate is controversial and likely varies considerably from person to person due to variable absorption.
- Lower calcium intake, which acts by increasing the intestinal absorption and subsequent urinary excretion of oxalate due to decreased calcium oxalate complex formation within the intestinal lumen [8]. The effect on oxalate more than counterbalances the decrease in calcium absorption and excretion.
- Excessive vitamin C and D supplementation.

The following medications are associated with increased risk of calcium stone formation:

- Loop diuretics
- Corticosteroids
- Vitamin D/calcium supplements
- Theophylline
- Acetazolamide
- Amphotericin B

Uric Acid Stones

Uric acid stones result from persistently acidic urine (pH <5.5), which promotes uric acid precipitation, as well as in the setting of uric acid overproduction and excretion, as seen in those with gout or on uricosuric medications. Uric acid stones may antedate gouty arthritis in up to 40% of patients with primary gout.

In patients with chronic diarrhoea, ongoing bicarbonate loss (from the pancreatic secretions) and volume depletion lead to the kidneys trying to conserve sodium and water avidly. Reclaiming of sodium is linked to tubular secretion of hydrogen. Bicarbonate loss in stool also leads to metabolic acidosis, which in turn leads to a compensatory increase in hydrogen secretion in urine. The net effect is concentrated and acidic urine that potentiates urate nephropathy. Apart from chronic metabolic acidosis, acidic urine may also be seen in patients with diabetes, insulin resistance, and obesity, possibly related to reduced ammoniagenesis [9]. Low urine volume due to inadequate fluid intake or excessive extra-renal fluid loss, as in diarrhoea or perspiration, can also lead to uric acid stones.

The following medications, by increasing urinary uric acid concentration, are associated with an increased risk of uric acid stone formation:

- Aspirin – high dosages (>3 g/day) can be uricosuric, whilst low dosages (1–2 g/day) cause uric acid retention
- Probenicid
- Allopurinol

Struvite Stones

Struvite (magnesium ammonium phosphate) stones develop in patients with chronic upper UTI due to urease-producing organism such as *Proteus*, *Pseudomonas* or *Klebsiella*. Women and individuals with a neurogenic bladder or urinary diversion are more likely to form pure struvite stones due to an increased predisposition to develop upper UTI. Occasional patients present with large branched (staghorn) calculi filling the collecting system and requiring surgical management.

Cystine Stones

Patients with cystinuria have decreased proximal tubular reabsorption of filtered cystine, resulting in increased urinary cystine excretion and cystine nephrolithiasis. Usually patients present in childhood or young adulthood and rarely patients present with staghorn calculi requiring surgical management. The pattern of inheritance may be autosomal dominant or autosomal recessive with incomplete penetrance. For some reason, male patients seem to have a more severe disease. Cystinuria is diagnosed amongst patients with nephrolithiasis and one or more of the following findings:

- Stone analysis showing cystine.
- Positive family history of cystinuria.
- Identification of pathognomonic hexagonal cystine crystals on urinalysis.

Patients should have 24-hour urinary cystine excretion measured. Whilst the normal rate of cystine excretion is 30 mg/day (0.13 mmol/day), these patients generally excrete more than 250 mg/day (approximately 1 mmol/day).

Medications Precipitating as Renal Stones

Urinary calculi can also be induced by medications when the drugs crystallize and become the primary component of the stones. Similar to the pathogenesis of calcium stones discussed earlier, urinary supersaturation of the agent may promote formation of the calculi. Drugs that induce calculi via this process include magnesium trisilicate, ciprofloxacin, sulphur-containing medications such as sulfamethoxazole-trimethoprim, triamterene, indinavir, and ephedrine, alone or in combination with guaifenesin.

Other Risk Factors

Other risk factors for developing renal stones include history of prior nephrolithiasis, family history of nephrolithiasis, obesity, and excessive physical exercise (e.g. marathon running), which could increase crystalluria and hence increase the risk of stones in predisposed individuals [10, 11]. Patients with hypertension have an approximately twofold higher risk of nephrolithiasis [10, 11].

Clinical Manifestations

Occasionally, patients are diagnosed with asymptomatic nephrolithiasis when they undergo radiological imaging of the abdomen for other reasons or surveillance imaging due to a prior history of stones. This asymptomatic phase is more likely to continue in patients who do not have a history of renal colic [12].

Symptoms and Signs

Symptoms develop when stones initially pass from the renal pelvis into the ureter. The most common symptom is pain, which varies from a mild ache to a severe pain requiring parenteral analgesics. The pain typically fluctuates in intensity and is related to movement of the stone in the ureter and associated ureteral spasm. Pain is thought to occur primarily from urinary obstruction with distention of the renal capsule, and the location of pain depends on the location of the obstruction. Obstruction in the upper ureter or renal pelvis causes flank pain or tenderness, whereas obstruction in the lower ureter leads to pain that radiates to the ipsilateral testicle or labium. The location of the pain may change as the stone migrates.

Gross or microscopic haematuria occurs in the majority of patients with symptomatic (with pain) nephrolithiasis, and often in asymptomatic patients as well. Other than passage of a stone or gravel, this is the discriminating sign of a kidney stone in patients presenting with unilateral flank pain. However, the absence of haematuria in the setting of acute flank pain does not exclude nephrolithiasis. In approximately 10–30% of patients with documented nephrolithiasis, haematuria is not detected [13, 14]. The sensitivity of haematuria is thought to be dependent on the interval from the onset of acute pain to the time of urine examination – haematuria is more likely to be detected on the first day of onset of acute pain compared to subsequent days [15].

Other symptoms that are commonly seen in patients with nephrolithiasis include nausea, vomiting, dysuria, and urgency. The last two symptoms typically occur when the stone is in the distal ureter.

Classic symptoms of nephrolithiasis are less common with struvite stones because of their smooth surface. Affected patients often present with symptoms of a UTI, mild flank pain, or haematuria and have a persistently alkaline urine pH (>8), often with multiple magnesium ammonium phosphate crystals in the urine sediment. The stone may grow rapidly over a period of weeks to months and, if not adequately treated, can develop into a staghorn or branched calculus involving the entire renal collecting system.

Complications

Patient with bilateral ureteric calculi may present with acute kidney injury (AKI). Nephrolithiasis can cause persistent renal obstruction, which may potentially lead to permanent kidney damage if left untreated. Staghorn calculi, which are classified as upper urinary tract stones that involve the renal pelvis and extend into calyces, do not typically produce symptoms unless the stone is big enough to result in urinary tract obstruction or is associated with infection. They may lead to progressive renal impairment over time if present bilaterally [16].

Investigation

Urine: Urinalysis, 24-Hour Urine Collection, and Urine Culture

A careful urinalysis should be performed, since certain findings point towards specific diagnosis (Figure 4.1). A urine pH >7 is suggestive of calcium phosphate or struvite calculi, depending on the presence of phosphate or struvite crystals in the urine sediment. The presence of hexagonal cystine crystals is diagnostic of cystinuria.

Although uric acid crystals and calcium oxalate crystals may be seen in individuals without nephrolithiasis, if seen in a patient with known stone disease they are likely to represent the composition of the stone.

At least two sets of 24-hour urine collections should be obtained to measure urine volume, pH and excretion of calcium, uric acid, citrate, oxalate, sodium, potassium, and creatinine (to ensure the completeness of the collection).

Urine culture may show growth of urease-producing organism such as *Proteus*, *Pseudomonas* or *Klebsiella* in those with struvite stones.

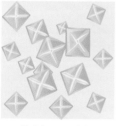
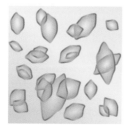
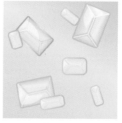
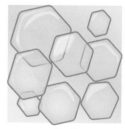

| Calcium oxalate crystals | Uric acid crystals | Struvite crystals | Cystine crystals |

Figure 4.1 Different types of urinary crystals.

Blood Biochemistry: Sodium, Potassium, Chloride, Bicarbonate, Urea, Creatinine, Calcium, Phosphate, and Uric Acid

Serum parathyroid hormone (PTH) should be measured if the serum calcium is raised. A low bicarbonate level may be suggestive of chronic acidosis leading to renal stones, as in distal RTA or chronic diarrhoea.

Radiological Evaluation: Non-Contrast Computed Tomography of the Abdomen and Pelvis or Ultrasound

The diagnosis of nephrolithiasis should be suspected in all patients with the acute onset of flank pain, particularly in the setting of haematuria and absent abdominal guarding.

Both non-contrast computed tomography (CT) of the abdomen and pelvis and ultrasonography are considered initial diagnostic studies of choice. CT of the abdomen and pelvis is useful to diagnose other conditions like appendicitis or diverticulitis mimicking renal stones. It is important to recognize that ureteral dilatation without a stone on the scan could represent recent passage of a stone. CT is more sensitive in detecting stone than ultrasonography, but is associated with radiation exposure, and cumulative radiation dose could be high in patients who undergo multiple CT scans for recurrent nephrolithiasis. Ultrasound (Figure 4.2) is the initial diagnostic test of choice in pregnant women, or if alternative diagnosis such as cholecystitis or gynaecological

pathology is highly suspected. The specificity of CT can be as high as 100% and therefore a positive study confirms the diagnosis of nephrolithiasis [17]. As with ultrasonography, CT can also detect secondary signs of urinary tract obstruction, namely ureteral dilatation, collecting system dilatation with or without frank hydronephrosis.

There is a growing interest in the use of low-dose non-contrast CT, which uses a significantly reduced radiation dose and still allows identification of renal and ureteral calculi with similar sensitivity and specificity as standard CT, with exceptions for small stones (less than 2 mm in diameter) or in obese patients (BMI >30) [18, 19].

Less Frequently Used Radiological Tests

Less frequently used radiological tests include plain X-ray, intravenous pyelography (IVP), and magnetic resonance imaging (MRI). A plain abdominal X-ray can detect sufficiently large radiopaque stones such as calcium, struvite, and cystine stones, but will miss radiolucent uric acid stones and may miss small stones or those overlying bony structures.

IVP has a higher sensitivity than plain X-ray and provides data about the degree of obstruction. It was previously the investigation of choice, but is no longer used much due to the potential for contrast reactions, lower sensitivity, and higher radiation exposure compared to non-contrast CT.

MRI is rarely used because it is not optimal for identifying stones; thus it is only utilized if there is a specific indication to reduce radiation exposure (e.g. a pregnant patient).

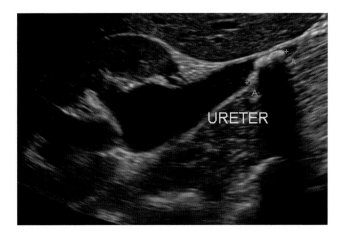

Figure 4.2 Ultrasound image of ureteric calculi.

Determination of Stone Composition on Computed Tomography

The stone composition may be suggested by density on CT scan as well as location and/or general appearance. Although struvite (magnesium ammonium phosphate) and cystine stones are often radiopaque, they are not as dense as stones composed of calcium oxalate or calcium phosphate. Struvite stones are more likely in the presence of large calculi in the renal pelvis, whereas the presence of nephrocalcinosis favours calcium phosphate stones. Bilateral calcifications at the corticomedullary junction are typically seen in MSK and this is suggestive of calcium oxalate or calcium phosphate stones.

In general, calcium stones can usually be distinguished from uric acid, cystine, and struvite stones. However, CT scans are not sensitive enough to distinguish calcium oxalate from calcium phosphate. Studies have suggested that dual-energy CT (DECT), which is a relatively new form of CT that utilizes two energy sources, may be more sensitive than standard helical CT for determining stone composition [20].

Management

Acute Therapy

Most patients with acute renal colic can be managed conservatively with analgesics. Forced intravenous hydration, compared with minimal intravenous hydration, does not appear to be more beneficial in reducing the amount of analgesics required or in facilitating stone passage [21].

Patients should be instructed to strain their urine for several days if possible and to bring in any stone that passes for analysis; this often enables clinicians to plan preventive therapy.

Urgent urological consultation should be sought in patients with urinary sepsis, significant obstruction causing AKI, anuria, and/or uncontrolled pain. Outpatient urology referral is indicated in patients with a stone greater than 10 mm in diameter and in those who fail to pass the stone after a trial of conservative management, including medical expulsive therapy (MET), particularly if the stone is >4 mm in diameter [21].

Pain Management

For patients with renal colic, both non-steroidal anti-inflammatory drugs (NSAIDs) and opioids are effective. Since it is thought that the pain is caused by ureteral spam, NSAIDs have the possible advantage of directly treating this mechanism by decreasing ureteral smooth muscle tone [22]. On the other hand, use of NSAIDs in patients with pre-existing renal disease or severe volume depletion can lead to acute kidney injury.

NSAIDs should be stopped three days before anticipated shock wave lithotripsy (SWL) to minimize the risk of bleeding. Standard doses of opiates will relieve pain in those who do not respond to NSAIDs.

Medical Expulsive Therapy

The likelihood of spontaneous stone passage depends on the size and location of the stone; smaller and more distal stones are more likely to pass without intervention. Most stones less than 5 mm in diameter pass spontaneously, but stones greater than 10 mm in diameter are unlikely to do so [23].

Calcium-channel blockers (usually nifedipine) and alpha-blockers (usually tamsulosin) have emerged as the most promising agents for MET [24]. Although studies directly comparing nifedipine with tamsulosin have reported similar rates of stone passage, a potential advantage of tamsulosin is somewhat faster stone passage and fewer hospitalizations and procedures.

Urological Intervention

Current options for therapy of stones that do not pass include SWL, ureteroscopic lithotripsy with electro-hydraulic or laser probes, percutaneous nephrolithotomy, and laparoscopic stone removal. Open surgical stone removal is rarely needed. SWL works best for stones in the renal pelvis and upper ureter, whilst ureteroscopy continues to be the treatment of choice for most middle and distal ureteral stones. Complications of SWL include obstruction by the stone fragments and UTI, occurring in less than 10% of cases. Both SWL and ureteroscopy are considered first-line management options for ureteral stones that require removal; ureteroscopy yields higher stone-free rates than SWL, but has an increased incidence of complications [25].

SWL is only successful in approximately 50% of cases for patients with larger renal calculi (e.g. >1.5 cm), renal stones of harder composition (e.g. cystine or calcium oxalate monohydrate) or stones in complex renal or ureteral locations (e.g. lower pole calyx or mid-ureter). In these settings, endoscopic stone fragmentation with a percutaneous or ureteroscopic approach is often preferred.

Further Evaluation and Subsequent Treatment

Since the chances of stone recurrence are quite high (35–40% in men), there is an argument for a complete metabolic evaluation in the first-time stone former. However, there are data suggesting that a comprehensive medical evaluation is not cost-effective for patients who have formed their first stone. Some therefore recommend only a limited evaluation after the first stone formation. This limited evaluation should include serum biochemistry including serum calcium, phosphate, and bicarbonate (the latter to rule out chronic acidosis leading to renal stones, as in distal RTA or chronic diarrhoea).

A complete metabolic evaluation should be performed in the following patients at moderate to high risk for recurrent disease:

- Middle-aged, white males with a family history of stones.
- Patients with chronic diarrheal states and/or malabsorption, pathologic skeletal fractures, osteoporosis, UTI, and/or gout.
- Patients with stones composed of cystine, uric acid or calcium phosphate.

In addition to the basic blood tests already discussed, a complete metabolic evaluation for renal stones involves 24-hour urine collection. The urine volume, pH, and excretion of calcium, uric acid, citrate, oxalate, phosphate, sodium, potassium and creatinine (to assess the completeness of the collection) should be measured. Furthermore, urinary supersaturation should be calculated for calcium oxalate, calcium phosphate, and uric acid. Once it has been determined that therapy to prevent new stone formation is required, the following guidelines can be used:

- Patients should increase their fluid intake, with the goal of producing at least 2 l of urine daily.
- Dietary recommendations tailored to the individual's habits and urine composition may be beneficial.
- Patients with calcium stones who cannot be managed solely with dietary modifications can be treated with a thiazide diuretic and low sodium diet to achieve lower urine calcium excretion.
- Patients with uric acid stones can be treated with potassium citrate to alkalinize the urine and occasionally with allopurinol (for patients with severe hyperuricosuria).
- Patients with cystine stones can be treated with a high fluid intake and urinary alkalinization, with many needing a thiol-containing drug (penicillamine or tiopronin).

- Struvite stones typically require complete stone removal with percutaneous nephrolithotomy, as well as aggressive prevention and treatment of future UTIs.

Recommendations for Specific Stone Types

Calcium Oxalate

Risk factors for calcium oxalate stones include higher urine calcium, higher urine oxalate, and low urine citrate. This stone type is insensitive to pH in the physiological range.

High Urine Calcium

Although the term hypercalciuria is used, there is no widely accepted cut-off level that distinguishes between normal and abnormal urine calcium excretion. Since the relation between urine calcium and stone risk appears to be continuous, the use of an arbitrary threshold should be avoided.

Patients with persistent stone disease and high urine calcium that is not due to hypercalcaemia (often referred to as idiopathic hypercalciuria) should be managed with a reduced animal protein and low salt diet plus a thiazide diuretic [26].

Restriction in dietary calcium intake is not recommended unless the intake is excessive (more than 2000 mg/day). Although urine calcium excretion may decrease with restriction, the decrease in free intestinal calcium leads to decreased binding of oxalate by calcium in the intestinal lumen, resulting in increased absorption of dietary oxalate and enhanced oxalate excretion. The net effect may be increased supersaturation of the urine with calcium oxalate and an increased tendency to stone formation.

Thiazide therapy can lower calcium excretion by as much as 50%, primarily by inducing mild volume depletion, which leads to a compensatory rise in the reabsorption of sodium in the thick ascending limb of loop of henle which in turn leads to a rise in passive calcium reabsorption. This results in a significant reduction in the number of new stone recurrences. Urinary calcium and sodium excretion should be monitored after the institution of thiazide therapy. In the case of ongoing hypercalciuria, sodium excretion of below 100 mEq (2300 mg) per day should be aimed at by further restricting salt intake. The potassium-sparing diuretic amiloride can also be added, since this drug may increase calcium reabsorption in the cortical collecting tubule, further lowering calcium excretion [27].

High Urine Oxalate

As for urine calcium, no definition of 'abnormal' urine oxalate excretion is widely accepted, and the relation between urine oxalate and stone risk is also continuous.

A low oxalate diet should be tried first in patients with hyperoxaluria. The primary foods to avoid are spinach and nuts. If the low oxalate diet alone is insufficient, increasing dietary calcium or adding calcium citrate supplement should be considered even if the urine calcium is high. However, the amount of urinary oxalate that is derived from the diet is variable. Thus, if the urine oxalate does not fall despite adherence to a low oxalate diet, then the oxalate restriction can be removed. Avoiding high-dose vitamin C supplements is also a known strategy that reduces endogenous oxalate production.

Low Urine Citrate

Urinary citrate inhibits calcium oxalate and calcium phosphate crystallization. Increased consumption of foods rich in alkali (e.g. fruits and vegetables) can increase urine citrate. If dietary modification alone is not adequate to increase urine citrate, the addition of supplemental citrate, typically potassium citrate, is recommended. Sodium salts such as sodium bicarbonate, whilst successful in raising urine citrate, are typically avoided due to the adverse effects of sodium on urinary calcium excretion. Rise in urinary sodium increases urinary sodium urate formation, which can serve as a nidus for calcium oxalate precipitation.

Calcium Phosphate

Calcium phosphate stones share risk factors with calcium oxalate stones, including higher urine calcium, and lower urine citrate concentrations. In addition, higher urine phosphate levels and higher urine pH (typically ≥6.5) are associated with an increased risk of calcium phosphate stone formation. Hence, calcium phosphate stones are more common in patients with distal RTA and primary hyperparathyroidism.

As for oxalate stones, thiazide diuretics with sodium restriction may be used to reduce urine calcium, and supplemental citrate (e.g. potassium citrate) can be used to increase urine citrate concentration. However, supplemental citrate will also increase the urine pH, thereby increasing the risk of stone formation, since calcium phosphate stones form more readily in alkaline urine. Hence, the urine pH should be monitored closely. Reduction of dietary phosphate may be beneficial by reducing urine phosphate excretion.

Uric Acid

The two main risk factors for uric acid stones are persistently low urine pH and high uric acid excretion. Bicarbonate loss and volume contraction in chronic diarrhoea lead to a concentrated and acidic urine which predisposes to uric acid stones. Urine pH is the predominant influence on uric acid solubility, and thus alkalinizing urine is the mainstay of prevention of uric acid stone formation. This can be readily achieved by increasing the intake of foods rich in alkali (e.g. fruits and vegetables) and reducing the intake of foods that produce acid (e.g. meat). If required, supplementation with bicarbonate or citrate salts can be used to reach the recommended pH goal of 6–7.

Urinary uric acid excretion is determined by uric acid production. Uric acid is the end product of purine metabolism, and therefore reduced consumption of purine-containing foods can reduce urine uric acid excretion. The indications for xanthine oxidase inhibitors such as allopurinol to reduce uric acid production are usually reserved for patients who continue to have stones despite urinary alkalinization and dietary modification.

Diabetes mellitus and metabolic syndrome are characterized by increased body weight, which is associated with both a more acidic urine pH and an increase in urinary uric acid excretion and supersaturation. Weight reduction and better control of diabetes mellitus are known to have a beneficial effect.

Cystine

Because the dietary precursor of cystine which is methionine, is an essential amino acid, it is impractical to reduce its intake. Treatment consists of high fluid intake, sodium and protein restriction, and urinary alkalinization (often with potassium citrate, as the sodium in sodium bicarbonate may increase cystine excretion). Most patients will need the addition of a thiol-containing drug (penicillamine or tiopronin), which converts urinary cystine into the soluble cysteine. The use of penicillamine is often limited by the high incidence of side effects such as fever, rash, abnormal taste, arthritis, leukopenia/aplastic anaemia, hepatotoxicity, pyridoxine (vitamin B6) deficiency, and nephrotic-range proteinuria (often due to membranous nephropathy). Although tiopronin use may be associated with similar adverse effects, the incidence of these effects is lower than with the use of penicillamine.

Struvite

Struvite stones often require surgical removal and new stone formation can be avoided by the prevention of UTIs. In patients with recurrent upper UTIs (e.g. individuals with surgically altered urinary drainage or spinal cord injury), the urease inhibitor acetohydroxamic acid can be considered; however, this agent should be used with caution because of potential side effects.

Long-Term Follow-Up

Typically, the recommendations provided should be followed for the patient's lifetime, and it is necessary to tailor them in a way that is acceptable to the patient. Long-term follow-up is imperative to ensure that the preventive measures have been implemented and are successful in reducing the risk of new stone formation.

Radiological Monitoring

Another management issue is radiological monitoring to determine whether new stones have formed or previous stones have increased in size. Some suggest that monitoring should be performed initially at one year and, if negative, every two to four years thereafter, depending upon the likelihood of recurrence. When choosing a modality for radiological monitoring, cumulative radiation exposure should be considered, particularly in women of childbearing age.

References

1. Coe, F.L., Parks, J.H., and Asplin, J.R. (1992). The pathogenesis and treatment of kidney stones. *N. Engl. J. Med.* 327 (16): 1141.
2. Andrew, P. (2010 May). Physiopathology and etiology of stone formation in the kidney and the urinary tract. *Evan. Pediatr. Nephrol.* 25 (5): 831–841.
3. Romero, V., Akpinar, H., and Assimos, D.G. (2010 Spring-Summer). Kidney stones: a global picture of prevalence, incidence, and associated risk factors. *Rev. Urol.* 12 (2–3): e86–e96.
4. Gault, M.H., Chafe, L.L., Morgan, J.M. et al. (1991). Comparison of patients with idiopathic calcium phosphate and calcium oxalate stones. *Medicine (Baltimore)* 70 (6): 345.
5. Pak, C.Y., Poindexter, J.R., Adams-Huet, B., and Pearle, M.S. (2003). Predictive value of kidney stone composition in the detection of metabolic abnormalities. *Am. J. Med.* 115 (1): 26.
6. Parks, J., Coe, F., and Favus, M. (1980). Hyperparathyroidism in nephrolithiasis. *Arch. Intern. Med.* 140 (11): 1479.
7. Yagisawa, T., Kobayashi, C., Hayashi, T. et al. (2001). Contributory metabolic factors in the development of nephrolithiasis in patients with medullary sponge kidney. *Am. J. Kidney Dis.* 37 (6): 1140.
8. von Unruh, G.E., Voss, S., Sauerbruch, T., and Hesse, A. (2004). Dependence of oxalate absorption on the daily calcium intake. *J. Am. Soc. Nephrol.* 15 (6): 1567.
9. Abate, N., Chandalia, M., Cabo-Chan, A.V. Jr. et al. (2004). The metabolic syndrome and uric acid nephrolithiasis: novel features of renal manifestation of insulin resistance. *Kidney Int.* 65 (2): 386.
10. Cappuccio, F.P., Strazzullo, P., and Mancini, M. (1990). Kidney stones and hypertension: population based study of an independent clinical association. *BMJ* 300 (6734): 1234.
11. Rodgers, A.L., Greyling, K.G., and Noakes, T.D. (1991). Crystalluria in marathon runners. III. Stone-forming subjects. *Urol. Res.* 19 (3): 189.
12. Taylor, E.N. and Curhan, G.C. (2006). Body size and 24-hour urine composition. *Am. J. Kidney Dis.* 48 (6): 905.
13. Bove, P., Kaplan, D., Dalrymple, N. et al. (1999). Reexamining the value of hematuria testing in patients with acute flank pain. *J. Urol.* 162 (3 Pt 1): 685.
14. Press, S.M. and Smith, A.D. (1995). Incidence of negative hematuria in patients with acute urinary lithiasis presenting to the emergency room with flank pain. *Urology* 45 (5): 753.
15. Kobayashi, T., Nishizawa, K., Mitsumori, K., and Ogura, K. (2003). Impact of date of onset on the absence of hematuria in patients with acute renal colic. *J. Urol.* 170 (4 Pt 1): 1093.
16. Ulahannan, D., Blakeley, C.J., Jeyadevan, N., and Hashemi, K. (2008). Benefits of CT urography in patients presenting to the emergency department with suspected ureteric colic. *Emerg. Med. J.* 25 (9): 569.
17. Matlaga, B.R., Shah, O.D., and Assimos, D.G. (2003 Fall). Drug-induced urinary calculi. *Rev Urol.* 5 (4): 227–223.
18. Zilberman, D.E., Tsivian, M., Lipkin, M.E. et al. (2011). Low dose computerized tomography for detection of urolithiasis – its effectiveness in the setting of the urology clinic. *J. Urol.* 185 (3): 910.
19. Zilberman, D.E., Ferrandino, M.N., Preminger, G.M. et al. (2354). In vivo determination of urinary stone composition using dual energy computerized tomography with advanced post-acquisition processing. *J. Urol.* 184 (6): 2010.
20. Curhan, G. (2014 Sep). Imaging in the emergency department for suspected nephrolithiasis. *N. Engl. J. Med.* 371 (12): 1154–1155.

21. Portis, A.J. and Sundaram, C.P. (2001). Diagnosis and initial management of kidney stones. *Am. Fam. Physician* 63 (7): 1329.

22. Parekattil, S.J., Kumar, U., Hegarty, N.J. et al. (2006). External validation of outcome prediction model for ureteral/renal calculi. *J. Urol.* 175 (2): 575.

23. Miller, O.F. and Kane, C.J. (1999). Time to stone passage for observed ureteral calculi: a guide for patient education. *J. Urol.* 162 (3 Pt 1): 688.

24. Preminger, G.M. (2000). The value of intensive medical management of distal ureteral calculi in an effort to facilitate spontaneous stone passage. Editorial comment. *Urology* 56 (4): 582.

25. Kumar, S., Jayant, K., Agrawal, M.M. et al. (2015). Role of tamsulosin, tadalafil, and silodosin as the medical expulsive therapy in lower ureteric stone: a randomized trial (a pilot study). *Urology* 85 (1): 59.

26. Borghi, L., Schianchi, T., Meschi, T. et al. (2002). Comparison of two diets for the prevention of recurrent stones in idiopathic hypercalciuria. *N. Engl. J. Med.* 346 (2): 77.

27. Fink, H.A., Wilt, T.J., Eidman, K.E. et al. (2013). Medical management to prevent recurrent nephrolithiasis in adults: a systematic review for an American College of Physicians Clinical Guideline. *Ann. Intern. Med.* 158 (7): 535.

Questions and Answers

Questions

1. Which is the most common stone type?
   a. Calcium phosphate
   b. Calcium oxalate
   c. Uric acid
   d. Struvite (magnesium ammonium phosphate)
   e. Cystine

2. Which one of the following is NOT a risk factor for calcium stones?
   a. Hypercalciuria
   b. Hyperoxaluria
   c. Hypercitraturia
   d. Persistently high urine pH
   e. High urine volume

3. Patients at high risk for recurrence do NOT include:
   a. Patients with recurrent renal calcium stones
   b. Patients with osteoporosis
   c. Middle aged white male with a family history of stone disease
   d. Patients with struvite stones
   e. Patients with chronic diarrhoea

4. In setting of metabolic evaluation, which one of following is NOT measured in 24 hour urine collection?
   a. Urine volume
   b. Urinary chloride excretion
   c. Urine oxalate excretion
   d. Urinary creatinine excretion
   e. Urinary sodium excretion

5. For patients with calcium stones and hypercalciuria, which one of the following is TRUE?
   a. Calcium intake more than 3 g/day is recommended
   b. Thiazide therapy should be avoided as it causes volume depletion
   c. Loop diuretic should be avoided
   d. Allopurinol is useful as most calcium stones form on top of uric acid stones
   e. Calcium intake recommended is less than 1 g/day

Answers

1. b. While calcium containing stones make up more than 75% of all renal stones, calcium oxalate stones are commoner than calcium phosphate stones.

2. c. Citrate inhibits urinary calcium oxalate (and calcium phosphate) stone formation by binding with calcium to form a soluble complex which is excreted in urine. Persistently elevated urine pH is a risk factor for calcium phosphate stones.

3. b. Osteoporosis does not have link with renal stones.

4. b. In the setting of metabolic evaluation for renal stones, the urine volume, pH, and excretion of calcium, uric acid, citrate, oxalate, phosphate, sodium, and creatinine (to assess the completeness of the collection) should be measured. In addition, urinary supersaturation should be calculated for calcium oxalate, calcium phosphate, and uric acid.

5. c. Thiazide therapy can lower calcium excretion primarily by inducing mild volume depletion which leads to a compensatory rise in the proximal reabsorption of sodium, and thus rise in passive calcium reabsorption. Loop diuretics decrease calcium reabsorption and raise the urinary calcium.

5

Kidney Cancer

Gowri Raman and Surjit Tarafdar

Summary

- More cases of renal cancer are being diagnosed now due to the availability of renal imaging
- Renal cancer can occur sporadically or in association with familial syndromes such as Von Hippel Lindau disease and tuberous sclerosis
- The majority of renal cancers arise in the cortex and are called are renal cell carcinomas (RCC)
- Clear cell renal cell carcinoma is the commonest type of RCC, accounting for 80–90% of cases
- followed by papillary, chromophobe, oncocytoma, collecting duct, and very rarely renal medullary carcinoma
- Surgery is first-line treatment for localized disease
- For advanced disease, immunotherapy, vascular endothelial growth factor (VEGF) pathway inhibitors, or mammalian target of rapamycin (mTOR) inhibitors can be considered

Of all cases of renal cancer, 85% arise in the renal cortex and are called renal cell carcinoma (RCC). Transitional cell carcinomas, which originate in the renal pelvis, are the next most common, accounting for about 8% of all cases. Less common renal parenchymal tumours include oncocytomas, collecting duct tumours, and renal sarcomas. Wilms' tumour is the commonest renal cancer in children <15 years old, accounting for about 95% of all paediatric cases, and is very rarely seen in adults. Secondary renal neoplasms are usually clinically insignificant and often discovered post mortem.

According to the Cancer Council of Australia, renal cancer is the seventh most common cancer diagnosed in Australian men and the eleventh most common cancer in women. The male to female ratio of renal cancer is 2 : 1, and patients usually present in the sixth to eighth decades of life. The inherited syndromes described later in this chapter are associated with 2% of RCCs.

More renal cancers are now being detected earlier due to the availability of renal imaging (Figure 5.1). However, despite this, 30% of patients present with advanced disease [1]. Up to 40% of patients treated with localized disease unfortunately present with a recurrence [1]. When patients present with localized RCC, surgery might be curative, whereas the median survival of patients with metastatic disease is 13 months.

Causative Factors

The following are known risk factors for RCC [2]:

- Smoking
- Obesity
- Hypertension
- Acquired cystic kidney disease associated with end-stage renal disease

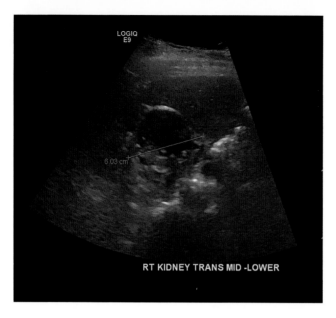

Figure 5.1 Incidental renal mass detected on ultrasound.

- Occupational exposure to toxic compounds such as cadmium, asbestos, and petroleum by-products
- Prolonged ingestion of non-steroidal anti-inflammatory drugs [3]
- Chronic hepatitis C infection
- Sickle cell trait and disease associated with increased risk of renal medullary carcinomas

RCC can also occur as part of the following familial syndromes:

- *Von Hippel Lindau (VHL) disease*: an autosomal-dominant familial cancer syndrome which manifests as retinal haemangioblastomas, haemangioblastomas of the spinal cord and cerebellum, pheochromocytomas, tumours of the middle ear, neuroendocrine tumours of the pancreas, clear cell RCC, and renal cysts (see Table 5.1). In this condition, mutation of the VHL gene (located on chromosome 3) leads to defective production of pVHL, which normally functions as a tumour suppressor protein. Hypoxia-inducible factor-1 alpha (HIF-1alpha) and hypoxia-inducible factor-1 beta (HIF-1beta) lead to production of erythropoietin and several proteins involved in angiogenesis, such as vascular endothelial growth factor (VEGF), transforming growth factor alpha (TGF-alpha) and GLUT-1 glucose transporter. Normally, under hypoxic conditions, pVHL leads to degradation of HIF-1alpha. When pVHL protein is defective, enhanced HIF-1alpha levels lead to overexpression of these angiogenic proteins, creating an environment favourable for epithelial cell proliferation (see Figure 5.2). The disease is not very rare (1 in 36 000

Table 5.1 Tumours associated with Von Hippel Lindau (VHL) disease

| Haemangioblastomas of the cerebellum and spine |
| Retinal haemangioblastomas |
| Clear cell renal cell carcinomas |
| Pheochromocytomas |
| Endolymphatic sac tumours of the middle ear |
| Serous cystadenomas and neuroendocrine tumours of the pancreas |
| Papillary cystadenomas of the epididymis and broad ligament |

live births) and the mean age of initial manifestations of the disease is 26 years. RCCs in this condition are often multicentric and bilateral [4, 5].
- Tuberous sclerosis is a disease characterized by multiple benign hamartomas of the brain, eyes, heart, lung, liver, skin, and kidney, along with renal cysts. It is discussed in Chapter 12.
- Familial clear cell renal cancer has been reported in patients with translocations of chromosome 3p. Patients with this histological variant tend to have a poorer prognosis when compared to the other types of RCC [2].
- Hereditary papillary RCC is an autosomal-dominant disorder with bilateral and multifocal papillary RCC with type 1 histology [2]. These tumours

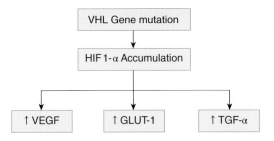

Figure 5.2 Pathogenesis of renal cell carcinoma in Von Hippel Lindau disease. A mutated VHL gene leads to enhanced HIF-1-alpha levels, which in turn lead to overexpression of angiogenic proteins (VEGF, TGF-alpha, and GLUT-1), creating an environment favourable for epithelial cell proliferation. GLUT-1, glucose transporter; HIF-1alpha, hypoxia-inducible factor-1-alpha; TGF-alpha, transforming growth factor alpha; VEGF: vascular endothelial growth factor.

occur earlier than the usual RCC (in the fourth to sixth decades) and can metastasize [4].

- Hereditary leiomyomatosis and renal cell cancer syndrome, which manifests as cutaneous and uterine leiomyomas, is associated with papillary RCC with type 2 histology. This autosomal-dominant condition involves the loss of an FH allele (encoding a protein fumarate hydratase, an enzyme involved in the Krebs cycle) [2]. The RCC in this syndrome is usually solitary and the most aggressive amongst the familial syndromes [2].
- Birt–Hogg–Dubé (BHD) syndrome is an autosomal-dominant condition characterized by cutaneous fibrofolliculomas, lung cysts, pneumothorax, and renal cancer. In this condition there is a mutation of the BHD gene, which encodes the tumour suppressor protein folliculin [2]. Up to 90% of these patients present with cutaneous and pulmonary lesions. The pulmonary cysts are usually asymptomatic, but can be associated with spontaneous pneumothorax [4]. The lifetime risk of developing renal cancer is up to 16% [6]. Patients often develop multiple bilateral renal tumours, which are most often chromophobe or mixed chromophobe and oncocytomas.

Renal Tumour Classification Based on Histology

Size should not be used as a marker to differentiate between benign and malignant renal masses, as small tumours are often malignant. The tumours are classified into the following sub-groups:

- Clear cell (80–90% of RCCs)
- Papillary (10–15%)
- Chromophobe (5–10%)
- Oncocytomas (3–7%)
- Collecting duct (<1%)
- Renal medullary carcinoma (rare)

Clear Cell Renal Cell Carcinoma

This is the most common type of RCC. Histologically, the high lipid content is dissolved during slide preparation, giving an appearance of clear cytoplasm [5]. Clear cell RCCs originate from the epithelial cells of the proximal renal tubule [7]. Macroscopically they are mostly solid and at times cystic.

They may occur sporadically or in association with VHL disease. In up to 80% of sporadic cases of clear cell carcinoma, the VHL gene on chromosome 3 is inactivated by deletion, mutation or methylation. As discussed with VHL disease, when the VHL protein is lost or defective, there is a lack of inhibition of several proteins that may promote tumour angiogenesis, growth, and metastasis.

Papillary Renal Cell Carcinoma

Like clear cell RCC, papillary RCC also originates from the proximal tubule [8]. However, these tumours have distinct morphological features and are further divided into two types based on their histological appearance. Type 1 tumours are characterized by small cells with pale cytoplasm and small oval nuclei with indistinct nucleoli. Type 2 tumours are characterized by large cells with abundant eosinophilic cytoplasm. Type 2 tumours are genetically more heterogeneous and tend to have a poorer prognosis [2].

As already discussed, papillary type 1 tumours are associated with hereditary papillary renal cell carcinomas, whilst type 2 tumours are associated with hereditary leiomyomatosis and renal cell cancer syndrome.

Papillary RCC metastasizes less frequently than clear cell carcinoma, but has a worse prognosis if it does.

There is an association between a duplicated chromosome 7 (which contains the MET proto–oncogene) and the development of papillary RCC [5].

Chromophobe Renal Cell Carcinomas and Oncocytomas

Both oncocytomas and chromophobe renal cell carcinomas (CRCCs) originate in the collecting duct.

Oncocytomas are benign tumours that are derived from type A intercalated cells in the collecting duct [9]. Oncocytomas that are sporadic are usually unilateral and single; bilateral and multiple oncocytomas may be seen in tuberous sclerosis or BHD syndrome.

CRCCs are derived from type B intercalated cells. Macroscopically these tumours tend to be larger than the other subtypes of RCC. Unlike oncocytomas, these tumours are not benign and can metastasize [10].

Both oncocytomas and CRCCs have abundant granular eosinophilic cells. When compared to oncocytomas, the eosinophilic cells in chromophobe tumours have a coarser cytoplasm and distinctive perinuclear clearing. Also, unlike oncocytomas, CRCCs also have more irregular nuclear contours and stain with Hale's colloidal staining [9]. CRCCs typically have sheets of cells aligned along thin fibrovascular septae.

Collecting Duct Renal Cell Carcinoma

Collecting duct carcinoma (CDC) accounts for less than 1% of all RCCs. CDC arises from the principal cells in the collecting ducts. It is an aggressive tumour with generally poor prognosis.

Renal Medullary Carcinoma

Renal medullary carcinoma (RMC) is a rare and extremely aggressive form of kidney cancer found almost exclusively in patients with sickle cell trait. RMC is considered to be a subtype of CDC. Affected patients tend to be young, with a median age of 19–22 years, and are almost always of African origin (though there are a few case reports in Hispanics, Brazilians and Caucasians) [8]. Metastatic disease is seen at presentation in 95% of patients and median survival is five months.

Presentation

The classic triad of flank pain, haematuria, and a palpable abdominal mass has now become uncommon due to earlier incidental discovery of the renal mass on radiographic examination.

The frequency of the individual components of the classic triad are as follows:

- Haematuria – 40%
- Flank pain – 40%
- A palpable mass in the flank or abdomen – 25%

Other signs and symptoms include:

- Weight loss (33%)
- Fever (20%)
- Left-sided varicocele due to obstruction of the testicular vein
- Paraneoplastic syndrome, which can manifest as hypertension, fatigue, weight loss, anaemia, raised erythrocyte sediment rate, abnormal liver function tests, hypercalcaemia, anaemia, and polycythaemia [2]

Investigations

Baseline investigations should include serum creatinine, glomerular filtration rate (GFR), complete cell blood count, erythrocyte sedimentation rate (ESR), liver function studies, lactate dehydrogenase (LDH), serum corrected calcium, coagulation study, and urinalysis.

If there are central renal masses abutting or invading the collecting system, urinary cytology and endoscopic assessment of the upper urinary tract should be considered to rule out the presence of urothelial cancer.

Imaging can include computed tomography (CT) of abdomen and pelvis, CT of chest and brain, bone scan (only in patients with bone pain and/or an elevated serum alkaline phosphatase), and magnetic resonance imaging (MRI) to evaluate renal vein and vena cava.

In CT imaging, enhancement is determined by comparing the pre and post contrast Hounsfield units (HU). A change in 15 HU or more post contrast is consistent with enhancement. If the CT is inconclusive, MRI can be used to further evaluate the lesion [2].

Biopsy of the renal tumour can be carried out using a core or fine needle aspirate. If the imaging is very suggestive and the patient requires surgery, a biopsy is generally not required [2]. However, percutaneous renal tumour biopsies are useful in the following settings [11, 12]:

- Histological diagnosis of radiologically indeterminate renal masses.
- To select patients with small renal masses for surveillance approaches.
- To obtain histology before ablative treatments.
- To select the most suitable form of targeted pharmacological therapy in the setting of metastatic disease.

Staging

TNM staging is generally used when evaluating a patient with RCC (Table 5.2). Further staging is done using the Fuhrman nuclear grade, identifying the

Table 5.2 TNM staging of renal cancer

Primary tumours (T)

TX	Primary tumour cannot be assessed
T0	No evidence of primary tumour
T1	Tumour ≤7 cm in greatest dimension, limited to the kidney
T1a	Tumour ≤4 cm in greatest dimension, limited to the kidney
T1b	Tumour >4 cm but ≤7 cm in greatest dimension, limited to the kidney
T2	Tumour >7 cm in greatest dimension, limited to the kidney
T2a	Tumour >7 cm but ≤10 cm in greatest dimension, limited to the kidney
T2b	Tumour >10 cm, limited to the kidney
T3	Tumour extends into major veins or perinephric tissues, but not into the ipsilateral adrenal gland and not beyond the fascia of Gerota
T3a	Tumour grossly extends into the renal vein or its segmental (muscle-containing) branches, or tumour invades perirenal and/or renal sinus fat but not beyond the fascia of Gerota
T3b	Tumour grossly extends into the vena cava below the diaphragm
T3c	Tumour grossly extends into the vena cava above the diaphragm or invades the wall of the vena cava
T4	Tumour invades beyond the fascia of Gerota (including contiguous extension into the ipsilateral adrenal gland)

Regional lymph node (N)

NX	Regional lymph nodes cannot be assessed
N0	No regional lymph node metastasis
N1	Metastasis in regional lymph node(s)

Distant metastasis (M)

M0	No distant metastasis
M1	Distant metastasis

RCC subtype, assessing for sarcomatoid features, microvascular invasion, tumour necrosis, and invasion of the collecting system [2].

Stage	T (tumour)	N (nodes)	M (metastasis)
I	T1	N0	M0
II	T2	N0	M0
III	T1–2	N1	M0
	T3	NX, 0–1	M0
IV	T4	Any N	M0
	Any T	Any N	M1

Treatment

The initial approach to treatment is guided by the staging of the disease, as well as the patient's age and comorbidities. Generally, stages I, II, and III are considered to be localized disease, whilst stage IV, which includes tumour invading beyond the fascia of Gerota or extending into the ipsilateral adrenal gland (T4) and metastatic disease (M1), is considered to be advanced disease.

In general, surgery is curative for most patients with localized disease, stages I, II, and III.

Surgery

Partial or radical nephrectomy is the treatment of choice for localized RCC [13]. Radical nephrectomy involves removal of the entire kidney, adrenal gland, Gerota's fascia, and regional lymph nodes.

Studies have shown that patients who have nephron-sparing surgery have a better quality of life with no difference in overall survival.

In a retrospective study, cytoreductive nephrectomy has been shown to prolong overall survival in selected patients with metastatic RCC who have received treatment with VEGF-targeted agents [14].

A less invasive option that could be considered is percutaneous ablation using thermal ablative techniques such as radiofrequency heat ablation and cryoablation. Patients with multiple comorbidities who may not tolerate surgical intervention, and who have tumours less than 3 cm in size, would be candidates for this approach [2].

Medical Therapy

Systemic therapy is initiated when unresectable disease, in the form of either metastatic or locally advanced disease, is present. In addition, systemic therapy is also considered in patients who have a recurrence after surgery. Immunotherapy and molecularly targeted therapy are the primary systemic modalities for the management of these two groups of patients. It must be borne in mind that the available evidence for use of these agents is predominantly for clear cell RCC.

Immunotherapy

There have been reports of spontaneous regression of the tumour and infrequent complete regression of metastatic disease with immunotherapy. It works by either boosting tumour antigenicity or host surveillance [2].

Immunotherapy consists of interleukin-2 (IL-2) or molecular targeted therapy such as nivolumab. Whilst high-dose IL-2 can induce durable, high-quality remissions in a minority of patients, it is associated with a significant risk of toxicity. The complications include hypotension, cardiac arrhythmias, metabolic acidosis, fever, nausea and vomiting, dyspnoea, oedema, oliguria and renal failure, neurotoxicity, and dermatological complications.

Nivolumab was approved by the US Food and Drug Administration for patients with advanced RCC whose disease has progressed following anti-angiogenic therapy. Nivolumab is a fully human immunoglobulin G4 monoclonal antibody that selectively inhibits programmed cell death-1 (PD-1) activity by binding to the PD-1 receptor. Diarrhoea or colitis is a common adverse effect, with other less common adverse effects being encephalitis, diabetes mellitus, adrenal insufficiency, dermatological toxicity, and hepatotoxicity [15].

Anti-Angiogenic and Targeted Therapy Targeting Vascular Endothelial Growth Factor and Transforming Growth Factor-Alpha Pathways

Drugs targeting angiogenesis are used for systemic treatment of patients who have metastatic RCC with a clear cell histological component [16].

Anti-angiogenic drugs targeting the VEGF pathway with proven benefit in RCC include tyrosine kinase (TK) inhibitors (sunitinib, sorafenib, pazopanib, and axinitib) and humanized monoclonal antibodies that bind VEGF (bevacizumab).

In patients who have failed VEGF-targeted therapy, everolimus, a mammalian target of rapamycin (mTOR) inhibitor, is recommended [17].

Sunitinib

Sunitinib is an oral TK inhibitor. It selectively inhibits platelet-derived growth factor receptor (PDGFR), vascular endothelial growth factor receptor (VEGFR), c-KIT, and FMS-like TK 3 (FLT-3), and has anti-tumour and anti-angiogenic activity [17].

Side effects of sunitinib include hypertension, vomiting, diarrhoea, and hand–foot syndrome.

Sorafenib

Sorafenib is a multiphase TK inhibitor which targets Raf-1 serine/threonine kinase, B-Raf, VEGFR-2, PDGFR, FLT-3, and c-KIT (16). Common side effects include hand–foot syndrome, dry and itchy skin, hypertension, diarrhoea, leucopenia, and hair thinning.

Pazopanib

Pazopanib is an oral angiogenesis inhibitor that targets VEGFR, PDGFR, and c-KIT (9). A phase 3 randomized controlled trial showed that both pazopanib and sunitinib had similar rates of progression-free survival [16].

Pazopanib is better tolerated than sunitinib, but can lead to significant liver function test derangement, weight loss, and change in hair colour [16].

Axitinib

Axitinib is a potent and selective second-generation inhibitor of VEGF receptors. It has been shown to have a longer progression-free survival when compared to sorafenib as second-line therapy.

Bevacizumab

VEGF is overexpressed in clear cell RCC tissue and may be the most important tumour angiogenic factor. In patients with good or intermediate risk, bevacizumab in combination with interferon alpha improves progression-free survival [17]. Adverse effects include severe or fatal haemorrhage (including haemoptysis, gastrointestinal bleeding, central nervous system haemorrhage or epistaxis), gastrointestinal perforation, and fistulas.

Mammalian Target of Rapamycin Inhibitors

Under normal conditions, mTOR regulates hypoxia-induced factors (HIF). Activation of mTOR by mutations causes disruption of tuberous sclerosis complex 1 and 2 genes (TSC1 and TSC2), which predisposes to the development of RCC. Temsirolimus and everolimus are selective inhibitors of mTOR and are used in patients with poor-risk metastatic RCC. Everolimus prolongs the progression-free survival in patients who have previously failed, or are intolerant of, VEGF-targeted therapy [17]. Adverse effects include gastrointestinal effects such as constipation or diarrhoea, hypercholesterolaemia, and bone marrow suppression.

Non-Clear Cell Carcinoma

Although sometimes VEGF inhibitors or mTOR inhibitors are used for these patients, there is no clear evidence supporting medical management of patients with non-clear cell RCC [17].

Additional Therapy

Chemotherapy and hormonal therapy have not shown any benefit for RCC so far. Although RCC is radio-resistant, there maybe some role for conventional and stereotactic radiation therapy to treat a single or limited number of metastases. The potential indications would include medically unfit patients, bilateral kidney malignancies, patients with chronic renal failure or patients with single functioning kidney [18].

References

1. Motzer, R.J., Hutson, T.E., Tomczak, P. et al. (2007). Sunitinib versus interferon alfa in metastatic renal-cell carcinoma. *N. Engl. J. Med.* 356 (2): 115–124.
2. Cohen, H.T. and McGovern, F.J. (2005). Renal cell carcinoma. *N. Eng. J. Med.* 353 (23): 2477–2490.
3. Cho, E., Curhan, G., Hankinson, S.E. et al. (2011). Prospective evaluation of analgesic use and risk of renal cell cancer. *Arch. Intern. Med.* 171 (16): 1487.
4. Marston Linehan, W., McClellan, M., Berton, Z. et al. (2003). The genetic basis of cancer of the kidney. *J. Urol.* 170: 2163–2172.
5. Rini, B., Campbell, S., and Escudier, B. (2009). Renal cell carcinoma. *Lancet* 373: 1119–1132.
6. Houweling, A.C., Gijezen, L.M., Jonker, M.A. et al. (2011). Renal cancer and pneumothorax risk in Birt–Hogg–Dubé syndrome: an analysis of 115 *FLCN* mutation carriers from 35 BHD families. *Br. J. Cancer* 105 (12): 1912–1919. https://doi.org/10.1038/bjc.2011.463.
7. Bodmer, D., Hurk, W., van Groningen, J.J.M. et al. (2002). Understanding familial and non familial renal cell cancer. *Hum. Mol. Genet.* 11 (20): 2489–2498.
8. Shetty, A. and Matrana, M.R. (2014). Renal medullary carcinoma: a case report and brief review of the literature. *Ochsner J.* 14 (2): 270–275.
9. Chao, D., Zisman, A., Pantuck, A. et al. (2002). Changing concepts in the management of renal oncocytoma. *Urology* 59 (5): 635–642.
10. Vera-Badillo, F.E., Conde, E., and Duran, I. (2012). Chromophobe renal cell carcinoma: a review of an uncommon entity. *Int. J. Urol.* 19 (10): 894–900. https://doi.org/10.1111/j.1442-2042.2012.03079.x.
11. Neuzillet, Y., Lechevallier, E., Andre, M. et al. (2004). Accuracy and clinical role of fine needle percutaneous biopsy with computerized tomography guidance of small (less than 4.0 cm) renal masses. *J. Urol.* 171 (5): 1802–1805. http://www.ncbi.nlm.nih.gov/pubmed/15076280.
12. Shannon, B.A., Cohen, R.J., de Bruto, H. et al. (2008). The value of preoperative needle core biopsy for diagnosing benign lesions among small, incidentally detected renal masses. *J. Urol.* 180 (4): 1257–1261. http://www.ncbi.nlm.nih.gov/pubmed/18707712.

13. Van Poppel, H., Da Pozzo, L., Albrecht, W. et al. (2011). A prospective, randomised EORTC inter-group phase 3 study comparing the oncologic outcome of elective nephron-sparing surgery and radical nephrectomy for low-stage renal cell carcinoma. *Eur. Urol.* 59 (4): 543.

14. Choueiri, T.K., Xie, W., Kollmannsberger, C. et al. (2011). The impact of cytoreductive nephrectomy on survival of patients with metastatic renal cell carcinoma receiving vascular endothelial growth factor targeted therapy. *J. Urol.* 185 (1): 60–66.

15. Xu J, Maher V.E , ZhangL, et al. (2017). FDA Approval Summary: Nivolumab in Advanced Renal Cell Carcinoma After Anti-Angiogenic Therapy and Exploratory Predictive Biomarker Analysis, The Oncologist. 22 (3): 311–317.

16. Motzer, R.J., Hutson, T.E., Cella, D. et al. (2013). Pazopanib versus sunitinib in metastatic renal-cell carcinoma. *N. Engl. J. Med.* 369 (8): 722–731.

17. Ljungberg, B., Bensalah, K., Canfield, S. et al. (2015). EAU guidelines on renal cell carcinoma: 2014 update. *Eur. Urol.* 67 (5): 913–924.

18. Kothari G., Louie A.V., Pryor D., et al. (2017). Stereotactic body radiotherapy for primary renal cell carcinoma and adrenal metastases. Chin Clin Oncol. 6 (2).

Questions and Answers

Questions

1. Regarding RCC, are the statements below true or false?
   a. Patients with RCC commonly present with haematuria, flank pain, and palpable abdominal mass
   b. More cancers are being detected due to widespread availability of imaging
   c. Obesity is a risk factor
   d. Papillary renal cell carcinoma is the most common type of RCC

2. A 65-year-old male smoker presents with painless haematuria. Urinalysis shows the presence of 2+ blood and no protein. Urine microscopy does not show any dysmorphic red cells. A renal tract USS shows the presence of a left cyst with an inhomogeneous appearance. His renal function is normal. What is the next most appropriate test?
   a. Renal biopsy
   b. Non-contrast CT/MRI
   c. CT with contrast
   d. PET scan

3. For localized RCC, the treatment of choice is:
   a. Partial/radical nephrectomy
   b. Chemotherapy
   c. Sunitinib
   d. Interferon alpha or high-dose interleukin 2

4. Patients with hereditary leiomyomatosis and renal cell carcinoma syndrome develop which histological type of RCC?
   a. Clear cell renal cell carcinoma
   b. Papillary cell renal cell carcinoma with type 1 histology
   c. Papillary cell renal cell carcinoma with type 2 histology
   d. Oncocytomas

5. Which of the following is not a tyrosine kinase inhibitor?
   a. Sunitinib
   b. Sorafenib
   c. Bevacizumab
   d. Axitinib

Answers

1. a. False. This presentation is now uncommon due to incidental detection of a renal mass via imaging.

   b. True. As discussed above, more renal cell cancers are being detected as incidental findings.

   c. True. Obesity, smoking, hypertension, and acquired cystic disease are risk factors.

   d. False. Clear cell carcinoma is the most common cause of RCC with an incidence of 80–90%. Papillary cell renal cell carcinoma has an incidence of 10–15%.

2. c. In most cases, CT can accurately diagnose RCC. It also provides information on the function and morphology of the kidneys, tumour extension, venous involvement, lymph node involvement, and surrounding structures. A change of more than 15 Hounsfield Units with contrast is significant and suggests a malignant process.

3. a. In localized RCC, partial/radical nephrectomy is the treatment of choice. RCC have minimal response to chemotherapy. Targeted treatments (tyrosine kinase inhibitors, VEGF-inhibitors) are used in treatment of naïve metastatic clear cell RCC. Interferon alpha and high-dose interleukin 2 were standard treatment prior to development of tyrosine kinase inhibitors.

4. c. This syndrome is associated with papillary cell carcinoma with type 2 histology. There are several inherited syndromes that are associated with RCCs. Some examples are: VHL disease, which is associated with clear cell RCC; hereditary papillary RCC, which is associated with papillary cell RCC with type 1 histology; and Birth Hogg Dube syndrome, which is associated with mixed chromophobe and oncocytomas.

5. c. Bevacizumab is a humanized monoclonal antibody that binds to VEGF. VEGF is overexpressed in clear cell renal cell carcinoma tissue and may be the most important tumour angiogenic factor. Sunitinib, sorafenib, and axinitib are tyrosine kinase inhibitors.

6

Acute Kidney Injury

Dipankar Bhattacharjee

Summary

- Acute kidney injury (AKI) is a clinical syndrome characterized by an abrupt decline in glomerular filtration rate (GFR), leading to the retention of toxic nitrogenous waste products such as urea and creatinine along with dysregulation of extracellular fluid volume
- In early AKI, the serum creatinine (SCr) may still be low despite the actual GFR being markedly reduced, as there may not have been sufficient time for the creatinine to accumulate
- Most cases of AKI are due to prerenal factors (>75%), whilst 10–15% are due to postrenal/obstructive causes and 5–10% are due to intrinsic renal causes
- AKI can be diagnosed by an acute increase in SCr as well as a decrease in urine output
- AKI secondary to contrast exposure is generally reversible and occurs within 24–48 hours of contrast administration, with improvement within 3–7 days
- Preventive strategy for contrast nephropathy consists of pre and post intravenous hydration with 0.9% saline or sodium bicarbonate and withdrawal of nephrotoxic drugs temporarily; N-acetylcysteine is no longer considered of value to prevent contrast nephropathy
- Atheroembolic renal disease causing renal failure usually occurs following manipulation of the aorta or other large arteries during angiography (commonest cause), angioplasty or cardiovascular surgery
- Gentamicin nephrotoxicity usually manifests as non-oliguric AKI, usually 5–10 days after exposure, and may be associated with hypokalaemia and hypomagnesaemia
- AKI can occur in patients who have rhabdomyolysis and less commonly in patients with haemolysis due to haem pigment nephropathy

Acute kidney injury (AKI) is a clinical syndrome characterized by an abrupt decline in glomerular filtration rate (GFR), leading to the retention of toxic nitrogenous waste products such as urea and creatinine, along with dysregulation of extracellular fluid volume.

The term AKI has evolved from what was previously known as acute renal failure (ARF) to reflect the fact that even small decrements in renal function, though not enough to cause overt organ failure, can be a predictor of adverse outcome if not detected and corrected in time. AKI can in fact be considered as a spectrum from 'increased risk' through 'damage' and 'low GFR' ending in 'ESRD' (end-stage renal disease) if unresolved. It is important to note that GFR does not decline in early stages of 'increased risk' or 'damage'. As early AKI is often a silent process, a high index of suspicion is necessary for diagnosis.

Lecture Notes Nephrology: A Comprehensive Guide to Renal Medicine, First Edition. Edited by Surjit Tarafdar.
© 2020 John Wiley & Sons Ltd. Published 2020 by John Wiley & Sons Ltd.

In early AKI, the serum creatinine (SCr) may still be low despite the actual GFR being markedly reduced, as there may not have been sufficient time for the creatinine to accumulate [1]. When the SCr is rising, estimates of GFR based on creatinine values will often overestimate the true GFR; just as GFR might be underestimated during the recovery phase of AKI, when the SCr is declining.

It is important to be aware that although AKI is defined by a reduction in GFR, the aetiology most of the time, as we shall discuss, involves prerenal or tubular factors rather than true glomerular defect.

Definition of Acute Kidney Injury

Until early 2000, there were 35 definitions of ARF in the literature [2]. An initial attempt to define AKI was made with the RIFLE criteria [3], which used the twin indicators of increment in SCr by >50% over <7 days or urine output (UO) of <0.5 ml/kg/h for >6 hours. Subsequently, the AKIN group modified the RIFLE criteria to propose an AKI definition and staging [4]. Following this, K-DIGO borrowed from both RIFLE and AKIN criteria and proposed the following definition of AKI:

Increase in SCr by >0.3 mg/dl (26.5 μmol/l) within 48 hours

or:

Increase in SCr by >50% within the prior 7 days

or:

UO <0.5 ml/kg/h for 6 hours

The reason for shifting to a relatively small SCr increment of 0.3 mg (26.5 μmol/l) to define AKI came from research indicating that even such a small rise can result in adverse outcomes [5, 6]. Although UO can vary widely in AKI depending on the integrity of renal tubules and fluid intake, it is still very useful early on when SCr has not started to rise; falling UO may be the only indicator of an impending AKI at that early stage [7].

Staging of Acute Kidney Injury

The mortality and length of hospital stay are directly proportional to the increasing stage of AKI [8–11]. K-DIGO AKI staging is described in Table 6.1.

Classification of Acute Kidney Injury as per the Anatomical Site of Pathology

Prerenal: Factors That Affect Renal Perfusion

1. Intravascular volume depletion:
   - Diarrhoea and vomiting, intraoperative bleed, excessive sweating, burns and excessive diuresis.
2. Vascular tone:
   - Vasodilatation from e.g. sepsis or drugs e.g. anaesthetic agents
   - Renal vasoconstriction like in Hepatorenal syndrome
3. Cardiac pump failure: e.g. MI, Arrhythmias, tamponade or heart failure
4. Drugs potentiating pre-renal AKI include Angiotensin converting enzyme inhibitors (ACEI), angiotensin receptor blockers (ARB), diuretics and nonsteroidal anti-inflammatory drugs (NSAID)

Table 6.1 Staging of AKI is based on two criteria: rise in serum creatinine (SCr) from baseline or a falling urine output (UO), whichever score is higher. A glomerular filtration rate calculation which relies on steady-state SCr is not reliable in acute kidney injury (AKI), as SCr tends to fluctuate in AKI

Stage	SCr criteria	UO criteria
1	Increase ≥26.5 μmol/l (0.3 mg/dl) within 48 h or increase ≥1.5–1.9 × reference SCr within 7 days	<0.5 ml/kg/h for >6 consecutive h
2	Increase ≥2–2.9 × reference SCr within 7 days	<0.5 ml/kg/h for >12 h
3	Increase ≥3 × reference SCr or increase ≥354 μmol/l within 7 days or commenced on renal replacement therapy irrespective of stage	<0.3 ml/kg/h for >24 h or anuria for 12 h

Renal: Intrinsic Renal Pathology

1. Glomerular: glomerulonephritis (GN); thrombotic microangiopathies, including thrombotic thrombocytopenic purpura/haemolytic uremic syndrome (TTP/HUS); vasculitis, e.g. antineutrophil cytoplasmic antibody (ANCA)-positive vasculitis.
2. Tubulointerstitial: acute tubular necrosis (ATN) from prolonged uncorrected hypoperfusion or nephrotoxins, acute interstitial nephritis (AIN) usually due to drugs such as penicillins, cephalosporins, PPIs, frusemide etc.
3. Intratubular obstruction: cast nephropathy (seen in myeloma), urate nephropathy, crystals due to drugs and toxins (acyclovir, sulphonamide, methotrexate, protease inhibitors, ethylene glycol).
4. Atheroembolic renal disease.

Postrenal: Any Cause of Obstruction to Urine Flow Downstream of Kidneys

1. Ureteric obstruction (e.g. bilateral stones), bladder neck or urethral obstruction, e.g. by stone, clot or more commonly enlarged prostate.
2. Ureteric obstruction of single functioning kidney.

Considerations

It is important to remember that more than 75% of all cases of AKI are due to prerenal factors, where the kidney is an innocent bystander. Prolonged and/or severe renal ischaemia due to any cause can lead to ATN. This is characterized by histological changes of necrosis with denudation of the tubular epithelium and occlusion of the tubular lumen by casts and cell debris.

About 10–15% of AKI are postrenal and only about 5–10% are due to an intrinsic renal cause; that is, pathology in the renal parenchyma itself. One must remember, though, that there may be multiple and various combinations of these factors (prerenal, renal or postrenal) in the same patient. For example, a patient being treated for heart failure might have prerenal AKI due to vigorous diuresis along with AKI secondary to intrinsic renal pathology due to AIN from frusemide.

A study in Madrid that evaluated all 748 cases of AKI in 13 tertiary-level hospitals concluded that the following were the causes of AKI:

- ATN – 45%
- Prerenal disease – 21%
- Acute superimposed on chronic kidney disease (CKD) – 13% (mostly due to ATN and prerenal disease)
- Urinary tract obstruction – 10% (most often older men with prostatic disease)
- GN or vasculitis – 4%
- AIN – 2%
- Atheroembolic renal disease – 1%

Pathophysiology

To achieve a GFR of 125 ml/min, the kidneys receive about 25% of the cardiac output, amounting to 1.1 l/min in a 70 kg adult male. Under adverse conditions, a constant renal blood flow (RBF) and perfusion are maintained by renal auto-regulation through adjustment of the vasomotor tone of afferent and efferent renal arterioles. This auto-regulation works across a wide range of mean arterial pressure (MAP), which is the tissue perfusion pressure, but fails when MAP is below 70 mmHg, as illustrated in Figure 6.1.

Therefore, it is important to maintain a MAP of at least 70 mmHg during the management of prerenal AKI. Otherwise renal tubules, which have high oxygen requirement (due to their high N^+-K^+-ATPase activity), suffer ischaemic injury resulting in ATN

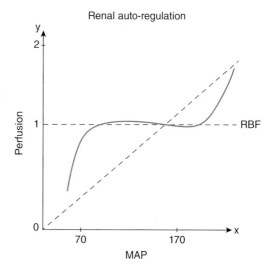

Figure 6.1 The relationship between mean arterial pressure (MAP) and renal blood flow (RBF) is not linear, which ensures a steady RBF over a wide range of blood pressures between a MAP of 70–170 mmHg, as shown by the curved line. However, this protective auto-regulation fails when MAP drops below 70 mmHg – RBF then starts to fall precipitously ushering in renal injury.

Table 6.2 Causes of acute tubular necrosis

Renal ischaemia	All causes of prerenal acute kidney injury if uncorrected, e.g. sepsis, diarrhoea, and vomiting, excessive diuresis, burns, etc.
Nephrotoxins	Aminoglycosides, haem pigment, radio-contrast media, foscarnet, cidofovir, tenofovir, mannitol

(see Table 6.2). Although renal tubules can regenerate and therefore ATN is reversible, it may take up to six weeks for recovery, sometimes leading patients to undergo dialysis treatment in the interim with its associated complications, cost and even mortality. Apart from severe and/or uncorrected prerenal causes, ATN can also occur with direct nephrotoxic injuries, for instance from radio-contrast dye, aminoglycosides or myoglobin pigment exposure.

Risk Factors

Although a consensus is still evolving, the following are generally agreed as risk factors for developing AKI [6]:

- Age >75 years
- CKD
- Diabetes mellitus
- Heart failure
- Nephrotoxic medication, e.g. non-steroidal anti-inflammatory drugs (NSAIDs), ACE inhibitors (ACEI) or angiotensin receptor blockers (ARB), aminoglycosides, e.g. gentamicin
- Liver disease
- Peripheral vascular disease

History Taking

Good history taking is very important in unearthing the presence of risk factors or nephrotoxin exposure, and also helps in evolving a management strategy. It is important to look back in the history or hospital notes for any events that could have a temporal relationship to the rise in SCr, such as recent radio-contrast exposure, diarrhoea, a period of hypotension or prolonged vomiting in the immediately preceding days. The history may also point

to an obstructive cause if lower urinary or prostatic symptoms are present.

Examination

Besides good general and systemic examination, the focus should to be look for the following findings which may indicate the cause:

1. Volume status is very important, as:
   - Hypovolaemia indicates prerenal AKI, necessitating quick correction of volume deficit. Usual indicators of hypovolaemia are hypotension or postural hypotension, tachycardia, reduced skin turgor, low jugular venous pressure and rapid weight loss.
   - Hypervolaemia with cardiac failure may point to cardio-renal syndrome, whereas ascites and liver stigmata may indicate hepato-renal syndrome.
2. Palpable bladder indicates obstructive uropathy from bladder neck pathology.
3. Skin rash may indicate renal vasculitis or allergic interstitial nephritis.

Investigation and Work-Up

Firstly, one needs to detect AKI as per the definition in the right clinical context; that is, a rise of 0.3 mg (26.5 μmol/l) of SCr from baseline or the required degree of oliguria. One must be aware, though, that it may take up to 48 hours for SCr to rise after injury – the 'silent period' (Figure 6.2), when low UO may be the only indicator (therefore included in the definition). The effort is on to find new biomarkers for early renal injury; serum cystatin C and urinary neutrophil gelatinase-associated lipocalin (NGAL) have been trialled for this purpose (Figure 6.3; see subsequent discussion).

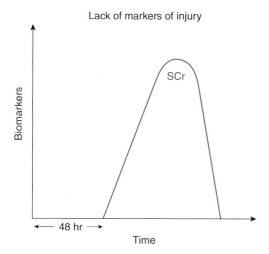

Figure 6.2 During the first 48 hours of renal injury, there is no biomarker (comparable to the early rise of troponin in acute coronary syndrome) that helps in early diagnosis. Serum creatinine (SCr) usually starts to rise after 48 hours (silent period) and falls again to baseline if there is full renal recovery.

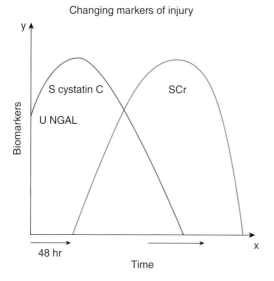

Figure 6.3 Serum cystatin C and urinary neutrophil gelatinase-associated lipocalin (U NGAL) may be helpful in diagnosing acute kidney injury in the first 48 hours of renal injury, as both are detectable in this early phase. SCr: serum creatinine.

The following investigations are advised in AKI:

- *Urine dipstick*: an extremely useful bedside investigation which gives highly valuable information. Presence of haematuria and proteinuria (with no

suspicion of urinary infection, tumour or stones), point towards an intrinsic renal cause of AKI like GN or renal vasculitis, which necessitates nephrology referral. A completely negative urine dipstick is a strong indicator of the absence of glomerular disease or vasculitis causing AKI.

- *Full blood count* (*FBC*): disproportionate anaemia may indicate underlying myeloma or microangiopathic haemolytic anaemia, for example HUS or TTP. If anaemia is associated with thrombocytopenia, the clinician should look for features of microangiopathic haemolysis; fragmented red blood cells (RBCs) in blood film. Leucocytosis or neutrophilia may indicate underlying sepsis.
- *C-reactive protein* (*CRP*): if high, suggests sepsis as a cause or contributor.
- *Urea, creatinine and electrolytes*: for diagnosis and monitoring the progress of AKI. Hyperkalaemia requires urgent medical therapy and/or dialysis, and if disproportionately high might be an indicator of cell lysis, suggesting rhabdomyolysis or tumour lysis syndrome.
- *Liver function tests* (*LFT*): if abnormal may indicate liver disease and the possibility of hepato-renal syndrome.
- *Coagulation profile*: if abnormal may indicate sepsis or thrombotic microangiopathy. A normal coagulation profile is a prerequisite for renal biopsy or central line insertion for dialysis.
- *Venous or arterial blood gas*: for assessing acid–base status, which may indicate a need for dialysis for refractory and severe metabolic acidosis.
- *Renal ultrasonography* (*USG*): unless the clinical suspicion of prerenal AKI is very high, renal USG is almost always done in the Emergency Department to rule out an obstructive cause. AKI in the inpatient setting is generally initially managed with fluid resuscitation and avoidance of nephrotoxic medications, and renal USG is done if no improvement is seen within the first 24 hours.

However, it is important to remember that obstruction may not be obvious in presence of dehydration and a repeat US may be necessary after fluid resuscitation. Cause of obstruction that can be missed by USG is Retroperitoneal fibrosis which requires a CT scan for diagnosis. Bilateral contracted kidneys on USG would signify underlying chronic kidney disease. Also, USG helps to ensure patient has two normal size kidneys which is generally a pre-requisite for performing a safe renal biopsy.

In the event of AKI and blood on the urinary dipstick with no evidence of urinary tract infection, stones or anatomical lesions on USG, urine should be sent to check for dysmorphic RBCs and RBC casts to investigate for GN.

When there is a suspicion of GN, the following additional investigations should be undertaken:

- Serum complements (low in infection related nephritis, lupus nephritis, mesangio-capillary glomerulonephritis, nephritis associated with endocarditis and cryoglobulinaemia).
- Blood and urinary cultures in case of suspicion of infection related GN and anti-streptococcal antibodies when there is a history of preceding pharyngitis or impetigo; anti-streptolysin, anti-hyaluronidase, anti-streptokinase, and anti-DNAse B antibodies.
- Anti-nuclear antibody (ANA), extractable nuclear antigen antibodies (ENA) and double-stranded DNA (ds-DNA) panels to exclude lupus nephritis.
- Hepatitis screen, to exclude cryoglobulinemic nephritis and mesangio-capillary GN.
- ANCA, to rule out vasculitis, for example PR3 (ANCA-positive granulomatosis with polyangiitis) and MPO (ANCA-positive microscopic polyangiitis).
- Anti-glomerular basement membrane (GBM) antibody to rule out Goodpasture's syndrome.
- Serum paraprotein, serum free light chains and urinary Bence-Jones protein if myeloma is suspected, for instance in patient with AKI and hypercalcaemia, anaemia, and/or bone pain/lesions.

Management

Immediate Management

- Fluid resuscitation to correct prerenal factors like hypovalaemia or sepsis-induced vasodilatory hypovolaemia.
- Monitoring of UO, fluid balance chart and daily weight to assess volume status.
- Withdrawal of all nephrotoxic and non-essential medications, such as ACE inhibitors, ARBs, diuretics, NSAIDS, aminoglycosides, and sometimes drugs that can cause interstitial nephritis. Metformin is in itself not nephrotoxic, but as it is renally cleared, it should be held to safeguard against the possibility of lactic acidosis given that many of these patients are acidotic. Dose adjustment of drugs according to changing renal function is required to avoid accumulation with resultant toxicity.
- Urinary catheter is required if bladder is palpable, if a large residual is found on bedside bladder scan or

if close monitoring is required and the patient might not be able to collect urine diligently.
- Urgent appropriate antibiotic treatment for suspected sepsis.
- Urgent management of hyperkalaemia: medical management with insulin/dextrose, salbutamol, and resonium; consider dialysis if patient is significantly hyperkalaemic (e.g. >6.5 mmol/l), particularly with electrocardiogram (ECG) changes and/or oliguanuric despite fluid resuscitation (urine is the main route of potassium excretion) and not responding to medical management.

The following are indications for referral to a nephrologist:

- Persistent oliguria and/or rising SCr despite supportive therapy and AKI in the context of poisoning
- Active urinary sediments; that is, haematuria and/or proteinuria.
- Suspected myeloma, for example accompanying hypercalcaemia and/or anaemia, presence of paraprotein or Bence–Jones protein.
- Suspected thrombotic microangiopathy; that is, presence of haemolysis or low platelet counts.
- Stage 3 AKI.
- Complications refractory to medical treatment, where dialysis is indicated:

  a) Hyperkalaemia (K^+ >6.5) with ECG changes
  b) Pulmonary oedema
  c) Acidosis (pH <7.15)
  d) Uremic encephalopathy
  e) Uremic pericarditis

If intrinsic renal disease is not suspected and prerenal factors are corrected, the usual course is for renal function to improve. The emphasis then shifts to maintaining an appropriate fluid balance, monitoring electrolytes and surveillance for any complications:

- Daily fluid balance chart.
- Daily weight.
- Daily monitoring of electrolytes, including bicarbonate.
- Review of the need for keeping the central lines, dialysis catheters or urinary catheters, since they increase infection risk.

Pharmacological Agents

There is no role for dopamine as a number of studies have not shown any benefit in recovery or outcomes [12]. Similarly, frusemide is not of much value in AKI, although theoretically it switches off the tubular ATPase pump and is supposed to reduce energy

AKI Management

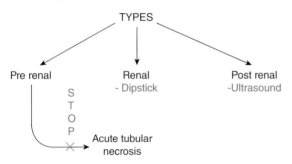

TYPES

Pre renal   Renal   Post renal
    - Dipstick   -Ultrasound

S T O P

Acute tubular necrosis

Figure 6.4 Most acute kidney injuries (AKIs) are due to prerenal factors and effort should be made to prevent progression to acute tubular necrosis. A renal cause of AKI is generally picked up by a simple urine dipstick test with active sediments, in contrast to prerenal AKI where the urine dipstick is bland. Postrenal causes usually need a renal ultrasound for diagnosis.

requirement and renal workload. It does not enhance renal recovery and does not reduce dialysis requirement or mortality either [13]. Frusemide may have a role in the treatment of fluid overload or pulmonary oedema associated with AKI.

Recovery Phase

This is ushered in by an increase in UO, improving biochemistry and sense of well-being. Sometimes patients go into a prolonged polyuric phase lasting up to weeks after ATN. This is because recovery of absorptive tubular function lags and can be a slow process. It is important at this stage to keep up with polyuric volume loss with sufficient fluid intake so that they do not get a second hit of AKI from dehydration. Electrolyte imbalance and new infections need to be watched closely.

Summary of Acute Kidney Injury Management

This can be summarized by the acronym **STOP**, which denotes early treatment of **S**epsis and volume correction, withdrawal of **T**oxic medications, excluding an **O**bstruction by ultrasound and seeking renal **P**arenchymal disease through a urine dipstick. As the clear majority of AKIs are due to prerenal factors, the expectation is that this will prevent progression to ATN (Figure 6.4).

It is now realized that not all patients with AKI will recover renal function to the previous baseline and some may progress to CKD in the long term. Also, the slope of GFR decline may worsen in pre-existing CKD patients who have an episode of AKI [14].

Therefore, there is an argument for following up AKI patients at least for some time to judge the GFR behaviour and then decide on the need for further follow-up and its frequency. One also needs to review the reintroduction of withdrawn medications or their

alternatives after an appropriate interval. Therefore, it is highly recommended that the discharge letter for an AKI patient from hospital should include advice on these matters [7, 15].

Oliguric versus Non-oliguric Acute Kidney Injury

The majority of AKI patients are oliguric. However, AKI from tubulo-toxic insults (e.g. aminoglycoside or chemotherapeutic agents like cisplatin) affects tubular absorption and therefore, even though a reduced amount of plasma is filtered in glomeruli, the major share of it appears in urine, giving rise to normal volume urine. There is some evidence that non-oliguric renal failure may indicate less severe disease [16]. Non-oliguric AKI has slightly better outcomes than oliguric AKI partly because it is easier to maintain fluid balance and consequently, there is less chance of pulmonary oedema and need for dialysis [17]. Biochemical clearance of waste products does not vary much between the two categories.

Specific Categories of Acute Kidney Injury

Contrast-Induced Acute Kidney Injury

Contrast nephropathy (contrast-induced or CI-AKI) is a generally reversible form of AKI that occurs soon after the administration of radio-contrast media.

CI-AKI typically occurs in patients with underlying renal impairment and is rarely seen in those with normal renal function. It may occur with both intravenous and intra-arterial contrast administration, but not oral contrast. Also, the presence of background risk factors like dehydration, diabetes, congestive cardiac failure (CCF), myeloma, and medications like NSAIDs, ACE inhibitors and ARBs enhance the risk further. A high-osmolar contrast is more nephrotoxic than a low-osmolar or iso-osmolar contrast.

Pathogenesis involves both renal medullary hypoxia due to vasoconstriction and direct tubular injury leading to ATN. However, unlike other types of ATN, contrast nephropathy is characterized by relatively rapid onset as well as recovery of renal function. AKI usually occurs within 24–48 hours of contrast administration and the creatinine tends to improve within 3–7 days.

The prevention strategy comprises of avoiding or delaying contrast imaging if possible, considering other modes of non-contrast imaging, pre and post intravenous hydration with 0.9% saline or sodium bicarbonate [18] and withdrawal of nephrotoxic drugs temporarily. Monitoring of renal function for up to one week post-contrast exposure is recommended. Administration of N-acetylcysteine is no longer considered of value to prevent contrast nephropathy.

Atheroembolic Renal Disease

Older patients with diffuse erosive atherosclerosis are susceptible to atheroembolic renal disease. Cholesterol crystal embolization to the kidneys is usually seen following manipulation of the aorta or other large arteries during angiography (commonest cause), angioplasty or cardiovascular surgery. Whilst the typical presentation is subacute kidney injury observed several weeks or more after a possible inciting event, at times patients present in AKI as early as one to two weeks after the event, suggesting massive embolization.

Cholesterol embolization to other organs may cause associated cyanosis or discrete gangrenous lesions in the toes with intact peripheral pulses (blue toes), livedo reticularis, and focal neurological deficits. Ophthalmological examination may reveal orange plaques in the retinal arterioles called Hollenhorst plaques.

Apart from worsening kidney function, patients may have eosinophilia, eosinophiluria, and hypocomplementaemia. There is no specific therapy for atheroembolic renal disease and treatment is supportive. All patients should be aggressively treated for secondary prevention of cardiovascular disease including introduction of statins and aspirin, avoidance of smoking and adequate control of hypertension and diabetes.

Gentamicin

Aminoglycosides are freely filtered across the glomerulus and partially taken up by the proximal tubular cells (PTC). The cationic charges on aminoglycosides (NH_4^+) cause them to bind to the abundant anionic charges on the cell membranes of the PTC. The drug accumulates in the PTC lysosomes and can reach levels 100–1000 times that in the serum. Intracellular aminoglycosides lead to defective protein synthesis and mitochondrial dysfunction, causing cellular damage in the PTC.

Non-oliguric AKI usually occurs 5–10 days after treatment with gentamicin. Involvement of the distal tubular cells may lead to hypokalaemia and hypomagnesaemia.

Gentamicin levels should be monitored to minimize nephrotoxicity and, where possible, a once-daily dosage schedule should be used, as it leads to less intracellular accumulation in the PTC.

Other Nephrotoxins Causing Acute Kidney Injury

Apart from ACE inhibitors and ARBs, which can cause AKI in the setting of reduced renal perfusion due to impaired vasoconstriction of the efferent arteriole, some of the other drugs known to potentiate AKI are discussed in the following sections.

Non-steroidal Anti-inflammatory Drugs

Prostaglandins help to maintain RBF by causing afferent arteriole vasodilatation. NSAID-mediated inhibition of cyclo-oxygenase enzymes with subsequent reduction in prostaglandin synthesis leads to inhibition of this prostaglandin-mediated afferent vasodilatation.

Although NSAIDs are unlikely to cause AKI in healthy individuals, they can be nephrotoxic in the following scenarios:

- Elderly patient with atherosclerotic disease
- Background of CKD
- State of renal hypoperfusion, e.g. hypotension, sepsis, use of diuretics, etc.
- Sodium-avid states, e.g. CCF, cirrhosis, and nephrotic syndrome

Calcineurin Inhibitors: Cyclosporine and Tacrolimus

Calcineurin inhibitors (CNIs) can cause AKI by causing renal vasoconstriction mediated by endothelin. This is usually reversible on dose reduction. Repeated and persistent renal ischaemia due to CNIs may lead to chronic interstitial fibrosis marked by a striped pattern.

CNIs may also rarely cause thrombotic microangiopathy, leading to an HUS-like clinical picture.

Amphotericin

Amphotericin is postulated to cause AKI by leading to both renal vasoconstriction and tubular toxicity. The risk of nephrotoxicity can be reduced by using lower doses of amphotericin and by avoiding concurrent therapy with other nephrotoxins. The incidence and severity of nephrotoxicity can also be minimized by administering amphotericin B in lipid-based formulations.

Crystal-Induced Acute Kidney Injury

Crystal-induced AKI is caused by the intratubular precipitation of crystals leading to tubular obstruction. The condition is most commonly seen because of acute uric acid nephropathy or following the administration of following drugs and toxins:

- Acyclovir
- Sulphonamide antibiotics
- Ethylene glycol (found in anti-freeze)
- Methotrexate
- Protease inhibitors

Urinalysis often reveals haematuria, pyuria, and crystalluria. Treatment consists of volume repletion with isotonic saline and administration of loop diuretic to wash out the obstructing crystals.

Haem Pigment Nephropathy

Myoglobin is released from muscle in patients with rhabdomyolysis, whilst haemoglobin is released from haemolysed RBCs in those with severe haemolysis. Both myoglobin and haemoglobin are filtered by the glomerulus into the urinary space, where they degrade and release haem pigment.

Haem can lead to AKI by three processes:

- Tubular obstruction, possibly in association with uric acid

- Direct proximal tubular cell injury
- Vasoconstriction leading to medullary hypoxia

In addition, patients with rhabdomyolysis are prone to volume depletion due to the sequestration of large amounts of fluid in the injured muscle.

New Horizons in Acute Kidney Injury

In the diagnostic field, two molecules (namely, serum cystatin C and urinary NGAL) are showing promise as early markers of renal injury (Figure 6.3).

Cystatin C is a low molecular weight protein (approx 13 kDa) which is filtered by the kidney serum level rises early in renal injury. In various studies, including a meta-analysis, it is found to be a useful early marker in AKI [19] and superior to SCr [20].

NGAL is a small polypeptide (25 kDa). It is isolated from secondary granules of human neutrophils and is readily detected in the urine. NGAL was detectable in the urine in the very first UO after ischaemia in both mouse and rat models of ARF. The appearance of NGAL usually precedes the appearance of other urinary markers and is related to the degree and duration of renal ischaemia. Various studies indicate that NGAL may represent a promising early, non-invasive, and sensitive urinary biomarker for prediction and monitoring of ischaemic and nephrotoxic renal injury [21]. NGAL seems to be emerging as a valuable troponin-like biomarker for the prediction of clinical outcomes in AKI [22].

References

1. Murray, P.T., Devarajan, P., Levey, A.S. et al. (2008). A framework and key research questions in AKI diagnosis and staging in different environments. *Clin. J. Am. Soc. Nephrol.* 3: 864–868.
2. Kellum, J.A., Levin, N., Bouman, C. et al. (2002). Developing a consensus classification system for acute renal failure. *Curr. Opin. Crit. Care* 8: 509–514.
3. Bellomo, R., Ronco, C., Kellum, J.A. et al. (2004). Acute renal failure-definition, outcome measures, animal models, fluid therapy and information technology needs: the Second International Consensus Conference of the Acute Dialysis Quality Initiative (ADQI) Group. *Crit. Care* 8: R204–R212.

4. Mehta, R.L., Kellum, J.A., Shah, S.V. et al. (2007). Acute kidney injury network: report of an initiative to improve outcomes in acute kidney injury. *Crit. Care* 11: R31.

5. Chertow, G.M., Burdik, E., Honour, M. et al. (2005). Acute kidney injury, mortality, length of stay, and costs in hospitalized patients. *J. Am. Soc. Nephrol.* 16 (11): 3365–3370.

6. Lewington, A. and Kanagasundaram, S. (2011). *Acute Kidney Injury Guidelines*. UK: Renal Association.

7. Kellum, J.A., Sileanu, F.E., Murugan, R. et al. (2015). Classifying AKI by urine output versus serum creatinine level. *J. Am. Soc. Nephrol.* 26 (9): 2231–2238. https://doi.org/10.1681/ASN.2014070724.

8. Hoste, E.A., Clermont, G., Kersten, A. et al. (2006). RIFLE criteria for acute kidney injury are associated with hospital mortality in critically ill patients: a cohort analysis. *Crit. Care* 10 (3): R73. Epub 2006 May 12.

9. Thakar, C.V., Christianson, A., Freyberg, R. et al. (2009). Incidence and outcomes of acute kidney injury in intensive care units: a veterans administration study. *Crit. Care Med.* 37 (9): 2552–2558.

10. Uchino, S., Bellomo, R., Goldsmith, D. et al. (2006). An assessment of the RIFLE criteria for acute renal failure in hospitalized patients. *Crit. Care Med.* 34 (7): 1913–1917.

11. Ostermann, M., Chang, R., Riyadh ICU programme user group et al. (2008). Correlation between the AKI classification and outcome. *Crit. Care* 12 (6): R144.

12. Friedrich, J.O., Adhikari, N., and Herridge, M.S. (2005). Meta-analysis: low-dose dopamine increases urine output but does not prevent renal dysfunction or death. *Ann. Intern. Med.* 142: 510–524.

13. Ho, K.M. and Sheridan, D.J. (2006). Meta-analysis of frusemide to prevent or treat acute renal failure. *BMJ* 333 (7565): 420–425.

14. Cerda, J., Lameire, N., Eggers, P. et al. (2008). Epidemiology of acute kidney injury. *Clin. J. Am. Soc. Nephrol.* 3 (3): 881–886.

15. NICE Guidelines [CG169] (2013). *Acute Kidney Injury: Prevention, Detection and Management*. National Institute for Health and Care Excellence.

16. Avila, M.O., Zanetta, D.M., Abdulkader, R.C. et al. (2009). Urine volume in acute kidney injury: how much is enough? *Ren. Fail.* 31: 884.

17. Oh, J., Shin, D.H., Lee, M.J. et al. (2013). Urine output is associated with prognosis in patients with acute kidney injury requiring continuous renal replacement therapy. *J. Crit. Care* 28: 379.

18. Hoste, E.A., De Waele, J.J., Gevaert, S.A. et al. (2010). Sodium bicarbonate for prevention of contrast-induced acute kidney injury: a systematic review and meta-analysis. *Nephrol. Dial. Transplant.* 25 (3): 747–758.

19. Herget-Rosenthal, S., Marggraf, G., Husing, J. et al. (2004). Early detection of acute renal failure by serum cystatin C. *Kidney Int.* 66: 1115–1122.

20. Dharnidharka, V.R., Kwon, C., and Stevens, G. (2002). Serum cystatin C is superior to serum creatinine as a marker of kidney function: a meta-analysis. *Am. J. Kidney Dis.* 40 (2): 221–226.

21. Mishra, J., Ma, Q., Prada, A. et al. (2003). Identification of neutrophil gelatinase-associated lipocalin as a novel early urinary biomarker for ischemic renal injury. *J. Am. Soc. Nephrol.* 14: 2534–2543.

22. Devarajan, P. (2010). Neutrophil gelatinase-associated lipocalin: a promising biomarker for human acute kidney injury. *Biomark. Med* 4 (2): 265–280.

Questions and Answers

Questions

1. An 86-year-old man with a history of hypertension had a road traffic accident leading to multiple fractures and a crush injury. He underwent prolonged surgery and required multiple blood transfusions. His peri-operative BP was 100/60 mmHg. He was oliguric postoperatively. His postoperative serum creatinine (SCr) was 200 μmol/l (Ref range 60–110 μmol/l), potassium was 6.8 mmol/l (Ref range 3.2–5 mmol/l), phosphate was 4 mmol/l (Ref range 0.75–1.5 mmol/l), and urinalysis showed positive dipstick for blood.

A. Which of the following statement is true?
   a. He has AKI
   b. He has CKD
   c. He has AKI on CKD
   d. Not certain

B. What are causative factors if it is AKI?
   a. AKI is from sepsis
   b. AKI is from prerenal factors like volume loss and hypotension
   c. Rhabdomyolysis
   d. b and c.

2. A. A 60 year-old man had an emergency repair of his supra-renal abdominal aortic aneurysm (AAA). His preoperative SCr was 125 μmol/l. He had a CT aortogram prior to surgery which showed aortic dissection. He had prolonged peri-operative hypotension. He was given 8 units of blood transfusion and 3 l of normal saline. He was given diclofenac postoperatively to control pain. He developed oliguria and pulmonary oedema 48 hours postoperatively and SCr rose to 305 μmol/l. Which of the following is not a factor in his AKI?
   a. Prolonged hypotension
   b. Non-steroidal anti-inflammatory drug
   c. Radio-contrast dye
   d. Supra-renal clamping of aorta
   e. Urinary obstruction

B. What is the stage of AKI?
   a. Stage I
   b. Stage 2
   c. Stage 3

C. His urinary spot sodium (Na) is 100 mmol/l. Does he have?
   a. Pre-renal AKI
   b. ATN
   c. Acute interstitial nephritis

D. What would be the correct management?
   a. Continue with cautious fluid challenge
   b. Continue IV fluid at UO+ 30 ml/h
   c. Stop IV fluid
   d. Arrange for dialysis treatment
   e. Try a Frusemide infusion

3. Dialysis as treatment in AKI is indicated in the following except:
   a. Pulmonary oedema
   b. Rising level of creatinine >500 μmol/l
   c. Metabolic acidosis
   d. Hyperkalaemia resistant to medical treatment
   e. Pericarditis presumed to be uremic

4. A 64-year-old man with history of hypertension, hypercholesterolaemia, and type 2 diabetes mellitus had a bare metal stent placement for a silent MI and was discharged on aspirin in addition to his usual medications. He was hemodynamically stable throughout the procedure and during his hospital stay. Three weeks later, he presented to the GP with gangrenous lesions on the tips of his toes, and investigation revealed a serum creatinine of 186 μmol/l. His serum creatinine prior to the procedure was normal. What is the likely cause of his acute kidney injury?
   a. Allergic interstitial nephritis (AIN)
   b. ATN
   c. Postrenal AKI
   d. Contrast nephropathy
   e. Atheroembolic disease

Answers

1. A. d) Not certain. As baseline SCr is not given, it is difficult to be certain. However, it is very likely that he has an element of AKI with such acute illness.

   B. d) There is no indication of sepsis here and rhabdomyolysis is a distinct possibility given the history of trauma and crush injury. Hyperkalaemia and hyperphosphataemia are often observed in rhabdomyolysis due to release of potassium and phosphorus from damaged muscle cells.

2. A. e) Urinary obstruction would have been picked up on CT. All other factors have probably contributed to his renal dysfunction.

   B. b) Stage 2 as SCr is two to three times of the baseline SCr.

   C. b) ATN is likely as high urinary spot Na signifies loss of tubular absorptive function. Acute interstitial nephritis is more likely to present 5–10 days after introduction of offending drugs like antibiotics, diuretics, PPIs, etc., while prerenal AKI is associated with increased tubular reabsorption of Na and thereby low urinary Na.

   D. d) Dialysis treatment. Further fluid infusion will worsen the pulmonary oedema as he remains oliguric despite sufficient fluid resuscitation, and clinical picture is that of ATN. If there is a delay in arranging dialysis treatment, one can try a frusemide infusion to see if some urine output can be obtained to help pulmonary oedema and buy time for arranging dialysis.

3. b) Creatinine level > 500 µmol/l. Dialysis treatment is not guided by absolute level of urea or creatinine although if there are uraemic features clinically, dialysis can be considered.

4. e) There is no new medication mentioned in the history that can lead to AIN or nephrotoxic ATN. There is no reason to suspect ischemic ATN as BP was stable throughout. Contrast nephropathy usually leads to AKI starting within 24–48 hours of the contrast administration and recovery is usual by seven days. Atheroembolic disease leads to more insidious onset of renal impairment than contrast nephropathy as is seen in this case. The blue toes are another pointer towards atheroembolic disease.

7

Chronic Kidney Disease

P.S. Priyamvada and R. Jayasurya

Summary

- Chronic kidney disease (CKD) is defined as abnormalities of kidney structure or function present for more than three months irrespective of the cause
- Diabetes mellitus and hypertension are responsible for up to two-thirds of the cases of CKD, followed by glomerulonephritis and autosomal-dominant polycystic kidney disease
- The glomeruli of all CKD patients go through a phase of glomerular hypertension, hyperfiltration, and hypertrophy due to activation of the renin–angiotensin–aldosterone system
- Patients often remain asymptomatic until the CKD is quite advanced
- Cardiovascular disease is the leading cause of mortality in patients with CKD
- Patients with CKD should be referred to a nephrologist when the estimated glomerular filtration rate (eGFR) is <30 ml/min/1.73 m² in order to manage the various complications of CKD and potentially plan for renal replacement therapy
- Living donor pre-emptive renal transplantation should be considered in patients with CKD when the GFR is <20 ml/min/1.73 m²

Chronic kidney disease (CKD) represents a state of irreversible damage to renal parenchyma leading to a loss of kidney function. CKD is a significant and growing public health issue, responsible for a substantial burden of illness and premature mortality. According to Kidney Health Australia, more than 40% of people over the age of 75 have an indicator of CKD. Whilst people with CKD have a two- to threefold greater risk of cardiac death than people without the disease, only 10% of them are aware that they have the condition.

A definition and classification scheme for CKD was proposed by the US National Kidney Foundation Kidney Disease Outcomes Quality Initiative (NKF KDOQI) in 2002, subsequently modified by Kidney Disease: Improving Global Outcomes (KDIGO) in 2012.

Definition

CKD is defined as abnormalities of kidney structure or function, present for >3 months, irrespective of the cause. CKD is diagnosed if the glomerular filtration rate (GFR) is less than 60 ml/min/1.73 m² and/or the markers of kidney damage listed in Table 7.1 are present for a period of more than 3 months [1].

- *Albuminuria*: 24-hour urinary albumin excretion of 30 mg or higher, or urine albumin/creatinine ratio (ACR) of 30 mg/g (or 3.4 mg/mmol) or higher.
- *Urinary sediment abnormalities*: red blood cell (RBC) or white blood cell (WBC) casts may indicate the presence of glomerular injury or tubular inflammation.

Lecture Notes Nephrology: A Comprehensive Guide to Renal Medicine, First Edition. Edited by Surjit Tarafdar.
© 2020 John Wiley & Sons Ltd. Published 2020 by John Wiley & Sons Ltd.

Table 7.1 List of markers of chronic kidney disease (CKD): CKD is defined by the presence of either kidney damage or decreased kidney function for three or more months irrespective of cause

- Glomerular filtration rate (GFR) <60 ml/min/1.73 m²
- Albuminuria (albumin excretion rate, AER ≥30 mg/24 hours; albumin creatinine ratio (ACR) ≥30 mg/g or or 3.4 mg/mmol)
- Urine sediment abnormalities, e.g. red blood cell or white blood cell casts
- Renal biopsy evidence of glomerular, vascular or tubulointerstitial disease
- Structural abnormalities detected by imaging, e.g. polycystic kidneys, hydronephrosis or small and echogenic kidneys
- History of kidney transplantation (irrespective of the GFR)

- *Imaging abnormalities*: kidney damage may be detected by the presence of imaging abnormalities such as polycystic kidneys, hydronephrosis, or small and echogenic kidneys.
- *Pathological abnormalities*: a kidney biopsy may reveal evidence of glomerular, vascular or tubulointerstitial disease.
- *Kidney transplantation*: patients with a history of kidney transplantation are assumed to have CKD irrespective of the presence or absence of abnormalities on kidney biopsy or markers of kidney damage.

CKD is further classified based on the combined indices of kidney function (measured or estimated GFR) and kidney damage (albuminuria/proteinuria), irrespective of the underlying diagnosis (Tables 7.2 and 7.3).

According to the Caring for Australasians with Renal Impairment (CARI) 2012 guidelines, when

Table 7.2 Glomerular filtration rate (GFR) categories in chronic kidney disease

Category	GFR (ml/min/1.73 m²)	Description
G1	>90	Normal or high
G2	60–89	Mildly decreased
G3a	45–59	Mildly to moderately decreased
G3b	30–44	Moderately to severely decreased
G4	15–29	Severely decreased
G5	<15	Kidney failure

Source: KDIGO 2012 Clinical Practice Guideline for the Evaluation and Management of Chronic Kidney Disease.

Table 7.3 Albuminuria categories in chronic kidney disease (CKD)

Kidney damage stage	Urine albumin/ creatinine ratio (mg/mmol)	Urine protein/ creatinine ratio (mg/mmol)	24-hour urine albumin (mg/day)	24-hour urine protein (mg/day)
Normoalbuminuria	<2.5 (M) <3.5 (F)	<4 (M) <6 (F)	<30	<50
Microalbuminuria	2.5–25 (M) 3.5–35 (F)	4–40 (M) 6–60 (F)	30–300	50–500
Macroalbuminuria	>25 (M) >35 (F)	>40 (M) >60 (F)	>300	>500

F, female; M, male. Source: CARI 2012 guidelines.

reporting kidney function, stage (stages 1–5) is combined with degree of proteinuria, for instance albuminuria/proteinuria (normo/micro/macro-albuminuria), and clinical diagnosis to fully specify the CKD stage (e.g. stage 2 CKD with microalbuminuria secondary to diabetic nephropathy).

End-stage renal disease (ESRD) represents a state of kidney failure where the metabolic disturbances are severe enough for the patient to need renal replacement therapy.

It is recommended to use the 2009 Chronic Kidney Disease Epidemiology Collaboration (CKD-EPI) creatinine equation for estimating GFR in adults. As discussed in Chapter 2, the CKD-EPI creatinine equation gives a more accurate estimation of GFR in comparison to the Cockcroft–Gault equation and the Modification of Diet in Renal Disease (MDRD) study equation in people with normal or near-normal GFR.

Aetiology and Risk Factors

According to the US-based National Kidney Foundation, diabetes mellitus and hypertension are responsible for up to two-thirds of cases of CKD, followed by glomerulonephritis and autosomal-dominant polycystic kidney disease (ADPKD). The contributions by each disease might vary depending on the geographical location. The presence of certain comorbid conditions is associated with a high risk of developing CKD. These include a history of acute kidney injury (AKI); structural renal diseases/calculi; long-term ingestion of nephrotoxic medications such as non-steroidal anti-inflammatory drugs (NSAIDs), calcineurin inhibitors or lithium; a family history of kidney disease; a past history or family history of cardiovascular disease (CVD); haematuria; and older age. Polymorphisms in the APOL1 gene are associated with higher rates of disease progression and ESRD in patients with African ancestry [2].

Consequences of Loss of Kidney Function

Irrespective of the disease process leading to CKD, the kidney can adapt to the initial damage by increasing filtration in the remaining normal nephrons, a process called adaptive hyperfiltration. Increased activation of the renin–angiotensin–aldosterone system (RAAS) due to loss of renal mass leads to a rise in glomerular pressure, which in turn leads to glomerular hyperfiltration and hypertrophy. This enables the patient with mild renal insufficiency to maintain a normal, or near-normal, serum creatinine concentration. The renal tubules also adapt themselves to maintain sodium, potassium, calcium, phosphorous, and total body water within the normal range, as is often seen in patients with mild to moderate renal failure.

Following unilateral nephrectomy, a 30–40% increment in single-nephron GFR is observed in the single kidney. As kidney disease progresses, homeostasis is maintained by a diminishing pool of hyperfunctioning nephrons. Because of compensatory mechanisms, patients can remain asymptomatic until around 70% of the kidney function is lost. Glomerular hyperfiltration and compensatory hypertrophy eventually lead to damage of functional nephrons, thus initiating a vicious cycle. The factors that contribute to renal loss include activation of the RAAS, intra-glomerular hypertension, ongoing aetiology of primary cause of CKD, proteinuria, acidosis, and oxidative stress (Figure 7.1) [3].

Complications

The metabolic derangements resulting from CKD can affect almost all organ systems of the body. Patients often remain asymptomatic until the renal failure is quite advanced.

Fluid, Electrolyte and Acid–Base Disorders

Sodium and Water Homeostasis

Whilst in most patients with stable CKD the total body content of sodium and water is modestly increased, this is usually not apparent on clinical examination. However, the patient with mild to moderate CKD, despite appearing clinically euvolaemic, is less able to respond to a sudden or increased intake of sodium and is therefore prone to fluid overload. Patients with CKD and volume overload generally respond to a combination of dietary sodium restriction and loop diuretic therapy. The 2012 KDIGO guidelines recommend that, amongst all adults with CKD, sodium intake should be restricted to <2 g/day.

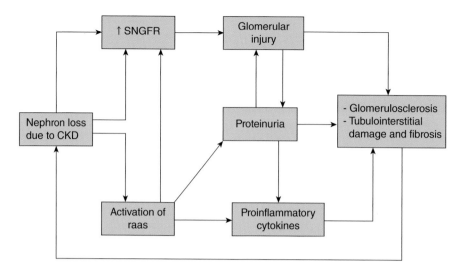

Figure 7.1 Consequences of loss of renal function. CKD, chronic kidney disease; RAAS, renin–angiotensin–aldosterone system; SNGFR, single-nephron glomerular filtration rate.

Potassium Balance

The ability to maintain potassium excretion at near-normal levels is generally maintained in patients with CKD as long as they pass urine. Patients with CKD also tend to have augmented potassium excretion in the gastrointestinal tract (GIT). Hyperkalaemia in CKD patients is usually seen in those who are oliguric or have an additional problem such as a high potassium diet, increased tissue breakdown, metabolic acidosis or hypoaldosteronism, due in some cases to the administration of an angiotensin-converting enzyme (ACE) inhibitor or angiotensin receptor blocker (ARB). Patients with diabetes mellitus and obstructive uropathy are prone to develop both metabolic acidosis and hyperkalaemia, due to type IV renal tubular acidosis (RTA) caused by hypoaldosteronism.

In the metabolic acidosis often seen in patients with advanced CKD, as hydrogen (H^+) enters the cells to be buffered, intracellular potassium (K^+) leaves the cells and moves into the extracellular fluid, tending to raise the plasma potassium concentration (Figure 7.2).

Metabolic Acidosis

There is an increasing tendency to retain H^+ ions amongst patients with CKD, leading to metabolic acidosis. In the early stages of CKD, patients can secrete H^+ ions but do not have enough urinary ammonium to buffer them, thus limiting H^+ excretion in the urine. Ammonium excretion begins to fall when the GFR is below 40–50 ml/min, and hyperkalaemia further reduces ammonium production (Figure 7.3).

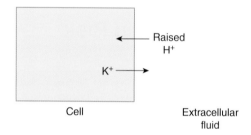

Figure 7.2 In metabolic acidosis, the excess extracellular hydrogen (H^+) enters cells; the cells as a compensation for the additional positive charge cause intracellular potassium (K^+) to move out, which in turn raises the serum K^+.

In advanced CKD, patients almost always have a high anion gap metabolic acidosis. However, in the early stages of CKD (stages 1–3), in patients with diabetic nephropathy, in those with predominant tubulointerstitial disease or obstructive uropathy, one can see a type IV RTA-like picture, leading to normal anion gap metabolic acidosis.

Cardiovascular System

CVD is a leading cause of mortality in patients with CKD. Patients with stage 3 CKD are more likely to die because of cardiac disease rather than progress to ESRD. The annual mortality rate amongst dialysis patients is around 20%, with more than half of deaths resulting from CVD. It is estimated that each 20% reduction in GFR carries a 50% increased risk for

$$H_2N-\overset{\underset{\|}{O}}{C}-CH_2-CH_2-\overset{\underset{|}{NH_2}}{CH}-COOH \xrightarrow[\text{Glutaminase}]{H_2O \quad\quad NH_4^+} HOOC-CH_2-CH_2-\overset{\underset{|}{NH_2}}{CH}-COOH$$

Glutamine   Glutamate

Figure 7.3 Role of glutaminase in generating ammonium from glutamine: In the kidneys, glutaminase generates ammonium from glutamine; the ammonium subsequently regenerates ammonia that helps to buffer the hydrogen (H^+) in urine. Hyperkalaemia has an inhibitory effect on glutaminase, leading to reduced ammonium synthesis and consequently a reduction in ammonia production. Lack of ammonia in the urine quickly saturates the urine with H^+, leading to failure of tubular excretion of H^+ and the resultant metabolic acidosis. CH_2: methylene; COOH: carboxyl; H_2N: amidogen; H_2O: water; NH_4^+: ammonium.

Table 7.4 Risk factors for cardiovascular disease in chronic kidney disease

Traditional risk factors	Non-traditional risk factors
Age	Anaemia
Male sex	Abnormal bone and mineral metabolism (hyperparathyroidism, hyperphosphatemia, high Ca × P product, vascular calcifications, elevated fibroblast growth factor-23 levels)
Hypertension	
Diabetes mellitus	
Dyslipidaemia	
Low HDL	
Physical inactivity	
Smoking	Hypoalbuminemia
Menopause	Activation of renin angiotensin systems
	Albuminuria
	Inflammation
	Oxidative stress
	Sympathetic overactivity
	Endothelial dysfunction

Ca, calcium; HDL, high-density lipoprotein; P, phosphorus.

major vascular events [4]. Cardiovascular risk starts at the micro-albuminuria stage, which is usually long before the GFR begins to decline. Apart from the traditional risk factors, a host of CKD-specific risk factors (Table 7.4) operate which contribute to the added burden of CVD [5]. Recent epidemiological evidence has shown a strong association between hyperphosphataemia and an increased cardiovascular mortality rate in patients even in early CKD. i.e. patients with GFR <60 mL/min/1.73 m².

Patients with CKD tend to have a higher prevalence of systemic hypertension, ischaemic heart disease, congestive heart failure (CHF), cardiac arrhythmias, peripheral vascular disease, strokes, and vascular and valvular calcifications [6]. The incidence of uraemic pericarditis has fallen significantly due to the improvements in medical care. CKD patients with CVD tend to have worse outcomes when compared to the general population.

Systemic Hypertension

Data from the MDRD study showed that the prevalence of hypertension rose progressively from 65% to 95% as the GFR fell from 85 to 15 ml/min/1.73 m². Multiple pathophysiological mechanisms including sodium retention, activation of RAAS, sympathetic overactivity, oxidative stress, endothelial dysfunction, elevated endothelin levels, and endogenous ouabain-like substances contribute to hypertension in CKD. In addition, erythropoiesis-stimulating agents can also result in hypertension. Hypertension is an independent risk factor for the progression of CKD.

Treatment of even mild hypertension is important in the CKD patient to protect against both progressive renal function loss and CVD.

Coronary Heart Disease

Coronary heart disease (CHD) accounts for 40–50% of mortality in dialysis patients. Patients often have diffuse multivessel involvement with coronary calcifications. Whilst traditional cardiovascular risk factors, such as hypertension often accompanied by left ventricular hypertrophy (LVH), smoking, diabetes, and dyslipidaemia are highly prevalent in CKD populations, non-traditional risk factors unique to patients with moderate to severe CKD include retention of uraemic toxins, hyperphosphataemia, anaemia, elevated levels of certain cytokines, increased calcium intake, abnormalities in bone mineral metabolism, and/or an increased 'inflammatory–poor nutrition state'. The chronic inflammatory milieu associated with CKD predisposes to enhanced oxidative stress and endothelial dysfunction. Uraemia-specific metabolites like cyanate, carbamylated low-density lipoprotein (LDL), asymmetric dimethyl arginine (ADMA), and p-cresyl sulphate can induce endothelial dysfunction.

Diagnosis and management of CHD can be challenging in the presence of CKD. The clinical presentation can often be atypical. Interpretation of electrocardiography (ECG) is often complicated by the presence of pre-existing ST-T changes resulting from LVH and strain, as well as electrolyte disturbances. Various enzyme markers like creatine kinase-MB and cardiac troponins, particularly Troponin T (Tn T), can be spuriously elevated secondary to reduced renal clearance. Investigations like dobutamine stress echocardiogram (DSE) and nuclear scintigraphy can be of prognostic value, but there is limited evidence to recommend them as routine screening tests. Invasive angiograms carry the risk of contrast-induced nephropathy in predialysis patients.

Congestive Heart Failure

CKD is associated with chronic volume overload, pressure overload, and structural myocardial changes, all of which predispose to cardiac failure. Whilst the volume overload is secondary to decreasing urine output with worsening CKD, the pressure overload is a result of long-standing hypertension and enhanced vascular stiffness. Structural myocardial changes such as myocyte hypertrophy and increased myocardial fibrosis result from a complex interplay of multiple factors including hypertension, vascular stiffness, chronic neurohumoral activation, increased aldosterone level, and extravascular calcifications. The various markers of myocardial damage, including B-type natriuretic peptides (BNP and NT-proBNP) and troponins, tend to be elevated in renal failure owing to reduced renal clearance, limiting their usefulness as screening tools.

Strokes, Arrhythmias and Sudden Cardiac Death

CKD is an independent risk factor for ischaemic and haemorrhagic stroke. Dialysis patients have a five- to tenfold higher relative risk of stroke when compared to the general population. Atrial fibrillation is seen in 15–20% of dialysis patients, which may contribute to embolic stroke. CKD patients are more prone to sudden cardiac death (SCD). Amongst dialysis patients, SCD accounts for about one-fourth of all deaths. Although CHD is an important cause of SCD, it is not the major one (unlike in the general population). In dialysis patients, 60–65% of cardiac deaths are attributed to arrhythmias. Factors contributing to SCD in these patients include structural alterations in the myocardium, electrophysiological remodelling, ischaemia, high sympathetic tone, electrolyte fluxes during dialysis and hypotension following dialysis.

Haematopoietic System

CKD is associated with anaemia and an increased risk of bleeding due to platelet dysfunction. The prevalence of anaemia increases with declining kidney function. Patients with diabetic kidney disease, chronic tubulointerstitial disease, African Americans, younger women, and older men tend to have particularly severe anaemia. On the other hand, patients with polycystic kidney disease have a lesser propensity for anaemia.

Anaemia

A normocytic, normochromic anaemia contributes to symptoms like fatigue, depression, reduced exercise tolerance and dyspnoea in patients with CKD [7]. Whilst LVH appears to be increasingly prevalent as the GFR falls, severe anaemia is associated with more frequent and severe LVH and an increase in all-cause as well as cardiovascular mortality.

The causes of anaemia in CKD are postulated to be as outlined in the following sections.

Erythropoietin deficiency

The primary cause of anaemia in patients with CKD is insufficient production of erythropoietin (EPO) by the diseased kidney. The peritubular fibroblasts produce EPO in response to hypoxia. EPO is an essential survival factor for RBC precursors ranging from colony-forming unit-erythroid (CFU-E) to late basophilic erythroblasts. Binding of EPO with the EPO receptor on the surface of erythroid precursors prevents the cells from undergoing apoptosis, and thus increases their survival. Loss of functioning renal mass leads to inappropriately reduced EPO levels. The uraemic state itself can depress erythropoiesis, in addition to reduced EPO levels.

Iron Deficiency

Regular erythropoiesis is dependent on a continuous supply of iron. The amount of iron absorbed from the GIT is usually around 1–2 mg/day, which constitutes around 5–10% of the iron ingested in the typical Western diet. Patients with CKD can have absolute, as well as functional, iron deficiency. Functional iron deficiency results from an inability of the body to mobilize iron from the storage pool. Absolute iron deficiency results from gastrointestinal blood loss, blood loss during dialysis, poor oral iron absorption, and use of drugs like proton pump inhibitors, calcium, lanthanum, and aluminium compounds. Haemodialysis is associated with blood loss, via blood sticking to the extracorporeal circuit; the annual loss amounts to approximately 1000–2000 ml. As each ml of blood contains 0.5 mg of iron, this alone would account for an annual requirement of around 500–1000 mg, which far exceeds the absorptive capacity of the gut. In addition, patients with CKD, especially ESRD patients on haemodialysis, have a significantly reduced capacity for iron absorption from the gut.

Role of Hepcidin

Depending on the iron needs of the body, iron absorbed by the duodenal cells is either stored as ferritin within the cells, or is released via the basolateral iron exporter ferroportin. Hepcidin, by causing internalization and degradation of ferroportin, prevents the release of the absorbed iron from the duodenal cells into the body. As the duodenal cells have a continuous turnover, the iron trapped within the cells is lost. Iron release from the macrophages is also dependent on ferroportin and hence inhibited by elevated hepcidin.

Hepcidin levels are increased by inflammation and CKD, leading to reduced iron absorption and anaemia [8].

Reduced Red Blood Cell mass

Both red cell life span and the rate of production of RBCs are reduced in uraemia, with the latter being a more important cause of reduced red cell mass. The circulating RBC mass can be further reduced due to blood loss in the dialysis circuit and occult loss from the GIT.

Inflammation

The inflammatory cytokines produced as a result of CKD lead to impaired production and a blunted response to EPO. Chronic inflammation of any cause contributes to functional iron deficiency by upregulating hepcidin, as discussed above.

Hyperparathyroidism

High parathyroid hormone (PTH) levels directly suppress the erythroid progenitors in bone marrow as well as renal EPO synthesis. High PTH also leads to

reduced red cell survival and resistance to EPO therapy as well as marrow fibrosis. There is recent evidence that vitamin D deficiency has a direct suppressive effect on erythropoiesis [9].

Drugs

RAAS inhibitors such as ACE inhibitors or ARBs lead to accumulation of N-acetyl-seryl-aspartyl-lysyl-proline (AcSDKP), which can downregulate erythropoiesis. Myelosuppressive agents such as cyclophosphamide used for the treatment of certain glomerulonephrites (e.g. ANCA positive vasculitis or Goodpasture's disease) can also contribute to anaemia by inducing bone marrow suppression.

Aluminium Overload

In the past, aluminium had been used as a phosphate binder. Currently there is a declining trend to use aluminium for phosphate control. Patients on haemodialysis can occasionally be exposed to aluminium through contamination of dialysate. High aluminium levels lead to altered iron metabolism, direct inhibition of erythropoiesis, and disruption of RBC membrane function.

Other Nutrient Deficiencies

Haemodialysis is associated with the loss of water-soluble vitamins including B-complex and folic acid, which can contribute to anaemia. The stringent dietary restrictions can also lead to multiple nutrient deficiencies.

Increased Risk of Bleeding and Platelet Dysfunction

Patients with CKD may have a prolonged bleeding time due to abnormal platelet aggregation and adhesiveness. An intrinsic dysfunction of glycoprotein IIb/IIIa (platelet membrane glycoprotein that plays a major role in both platelet aggregation and adhesion with fibrinogen) and von Willebrand factor contribute to the platelet dysfunction.

In CKD, increased endothelial nitric oxide (NO) synthesis leads to increased cyclic guanosine monophosphate (cGMP) levels, which also causes defective platelet aggregation and adhesion. Other contributory factors to platelet dysfunction are altered release of adenosine diphosphate (ADP) and serotonin from platelet alpha-granules, faulty arachidonic acid and prostaglandin metabolism, decreased platelet thromboxane A2 generation, and abnormal platelet cytoskeletal assembly due to low actin levels.

Bone and Mineral Metabolism

CKD is characterized by abnormalities of bone and mineral metabolism. Traditionally the associated disorders were called renal osteodystrophy [10]. The recent trend is to use the term renal osteodystrophy exclusively to define bone pathology associated with CKD. In view of the fact that mineral and bone disorders contribute to CKD-associated CVD and high mortality rates, KDIGO recommended that the new term chronic kidney disease–mineral and bone disorder (CKD–MBD) be used to describe the broader systemic disorder that occurs as a result of CKD.

The main abnormalities that contribute to the pathogenesis of secondary hyperparathyroidism are [11]:

- Phosphate retention
- Decreased free ionized calcium concentration
- Decreased 1,25-dihydroxyvitamin D (calcitriol) concentration
- Increased fibroblast growth factor 23 (FGF-23) concentration leading to decreased calcitriol production by inhibiting proximal tubular expression of 1-alpha-hydroxylase

- Repression of calcium-sensing receptors (CaSRs), fibroblast growth factor receptors and klotho in the parathyroid glands

Reduction of GFR to less than 70 ml/min leads to a decrease in renal phosphate clearance. The resultant phosphate retention is postulated to be the trigger for the development of CKD–MBD (Figure 7.4).

Phosphate retention leads to hypocalcaemia and the resultant increase in PTH secretion by different mechanisms:

- *Hypocalcaemia*: whenever the calcium × phosphate product is excessively high, both calcium and phosphate begin to get deposited at various sites all over the body including inside blood vessels, leading to lowering of serum calcium levels.
- *Decreased formation of calcitriol* (1,25-dihydroxyvitamin D, the active form of vitamin D): decreased activity of 1-alpha hydroxylase in the deceased kidney leads to reduced formation of calcitriol, and hence reduced intestinal absorption of calcium.
- *Increased PTH gene expression*: increased serum phosphate has a direct effect in increasing PTH secretion.

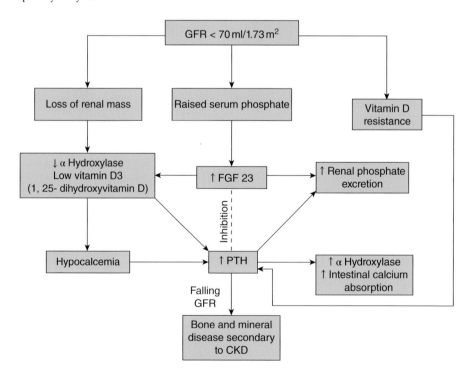

Figure 7.4 Mechanisms of genesis of chronic kidney disease–mineral and bone disorder (CKD-MBD). FGF23, fibroblast growth factor-23; GFR, glomerular filtration rate; PTH, parathyroid hormone.

The CaSR on the surface of the chief cells of the parathyroid glands senses minute-to-minute serum calcium levels and modulates PTH secretion accordingly. In CKD patients, the number of CaSRs is reduced. This reduced number of CaSRs hinders serum calcium's ability to suppress PTH secretion, resulting in inappropriately high PTH concentrations. The phosphaturic FGF-23 is secreted by bone osteocytes and osteoblasts in response to elevated phosphate levels in CKD [12]. FGF-23 helps to maintain a normal serum phosphate concentration by reducing renal phosphate as well as intestinal phosphate absorption. In renal proximal tubular cells, FGF-23 binds to the FGF receptor (FGFR) and its coreceptor, klotho, causing inhibition of the expression of the sodium/phosphate (Na/Pi) IIa cotransporter and thus inhibiting reabsorption of phosphate. FGF-23 also inhibits 1-alpha-hydroxylase, leading to decreased calcitriol synthesis and hence reduced intestinal calcium absorption. Under normal circumstances, FGF-23 suppresses PTH secretion by the parathyroid gland. However, amongst CKD patients, markedly decreased expression of FGFR-1 and klotho protein in the hyperplastic parathyroid gland causes the parathyroid gland to become resistant to the elevated FGF-23 levels. Thus, an elevated level of FGF-23 is not able to suppress PTH production in the CKD patient as it would do in a non-CKD patient.

Ongoing high PTH levels cause downregulation of the PTH receptors on the bones, which in turn leads to further increase in PTH secretion.

Ongoing uncontrolled secondary hyperparathyroidism can eventually lead to tertiary hyperparathyroidism, where the hyperplastic parathyroid gland continues to secrete high levels of PTH independent of the serum calcium levels. Patients often develop unexplained hypercalcaemia. Patients with tertiary hyperparathyroidism fail medical therapy and generally require parathyroidectomy. Prevalence of CKD–MBD in CKD stages 4 and 5 ranges from 62 to 100%.

Classification of Bone Disease in Chronic Kidney Disease

High Turnover Bone Disease

Hyperparathyroidism leads to increased bone turnover and osteitis fibrosa cystica. Before 1950, more than half of those who developed ESRD developed osteitis fibrosa cystica. With better management of serum phosphate and PTH levels in CKD patients, this condition is seen much less now.

High turnover bone disease is characterized by increased osteoclastic activity leading to bone resorption. Bone histology shows abnormal osteoid, bone marrow fibrosis, and the formation of bone cysts, sometimes with haemorrhagic elements so that they appear brown in colour; hence the term brown tumour. Clinical manifestations may include bone pain and fractures, brown tumours, compression syndromes by brown tumours, and EPO resistance in part related to the bone marrow fibrosis. Whilst routine X-ray of the skeleton is relatively insensitive for diagnosis, sub-periosteal erosions are often present in severe hyperparathyroidism, especially in the hands.

Low Turnover Bone Disease (Adynamic Bone Disease)

Adynamic bone disease is characterized by a low or absent bone formation with a paucity of bone cells (both osteoblast and osteoclast) and severely reduced osteoid volume. Over the last few decades, the prevalence of adynamic bone disease has been increasing, whilst the other forms of renal bone disease are on a decreasing trend. The principal causative mechanism of this disease seems to be over-suppression of PTH by zealous clinicians. Sometimes it can occur due to skeletal resistance to the effect of PTH. In patients with CKD stage 5, as well as those on dialysis, adynamic bone disease is now the commonest form of CKD renal bone disease. Though most patients are asymptomatic, they are at increased risk for fractures, hypercalcaemia, and vascular calcification; all of which have been shown to be associated with increased mortality. Treatment focuses on allowing the PTH levels to rise by decreasing the doses of calcium-based phosphate binders, decreasing or stopping active vitamin D analogues and by using non-calcium-based phosphate binders.

Dialysis-Related Amyloidosis

Dialysis-related amyloidosis (DRA) is characterized by the tissue deposition of amyloid, particularly in bone, articular cartilage, synovium, muscle, tendons, and ligaments. In contrast to fragments of immunoglobulin light chains in primary amyloidosis and serum amyloid A in secondary amyloidosis, the amyloid protein in DRA is derived primarily from beta2-microglobulin (beta2-m). It is almost exclusively seen in patients on dialysis. With the use of high-flux biocompatible membranes that provide better clearance of beta2-m, the condition is seen much less now. Affected patients most commonly complain of shoulder pain related to scapulo-humeral periarthritis and rotator cuff infiltration by amyloid, and/or symptoms of carpal tunnel syndrome. Diagnosis is often suspected with a combination of typical clinical features and characteristic radiographic findings of multiple bone cysts that rapidly enlarge over time. Treatment consists of optimization of dialysis therapy with high-flux biocompatible membranes to maximise the clearance of beta2-m. Renal transplantation is the definitive cure.

Osteomalacia

Osteomalacia is characterized by defective bone mineralization with markedly increased osteoid volumes. Aluminium toxicity used to be the most common cause of osteomalacia in patients with CKD, but is rarely seen now with the strict removal of aluminium from dialysis water and diminishing use of aluminium-based phosphate binders.

In conclusion, bone disease is often diagnosed on clinical grounds. Monitoring serum levels of calcium, phosphate, and PTH should begin when the GFR is less than 60 ml. Atraumatic bone fractures in the presence of a serum PTH that is lower than two times the upper limit of normal is suggestive of the commonly seen low turnover bone disease - adynamic disease. Although bone biopsy is the gold standard to distinguish between the different histological types, it is recommended only in selected patient populations (Table 7.5). Many times, the histological picture shows overlapping features of both high and low turnover diseases.

Table 7.5 Indications for bone biopsy in chronic kidney disease-mineral and bone disorder (CKD-MBD)

- Unexplained fractures
- Persistent bone pain
- Unexplained hypercalcaemia
- Unexplained hypophosphataemia
- Suspected aluminium toxicity
- Before therapy with bisphosphonates in patients with CKD–MBD

Neurological Manifestations

The neurological manifestations of CKD include various delirium syndromes, such as uraemic encephalopathy, dialysis disequilibrium syndrome (DDS), dialysis dementia, and chronic cognitive dysfunction; peripheral neuropathy; and sleep disorders, including sleep apnoea, restless leg syndrome , and periodic limb movement disorders [13].

Uraemic Encephalopathy

Uraemic encephalopathy occurs in patients with untreated or inadequately treated uraemia. The clinical manifestations can range from mild cognitive disturbance to delirium, seizures, coma, and death. Patients often have asterixis and hyperreflexia. Multiple pathophysiological mechanisms have been proposed for uraemic encephalopathy. These include activation of the excitatory N-methyl-D-aspartate (NMDA) receptors with concomitant inhibition of GABAergic neurotransmission due to accumulation of guanidino compounds, neuronal depression secondary to high PTH levels, accumulation of tryptophan metabolites like kynurenine and 3-hydroxy-kynurenine, increased nitrotyrosine levels, and disturbances of intermediary metabolism leading to reduced energy reserve in the brain.

Structural, infectious, and toxic brain pathologies should be ruled out before making a diagnosis of uremic encephalopathy.

Dialysis Disequilibrium Syndrome

DDS is discussed in Chapter 18.

Dialysis Dementia

Dialysis dementia is a progressive neurological disorder seen exclusively in haemodialysis patients. Its pathogenesis is linked to aluminium intoxication. With aluminium-free water used in haemodialysis and avoidance of aluminium-containing phosphate binders, it is rarely seen nowadays. The signs and symptoms of dialysis dementia include dysarthria, mental changes, hallucinations, myoclonus, and seizures.

Neuropathy

Uraemic neuropathy is a symmetrical, distal sensorimotor polyneuropathy with the lower limbs affected initially and sensory symptoms usually preceding the motor manifestations. Mononeuropathy typically results from the entrapment of median or ulnar nerves resulting from dialysis-associated amyloidosis. Sometimes patients develop ischaemic mononeuropathy as a complication of vascular access surgery. Autonomic neuropathy can lead to orthostatic hypotension.

Sleep Disorders

Sleep apnoea is more common amongst ESRD patients than in the general population, with a reported prevalence of more than 50%. The prevalence of sleep apnoea is similar amongst patients who are treated with peritoneal dialysis or haemodialysis.

Restless leg syndrome (RLS) is characterized by an irresistible urge to move one's legs, associated with feelings of discomfort or paraesthesia. Factors thought to be associated with the development of RLS include anaemia, iron deficiency, elevated serum calcium and uraemic peripheral neuropathy. Symptoms are precipitated by inactivity and alleviated by leg movements. RLS is associated with difficulty in initiating sleep, poor sleep quality, and impaired quality of life, along with increased risk of depression. Mild symptoms can be managed by good sleep hygiene and avoidance of dopamine-blocking anti-emetics such as metoclopramide, antidepressants, caffeine, alcohol, and nicotine. Levodopa and the dopamine receptor agonists pergolide, pramipexole, and ropinirole are effective in reducing the severity of symptoms in patients with RLS.

Endocrine Manifestations

Insulin

Insulin requirements typically show a biphasic course in diabetic patients with CKD. Whilst in the early stages there is an increased insulin requirement due to insulin resistance, as the GFR falls below 15–20 ml/min, reduction in renal clearance of insulin means that patients either need smaller doses of insulin/oral hypoglycaemics or sometimes do not need them any longer.

In mild to moderate CKD, uraemic toxins and excess PTH are postulated to lead to insulin receptor defects, especially in the skeletal muscles. The resultant insulin resistance leads to a requirement for increased doses of insulin. Insulin resistance is an independent risk factor for increased cardiovascular

morbidity and mortality. Insulin is freely filtered across the glomeruli as well as actively extracted from the peritubular capillaries and secreted into the proximal convoluted tubule (PCT) lumen, leading to a renal clearance of insulin of 200 ml/min that significantly exceeds the normal GFR of 120 ml/min. As the GFR falls to less than 15–20 ml/min, there is a dramatic reduction in the renal clearance of insulin, and patients at this stage often need much lower doses of insulin than previously [14].

Abnormalities of Thyroid Hormone

CKD is associated with alterations in the synthesis, secretion, metabolism, and elimination of thyroid hormones [15]. Epidemiological evidence suggests that there is increased prevalence of hypothyroidism in patients with CKD. The kidney normally contributes to the clearance of iodide by glomerular filtration. Thus, decreased iodide clearance in advanced CKD leads to elevated plasma inorganic iodide concentration, which in turn inhibits thyroid iodide organification and thus causes decreased thyroid hormone production (Wolff–Chaikoff effect). This may explain the increased incidence of hypothyroidism seen in patients with CKD.

Most patients with ESRD have decreased plasma levels of free triiodothyronine (T3), resulting from a decreased peripheral conversion of thyroxine (T4). Persistent inflammation and metabolic acidosis may be responsible for the reduced peripheral conversion. However, the inactive reverse T3 (rT3) remains normal, thus differentiating it from the sick euthyroid syndrome. Low T3 concentrations are believed to be associated with increased all-cause as well as cardiovascular mortality in uraemic patients.

Growth Hormone

Growth hormone (GH) secreted from the pituitary acts on hepatic GH receptors and upregulates the synthesis and release of insulin-like growth factor-1 (IGF-1) from the liver. IGF-1 circulates in the free form as well as bound to a family of IGF binding proteins (IGFBP 1–6). CKD is associated with low GH receptor density in peripheral tissues, low IGF-1, and elevated IGFBPs, which leads to peripheral resistance to the actions of GH. There is evidence that GH supplementation improves anabolic function, stimulates protein synthesis, decreases urea generation, and improves nitrogen balance in adult patients with CKD [15].

Dermatological Manifestations

Dermatological manifestations of CKD have a profound impact on the quality of life. Table 7.6 lists the common CKD-associated dermatological manifestations [16].

Uraemic Pruritus

Uraemic pruritus is found to affect approximately half of the patient population with CKD. It can be focal or generalized, and can be precipitated by external heat, sweat and stress. Whilst the actual mechanism of uraemic pruritus is not clearly elucidated, there are two major hypotheses. The immune hypothesis considers it to be an inflammatory systemic disease resulting from high levels of inflammatory cytokines and chemokines induced by uraemia. The opioid theory proposes that uraemic pruritus is due to changes in the endogenous opioidergic system resulting from hyperactivity of opioid μ receptors and concomitant downregulation of opioid κ receptors. The disorder seems to have an association with hyperparathyroidism as well. Itching frequently occurs in patients with elevated PTH levels and high calcium × phosphorus product (Ca × P).

Table 7.6 Dermatological manifestations of chronic kidney disease

Pruritis

Xerosis

Icthyosis

Pigmentary alterations

Skin infections

Purpura

Acquired perforating dermatosis (Kyrles disease)

Calcific uremic arteriopathy (Calciphylaxis)

Blistering disorders like porphyria cutanea tarda, pseudoporphyria

Eruptive xanthomas

Kaposi's sarcoma

Uraemic frost

Nephrogenic systemic fibrosis

Dialysis-associated steal syndrome

Dialysis-related amyloidosis

AV shunt dermatitis

Treatment consists of optimising dialysis using the generally accepted Kt/V targets and optimizing nutrition. Topical treatments, including skin emollients and capsaicin cream might be helpful. Patients who do not respond to topical therapy are candidates for systemic therapy including antihistamines, gabapentin, μ opioid receptor antagonists such as naltrexone, oral activated charcoal, 5-HT$_3$ antagonists, ultraviolet light, and short courses of immunomodulators such as thalidomide or tacrolimus.

Calcific Uraemic Arteriopathy (Calciphylaxis)

Calcific uraemic arteriopathy (CUA) is a serious complication of CKD. Once thought to be rare, it is now being increasingly recognized and reported on a global scale. The estimated prevalence is reported to be up to 4% of all patients on dialysis, although it may also be seen in the non-dialysis population. It is characterized by systemic medial calcification of the arterioles leading to ischaemia and subcutaneous necrosis. Histological inspection reveals small vessel mural calcification with or without endovascular fibrosis, extravascular calcification, and thrombotic vaso-occlusion.

Although the pathogenesis of CUA is not very well understood, it is probably part of the spectrum of CKD–MBD, where changes in serum calcium, phosphate, PTH, and vitamin D metabolism lead to vascular and soft tissue calcification, along with the bone disorders.

Apart from hyperparathyroidism, active vitamin D administration, hyperphosphataemia, and an elevated plasma Ca × P, deficiency of the following two inhibitors of vascular calcification is considered to play a role in the pathogenesis of CUA:

- Fetuin-A is a serum glycoprotein that binds calcium and phosphate in the circulation, thereby forming 'calciprotein particles' that help to clear the circulation of excess calcium and phosphate. Thus, Fetuin-A is postulated to prevent soft tissue calcification, including vascular calcium deposition. Fetuin-A levels are low in patients on haemodialysis, and their effectiveness in binding calcium and phosphate is also reduced.
- Matrix GLA protein (MGP) is synthesized by vascular smooth muscle and chondrocytes and inhibits calcification of arteries and cartilage. Since its activity depends upon vitamin K-dependent carboxylation, it can be inhibited by warfarin.

The risk factors include obesity, diabetes mellitus, female sex, white ethnicity, increased serum phosphate and PTH, hypercoagulable states such as protein C and S deficiency and antiphospholipid syndrome, hypoalbuminaemia, and the use of drugs such as warfarin, vitamin D, calcium-based phosphate binders, and systemic glucocorticoids. These excruciatingly painful lesions tend to occur in areas with large amounts of subcutaneous fat such as the thigh, abdomen and buttock. They start as livedo reticularis-like lesions that become painful, purpuric, and violaceous plaques or nodules, with subsequent ulceration and eschar formation. The necrotic areas can extend to deeper tissues and get secondarily infected. Systemic involvement has been rarely reported. It is associated with a high mortality, with death usually occurring because of infectious complications. Skin biopsy shows epidermal ulceration, dermal necrosis, vascular medial wall calcifications with subintimal or intimal hyperplasia and fibrosis of small and medium-sized blood vessels in the dermis and subcutaneous tissues. Management includes wound care, control of infection, treatment of bone mineral disorders by use of non-calcium-containing phosphate binders and discontinuation of vitamin D. Warfarin and systemic glucocorticoids should also preferably be discontinued.

Definitive therapy consists of hyperbaric oxygen and sodium thiosulphate. Intravenous sodium thiosulphate is used for the management of calciphylaxis. It chelates calcium and induces endothelial nitric oxide synthesis, which helps to improve tissue oxygenation. Many consider hyperbaric oxygen as a second-line therapy for recalcitrant calciphylaxis wounds that are unresponsive to therapy with sodium thiosulphate for three months. Hyperbaric oxygen therapy is believed to improve tissue perfusion. Those patients with raised PTH are treated with cinacalcet and in case of failure of medical therapy, offered parathyroidectomy. Both haemodialysis and peritoneal dialysis should be optimized to achieve dialysis adequacy.

Nephrogenic Systemic Fibrosis

- Nephrogenic systemic fibrosis (NSF) is a scleroderma-like disorder seen in patients with CKD, AKI, and failing kidney transplant following exposure to gadolinium (Gd)-containing agents used in magnetic resonance imaging (MRI) scans.
- Additional risk factors are believed to be high-dosage EPO therapy, hyperparathyroidism, hypothyroidism, and antiphospholipid syndrome.
- As a free ion, Gd is highly toxic, but MRI contrast agents are chelated compounds that are excreted unchanged, almost exclusively by the kidney.

Free Gd^{3+} may dissociate from the chelate with prolonged exposure to Gd in those with CKD.

- Subsequently the free Gd^{3+} ion can be absorbed into tissues via transmetallation, wherein Gd^{3+} swaps places with endogenous metals such as zinc and copper. As Gd^{+3} closely approximate Ca^{2+} ions in size, it behaves as an effective calcium channel blocker, which is postulated to play a role in the pathogenesis.
- Inside the tissues, Gd is phagocytized by macrophages, which in turn attracts circulating fibrocytes positive for CD34. These fibrocytes transform to fibroblasts and subsequently cause fibrosis. Skin biopsy shows characteristic thick collagen bundles with surrounding clefts and a variable increase in dermal mucin and elastic fibers. Immunohistochemical staining of skin biopsy specimen reveals abundance of CD34+ dermal dendritic cells, with the dendritic processes aligning along elastic fibers and around collagen bundles in a dense network.
- Although the usual latent period between exposure to Gd and the manifestation of NSF is two to four weeks, cases have presented years after the exposure. The skin involvement is typically bilateral and the fibrotic features develop in a distal to proximal pattern in both upper and lower limbs. Fibrosis can affect internal organs like the lung and heart.
- Currently there is no effective treatment for NSF, and Gd-containing contrast agents should be avoided in CKD patients with GFR <30 ml and in AKI. Although there is no clear-cut evidence that haemodialysis after exposure diminishes the risk of NSF, if the use of Gd is indicated very strongly, the patient should have a session of haemodialysis immediately after exposure and preferably a repeat haemodialysis within 24 hours. Gd is removed poorly by peritoneal dialysis and these patients should have haemodialysis if exposed to Gd.

Management of Chronic Kidney Disease

Although CKD is not reversible and invariably progresses to ESRD, patients with a recent decrease in renal function may be suffering from an underlying reversible process, which, if identified and corrected, may result in some recovery of function. In general, management strategies aim at slowing the progression and management of complications that occur because of CKD.

Reversible Factors

- *Renal hypoperfusion*: hypovolaemia due to diarrhoea or vomiting, hypotension due to sepsis or cardiac event, infection or drugs that lower GFR (such as ACE inhibitors, ARBs, NSAIDs and diuretics) can all cause a reversible decline in renal function. Diagnosis often rests on history and clinical examination, and removal or correction of the underlying factor often leads to recovery of renal function.
- *Underlying urinary tract obstruction*: urinary tract obstruction should always be considered in a sudden unexplained rise in creatinine. Patients would have no changes in their urinalysis and initially may maintain their urine output. Ultrasound is usually the investigation of choice to rule out an obstruction.
- *Prevention of AKI*: patients with CKD are more susceptible to AKI. AKI can also accelerate the progression of CKD. Hence, the utmost care should be taken to avoid AKI in patients with CKD. All CKD patients should be counselled to refrain from intake of nephrotoxic medications. Administration of potentially nephrotoxic agents like iodinated contrast media should preferably be avoided. Phosphate-containing bowel cleansing agents should be avoided in patients with CKD. Any intercurrent illness that could possibly lead to AKI should be adequately addressed.

Slowing the Progression of Chronic Kidney Disease

Therapeutic Lifestyle Changes

Therapeutic lifestyle changes are advised for patients with CKD as well as those who are at high risk of CKD. All patients should be counselled regarding maintaining a body mass index (BMI) <25 kg/m², smoking cessation, moderate exercise, and reduced salt intake. A high-protein diet can lead to hyperfiltration and worsen the intraglomerular hypertension. Once the GFR is <30 ml/min/1.73 m², protein intake should be lowered to 0.8 g/kg/day. However, once patients are established on dialysis they are advised to have more protein, usually 1.2 g/kg/day for haemodialysis and slightly more for those on peritoneal dialysis.

All patients should receive expert counselling and individualized advice on nutrition depending on the stage of CKD. Malnutrition should be avoided as it can contribute to adverse outcomes, especially in the later stages of CKD and ESRD. Additional dietary restrictions for fluid and electrolytes are often required with the progression of CKD.

When to Refer to a Nephrologist

Referral to a nephrologist is not uniform across healthcare systems, even within countries. However, most authorities agree that referral to a nephrologist is warranted when eGFR is less than 30 ml/min/1.73 m². Patients at or below this level of eGFR are at increased risk of ESRD, and late referral in this group is associated with increased morbidity and mortality.

Control of Hypertension

In addition to lifestyle changes and salt restriction, pharmacotherapy should be employed for the reduction of blood pressure (BP). Lowering BP reduces the rate of progression to CKD as well as cardiovascular risk.

In patients with CKD who have proteinuria of more than 500 mg/day, an ACE inhibitor or ARB is recommended as the first-line therapy for hypertension because of their combined anti-hypertensive and anti-proteinuric effect. One would have to monitor these patients for worsening GFR and hyperkalaemia when started on an ACE inhibitor or ARB. Diuretics and non-dihydropyridine calcium channel blockers (e.g. diltiazem and verapamil) are possible second- and third-line agents. Thiazide diuretics become less effective when the GFR is less than 30 ml/min and in these patients loop diuretics are preferred as initial therapy.

In patients with CKD who have proteinuria and oedema, initial therapy usually consists of both an angiotensin inhibitor for renal protection and a loop diuretic for oedema. The addition of a thiazide diuretic to loop diuretic is useful in resistant cases.

In contrast to their renoprotective effects in proteinuric CKD, angiotensin inhibitors do *not* appear to be more beneficial than other anti-hypertensive agents in patients with non-proteinuric CKD.

The current evidence does not recommend combination therapy with ACE inhibitors and ARBs, as it is associated with a high risk for hyperkalaemia, SCD, and AKI. In elderly patients with CKD, a gradual escalation of anti-hypertensive agents is recommended, with due consideration for age, comorbidities, and drug tolerability [17, 18].

Glycaemic Control

Strict glycaemic control in diabetes patients can delay the onset of microvascular complications. In patients with diabetes mellitus, Haemoglobin A1c (HbA1c) should be kept to <7.0% to prevent or delay the progression of microvascular complications, including diabetic nephropathy [17]. HbA1c levels can sometimes be erroneously low in CKD due to the reduced life span of RBCs. As discussed previously, insulin often requires dose reductions in advanced renal failure. Sulfonylurea derivatives, like gilbenclamide and glimepiride, carry a higher risk of hypoglycaemia. Glipizide is the sulfonylurea of choice in diabetic patients with CKD. Metformin should not be used when the GFR is less than 30 ml/min/1.73m². In patients with GFR between 30 and 45 ml/min/1.73 m², metformin can be considered after assessing an individual patient's risk profile. Thiazolidinediones do not require dose modification, but may lead to troublesome salt and water restriction. Dipeptide peptidase-4 (DPP-4) inhibitors, except linagliptin, need dose modification in renal failure. Insulin secretagogues, like repaglinide and mitiglinide, are considered safe, whereas nateglinide might require dose modification due to renal excretion. Alpha glucosidase inhibitors should be avoided in patients with GFR less than 30 ml/min/1.73 m².

Dyslipidaemia

The primary aim of the treatment of dyslipidaemia is to reduce the morbidity and mortality from atherosclerosis. It is recommended to add a statin with or without ezetimibe for all CKD patients aged over 50 years who are not yet on dialysis. In adults aged 18–49 with CKD, statin therapy is recommended for patients with a history of coronary artery disease, diabetes mellitus and prior stroke and when the estimated 10-year incidence of coronary death or non-fatal myocardial infarction is >10%. Statin therapy should be continued even after transfer to dialysis. But it is not recommended to start statins afresh for dialysis patients if they had not received the same prior to initiation of dialysis. The current guidelines do not recommend any specific targets for cholesterol in patients with CKD [17]. Markedly elevated triglyceride levels warrant treatment with a fibrate, with doses adjusted for renal failure.

Cardiovascular Risk Reduction

Even though patients with CKD are at high risk for CVD, they often receive suboptimal cardio-protective strategies. There is a lack of data from randomized controlled trials, as most of these trials have excluded CKD patients owing to the high risk. Control of hypertension and dyslipidaemia leads to risk reduction; even though the therapeutic effects of statins might be attenuated in advanced CKD. Use of antiplatelet agents carries a higher risk of bleeding and hence is reserved for secondary prophylaxis. Use of beta-blockers is associated with a reduced mortality in CHF. The non-traditional risk factors are most often non-amenable to correction. Drugs like cinacalcet and paricalcitol have been tried to improve vascular calcifications and LVH, but the results are not entirely promising [17, 18, 19].

Management of Complications

Management of Haematological Complications

Anaemia

A baseline haematological workup should include complete blood count, reticulocyte count, iron studies, folate and B_{12} levels. However, it must be remembered that ferritin is an acute phase reactant and may be increased by inflammation. All correctable causes including iron and vitamin deficiencies should be identified and corrected [7, 20].

All adult CKD patients with serum ferritin <200 ng/ml and transferrin saturation <20% should receive oral or parenteral iron. Oral iron is relatively ineffective in patients on haemodialysis and peritoneal dialysis, partly because higher levels of hepcidin in these patients impede the absorption from the gut. The dialysis-associated iron losses usually exceed the absorptive capacity of the intestines. Erythropoiesis-stimulating agents (ESAs) should be started after ensuring adequate iron stores in patients with advanced CKD with haemoglobin levels less than 100 g/l. The various iron preparations and ESAs used for management of anaemia in CKD are given in Tables 7.7 and 7.8, respectively. As per the 2012 KDIGO guidelines, the ESA dose should be adjusted to maintain a haemoglobin concentration of 100–115 g/l. Caution should be exercised whilst prescribing ESA to patients with active/prior malignancy and stroke [7, 17, 20].

Complications of EPO or ESA Therapy

Patients receiving EPO therapy who have haemoglobin concentrations >130 g/l are at higher risk for increased cardiovascular mortality and stroke. EPO can lead to worsening of hypertension, as well as increased arteriovenous graft thrombosis, seizures, and probably accelerated progression of diabetic

Table 7.7 Parenteral iron preparations in chronic kidney disease

Name	Standard dose	Infusion rate	Adverse events
HMW iron dextran	1–3 g	2–4 hours	Anaphylactic reactions, hypotension, nausea, vomiting, cardiac arrest Life-threatening adverse drug events – 11.3 per million
LMW iron dextran	1–3 g	2–4 hours	Allergic reactions Life-threatening adverse drug events – 3.3 per million
Iron sucrose	200–300 mg	2–3 hours	Higher doses – associated with hypotension, nausea, low back ache
Ferric gluconate	125–250 mg	1–4 hours	Higher doses – associated with hypotension, acute onset of diarrhoea, swelling of extremities
Ferric carboxymaltose	750–1000 mg	15 minutes	Hypophophataemia Increased number of cardiovascular events and death rates in treated patients compared to controls
Ferumoxytol	510 mg	17–60 seconds	Well tolerated Rarely anaphylactic reactions Paramagnetic properties Can alter MRI signals up to 3 months
Iron isomaltoside	1.5–1.7 g	1 hour	Low incidence of adverse events Nausea, abdominal pain

HMW, high molecular weight; LMW, low molecular weight; MRI, magnetic resonance imaging.

Table 7.8 Erythropoiesis-stimulating agents in chronic kidney disease

Agent	Dose	Route and frequency of administration	$t_{1/2}$
Erythropoietin	50–100 units/kg	Thrice weekly IV/SC	4–11 hours (IV) 8 hours (SC)
Darbopoietin	0.45–0.75 mcg/kg	Once weekly/ every 2 weeks IV/SC	48 hours (SC) 25.3 hours (IV)
Methoxypolyethylene glycol epoietin-beta	0.6 mcg/kg	2–4 weeks IV/SC	130 hours (IV/SC)

IV, intravenous; SC, subcutaneous.

retinopathy. Pure red cell aplasia (PRCA) is a rare complication of EPO therapy, which was initially reported with a particular brand of EPO-alpha (Eprex), though subsequently it was reported with other formulations including EPO-beta [21]. The diagnostic criteria for PRCA are given in Table 7.9. Treatment usually includes cessation of EPO and sometimes immunosuppressants including steroids alone or in combination with cyclosporine, cyclophosphamide or intravenous immunoglobulin. Haematological recovery rates are 2% without immunosuppressive treatment, 52% following immunosuppressive treatment, and 95% following renal transplantation [21].

Table 7.9 Diagnostic criteria for epoetin-associated pure red cell aplasia

Major criteria (each of the major criteria should be identified in all cases)

- Treatment with epoetin for at least 3 weeks
- Drop of haemoglobin level of about 1 g/l/day without transfusions or transfusion need of about 1 unit/week to keep haemoglobin level stable
- Absolute reticulocyte count <10,000/microL (or reticulocyte percentage <0.5 percent; typically <0.2 percent)
- No major drop of white blood cell or platelet counts

Minor features: Skin and systemic allergic features

Confirmational investigations

- Bone marrow aspirate with normal cellularity and less than 5% erythroblasts with evidence of maturation block
- Serum assay shows presence of antierythropoietin antibodies and evidence of neutralizing ability

Table 7.10 Management of uraemic bleeding

- Desmopressin (0.3–0.4 mcg/kg IV or SC; single dose- effect begins in an hour and lasts for four to eight hours)
- Cryoprecipitate (10 bags IV every 12–24 hours)
- Conjugated oestrogens (0.6 mg/kg IV over 30–40 minutes once daily for 5 consecutive days)[a]
- Treatment of anaemia with recombinant human erythropoietin

[a]Action starts only after 5–7 days. IV, intravenous; SC, subcutaneous.

Uraemic Bleeding

The advent of ESA and modern dialysis techniques have reduced the incidence of uraemic bleeding, but it can sometimes be troublesome in patients undergoing surgery and other invasive procedures including renal biopsy. The management strategies of uraemic bleeding are summarized in Table 7.10 [22].

Treatment of CKD–MBD

The goals of therapy include prevention or reversal of hyperphosphataemia, optimizing vitamin D and calcium balance, prevention of hyperparathyroidism and vascular calcification, and maintenance of bone health. Hyperphosphataemia should be controlled by limiting dietary phosphate intake and administration of oral phosphate binders. Serum calcium should be corrected to the normal range. The therapy for adynamic bone disease involves stopping or decreasing drugs that cause PTH suppression. As per KDIGO guidelines, PTH values in ESRF patients should be maintained at two to nine times the upper limit of normal [17].

Major classes of drugs used to manage CKD–MBD include:

- Phosphate-binding resins
- Vitamin D analogues
- Calcimimetic agents

Phosphate-Binding Agents

The ability for phosphate restriction is at times limited by the need for adequate protein intake. The following phosphate-binding agents should be added if dietary restriction fails to control serum phosphate [23]:

- Calcium-containing binders
- Non-calcium-containing binders such as sevelamer, lanthanum carbonate, aluminium-containing binder (limited use as discussed below), magnesium salts, and iron compounds

Calcium-Containing Binders

Calcium-containing binders are effective and relatively inexpensive. Calcium acetate is more effective in binding intestinal phosphate than calcium carbonate and causes less hypercalcaemia. The major disadvantage of calcium-containing phosphate binders is the potential for hypercalcaemia and soft tissue calcification, CUA, and an increased chance of developing adynamic bone disease. The total calcium intake including medicinal sources should be limited to 1500–2000 mg/day.

Non-Calcium-Containing Binders

Sevelamer
Sevelamer hydrochloride (Renagel) and sevelamer carbonate (Renvela) are non-absorbable cationic polymers that bind phosphate in the intestinal lumen through ion exchange. Sevelamer hydrochloride, but not sevelamer carbonate, may induce metabolic acidosis due to the release of protons from the resin during phosphate binding.

Lanthanum Salts
Lanthanum carbonate is a potent phosphate binder with a lower incidence of hypercalcaemia and oversuppression of PTH in comparison to calcium-based

binders. It retains its ability to bind phosphate through a pH range of 3–7.

Aluminium Salts

Aluminium-containing binders, including aluminium hydroxide and aluminium carbonate, have a short disintegration time. Unlike calcium-containing binders, aluminium is active over a wider pH range. When used, their use should be limited to less than two to three months, the dose should be as low as possible, and concurrent administration of citrate-containing compounds avoided. Plasma aluminium concentrations should regularly be monitored because of the risk of aluminium toxicity, which may manifest as vitamin D-resistant osteomalacia, microcytic anaemia, and dementia.

Other Phosphate-Binding Agents: Magnesium and Iron Compounds

Magnesium-containing medications and polymeric compounds of iron and starch have also been shown to be useful as phosphate binders. Magnesium is believed to improve cardiovascular outcomes as well as inhibit vascular calcifications.

Ferric citrate and sucroferric oxyhydroxide are the two iron-based binders found to be safe and effective in decreasing serum phosphate. Sucroferric oxyhydroxide has a similar therapeutic efficacy to sevelamer carbonate, but with a lower pill burden and better adherence. It retains phosphate-binding capacity through the entire range of physiological pH. A potential advantage of using ferric citrate as a phosphate binder is that iron from the drug is partly absorbed and could lead to a 20% reduction in EPO need and a 40% reduction in intravenous iron need [24].

Vitamin D Sterols

Calcitriol, the active form of vitamin D (1,25-hydroxy-vitamin D3), and other synthetic analogues of vitamin D are used to reduce PTH, but they are associated with a risk of hypercalcaemia and hyperphosphataemia.

Calcimimetics

Calcimimetics mimic the action of serum calcium on the CaSR and therefore inhibit PTH secretion. Cinacalcet is the only drug approved for this class for use in patients on dialysis. A study involving 404 participants showed that although cinacalcet decreased PTH levels in predialysis CKD patients, its use was associated with hypocalcaemia and hyperphosphataemia. However, cinacalcet is sometimes used in predialysis patients with severe secondary hyperparathyroidism that is refractory to therapy with calcitriol or synthetic vitamin D analogues.

Even though cinacalcet is theoretically postulated to have beneficial effects on vascular calcification, this effect has not been conclusively proven so far [25].

Parathyroidectomy

Parathyroidectomy is indicated only in selected patients. The indications for parathyroidectomy are given in Table 7.11.

Treatment of Acidosis

Metabolic acidosis, which is common with GFR below 30 ml/min, increases the rate of progression of CKD and mortality. In addition, it potentiates bone demineralization and muscle catabolism. All patients with serum bicarbonate levels less than 20 mEq/l should receive alkali supplementation. Alkali supplementation is associated with less decline of GFR and improvement in nutritional indices and muscle strength [26, 27].

Vaccination

Whilst infections are a leading cause of hospitalizations and mortality in CKD patients (especially those with ESRD), these patients have a reduced response to vaccination because of the general suppression of the immune system associated with uraemia.

All CKD patients should be vaccinated against pneumococci, hepatitis B, and influenza [28]. Response to the influenza vaccine is somewhat comparable to that

---

Table 7.11 Indications of parathyroidectomy in chronic kidney disease

- Persistent hypercalcaemia
- Persistent hyperphosphataemia
- Persistently elevated parathyroid hormone (PTH) despite adequate treatment
- Progressive extra-skeletal calcifications including calciphylaxis
- Persistent pruritus
- Kidney transplant candidates with persistently elevated PTH and parathyroid hyperplasia; persistently elevated PTH with hypercalcaemia and unexplained worsening of allograft function

of the general population. The serological response to hepatitis B and the pneumococcal vaccine is inferior, characterized by lower seroconversion rates, lower peak antibody response, and accelerated loss of immunological response.

All CKD patients should receive annual vaccinations with inactivated influenza vaccine, before the start of the influenza season. Live influenza vaccine is contraindicated in CKD.

All patients on dialysis or with GFR <30 ml/min/1.73 m² and high risk of pneumococcal infection (patients with nephrotic syndrome, diabetes mellitus, solid organ transplant, HIV infection, receiving immunosuppression) should receive pneumococcal vaccination. These patients should receive a single injection of 13-valent pneumococcal conjugate vaccine (PCV13) followed by 23-valent pneumococcal polysaccharide vaccine (PPSV23) after eight weeks. Revaccination with PPSV23 should be done every five years.

The hepatitis B vaccination schedule is somewhat different from the general population. The seroconversion rates are extremely variable and may range from 60 to 90.5%. Patients should receive double the standard dose (40 μg) administered at 0, 1, 2, and 6 months (rather than 0, 1, and 6 months as in the general population). A special formulation of hepatitis B vaccine designed for haemodialysis patients and other immunocompromised adult patients contains an increased dosage and can be administered in a three-dose schedule (Recombivax HB, 40 μg/ml). Antibody titres should be monitored annually; booster doses will be required if the anti-HBs titres fall to less than 10 mIU/ml. It may be preferable to give hepatitis B vaccination earlier to maximize the chances of achieving protective immunity.

Preparation for Renal Replacement Therapy

Patients with progressive and irreversible CKD should be managed in a multidisciplinary care setting with access to dietary counselling, counselling about different dialysis modalities, transplant, vascular access surgery, and psychosocial care. For patients who opt for haemodialysis, the forearm veins should be preserved by avoiding venepunctures and cannulations. Arteriovenous fistula is the preferred access and might require four to eight weeks for maturation; it should be planned sufficiently early to allow time for maturation. Living donor preemptive renal transplantation in adults should be considered when the GFR is <20 ml/min/1.73 m², with evidence of progressive CKD. A multidisciplinary approach to pre-ESRD

care has been found to be associated with better quality of life, better preservation of GFR and improved nutritional status.

References

1. (2011). 2013 Jan). Chapter 1.Definition and classification of CKD. *Kidney Int. Suppl.* 3 (1): 19–62. Available from http://kdigo.org/home/guidelines/ckd-evaluation-management/.
2. Parsa, A., Kao, W.H., Xie, D. et al. (2013). APOL1 risk variants, race, and progression of chronic kidney disease. *N. Engl. J. Med.* 369 (23): 2183–2196.
3. Taal, M.W. and Brenner, B.M. (2012). Adaptation to NephronLoss and mechanisms of progression in chronic kidney disease. In: *Brenner and Rector's the Kidney* (eds. M.W. Taal, G.M. Chertow, P.A. Marsden, et al.), 1918–1927. Philadelphia: Elsevier Saunders.
4. Collins, A.J., Foley, R.N., Herzog, C. et al. (2013). US renal data system 2012 annual data report. *Am. J. Kidney Dis.* 61: 1–476.
5. Kendrick, J. and Chonchol, M.B. (2008 Dec). Nontraditional risk factors for cardiovascular disease in patients with chronic kidney disease. *Nat. Clin. Pract. Nephrol.* 4 (12): 672–681.
6. Cai, Q., Mukku, V.K., and Ahmad, M. (2013 Nov). Coronary artery disease in patients with chronic kidney disease: a clinical update. *Curr. Cardiol. Rev.* 9 (4): 331–339.
7. Babitt, J.L. and Lin, H.Y. (2012). Mechanisms of anemia in CKD. *J. Am. Soc. Nephrol.* 23 (10): 1631–1634.
8. Tsuchiya, K. and Nitta, K. (2013 Feb). Hepcidin is a potential regulator of iron status in chronic kidney disease. *Ther. Apher. Dial.* 17 (1): 1–8.
9. Icardi, A., Paoletti, E., De Nicola, L. et al. (2013 Jul). Renal anaemia and EPO hyporesponsiveness associated with vitamin D deficiency: the potential role of inflammation. *Nephrol. Dial. Transplant.* 28 (7): 1672–1679.
10. Moe, S., Drüeke, T., Cunningham, J. et al. (2006). Kidney disease: improving global outcomes (KDIGO) definition, evaluation and classification of renal osteodystrophy; a position statemet from KDIGO. *Kidney Int.* 69: 1945–1953.
11. Lewis, R. (2012 Sep). Mineral and bone disorders in chronic kidney disease: new insights into mechanism and management. *Ann. Clin. Biochem.* 49 (Pt 5): 432–440.
12. Moe, S.M. and Sprague, S.M. (2012). Chronic kidney disease – mineral bone disorder. In: *Brenner and Rector's the Kidney* (eds. M.W. Taal, G.M.

Chertow, P.A. Marsden, et al.), 2021–2051. Philadelphia: Elsevier Saunders.

13. Tamura, M.K. (2012). Neurologic aspects of kidney disease. In: *Brenner and Rector's the Kidney* (eds. M.W. Taal, G.M. Chertow, P.A. Marsden, et al.), 2138–2156. Philadelphia: Elsevier Saunders.

14. Mak, R.H. and DeFronzo, R.A. (1992). Glucose and insulin metabolism in uremia. *Nephron* 61 (4): 377.

15. Carrero, J.J., Stenvinkel, P., and Lindholm, B. (2012). Endocrine aspects of chronic kidney disease. In: *Brenner and Rector's the Kidney* (eds. M.W. Taal, G.M. Chertow, P.A. Marsden, et al.), 2122–2137. Philadelphia: Elsevier Saunders.

16. Kuypers, D.R.J. (2009). Skin problems in chronic kidney disease. *Nat. Clin. Pract. Nephrol.* 5: 157–170.

17. (2013). Chapter 3: Management of progression and complications of CKD. *Kidney Int. Suppl.* 3: 73–90. http://kdigo.org/home/guidelines/ckd-evaluation-management.

18. (2012). KDIGO clinical practice guideline for the management of blood pressure in chronic kidney disease. *Kidney Int. Suppl.* 2: 405–414. http://kdigo.org/home/guidelines/blood-pressure-in-ckd.

19. Elliott, M.K., McCaughan, J.A., and Fogarty, D.G. (2014). Do patients with chronic kidney disease get optimal cardiovascular risk reduction? *Curr. Opin. Nephrol. Hypertens.* 23 (3): 267–274.

20. Brugnara, C. and Eckardt, K.U. (2012). Hematologic aspects of kidney disease. In: *Brenner and Rector's the Kidney* (eds. M.W. Taal, G.M. Chertow, P.A. Marsden, et al.), 2081–2120. Philadelphia: Elsevier Saunders.

21. Bennett, C.L., Cournoyer, D., Carson, K.R. et al. (2005 Nov 15). Long-term outcome of individuals with pure red cell aplasia and antierythropoietin antibodies in patients treated with recombinant epoetin: a follow-up report from the research on adverse drug events and reports (RADAR) project. *Blood* 106 (10): 3343–3347.

22. Hedges, S.J., Dehoney, S.B., Hooper, J.S. et al. (2007 Mar). Evidence-based treatment recommendations for uremic bleeding. *Nat. Clin. Pract. Nephrol.* 3 (3): 138–153.

23. Emmett, M. (2004 Sep). A comparison of clinically useful phosphorus binders for patients with chronic kidney failure. *Kidney Int. Suppl.* (90): S25–S32.

24. Negri, A.L. and Ureña Torres, P.A. (2015 Apr). Iron-based phosphate binders: do they offer advantages over currently available phosphate binders? *Clin. Kidney J.* 8 (2): 161–167.

25. Drüeke, T.B. and Ritz, E. (2009 Jan). Treatment of secondary hyperparathyroidism in CKD patients with cinacalcet and/or Vitamin D derivatives. *Clin. J. Am. Soc. Nephrol.* 4 (1): 234–241.

26. Yaqoob, M.M. (2013 Mar). Treatment of acidosis in CKD. *Clin. J. Am. Soc. Nephrol.* 8 (3): 342–343.

27. Alcázar Arroyo, R. (2008). Electrolyte and acid-base balance disorders in advanced chronic kidney disease. *Nefrologia* 28 (Suppl 3): 87–93. [Article in Spanish].

28. Centers for Disease Control and Prevention (2012). *Guidelines for vaccinating kidney dialysis patients and patients with chronic kidney disease.* Atlanta, GA: CDC. Available from http://www.cdc.gov/dialysis/PDFs/Vaccinating_Dialysis_Patients_and_patients_dec2012.pdf.

Questions and Answers

Questions

1. Which of the following is not responsible for hyperkalaemia in a patient with advanced CKD secondary to diabetic nephropathy?
   a. High potassium diet
   b. Metabolic acidosis
   c. Treatment with ACE-I
   d. Hypoaldosteronism
   e. Low K clearance due to CKD

2. Dialysis related amyloidosis (DRA) classically presents with:
   a. Heart failure
   b. Back pain
   c. Non-traumatic fractures of small bones of hands
   d. Peripheral neuropathy
   e. Shoulder pain

3. Which among the following vaccines is contraindicated in patients with CKD?
   a. Pneumococcal conjugate vaccine
   b. Varicella vaccine
   c. Injectable polio vaccine
   d. Live attenuated Influenza vaccine

4. Identify the correct statement regarding anaemia of CKD:
   a. Hepcidin causes mobilization of iron from reticuloendothelial system
   b. Erythropoietin deficiency leads to decreased recruitment of RBC precursors
   c. Hepcidin can decrease iron absorption from the intestine
   d. RBC survival is normal in uraemia

5. It is thought that the initial event that triggers the development of CKD MBD is:
   a. Hyperparathyroidism
   b. Low serum calcium
   c. Hyperphosphataemia
   d. Low potassium
   e. High potassium

Answers

1. e. The ability to maintain potassium excretion at near-normal levels is generally maintained in patients with CKD and they tend to have augmented potassium excretion in the GI tract. High potassium diet, metabolic acidosis, increased tissue breakdown, and hypoaldosteronism due to ACE-I or renal tubular acidosis type IV (which is common in diabetics) can all contribute to hyperkalaemia in these patients.

2. e. Patients affected with DRA most commonly present with shoulder pain. The amyloid protein in DRA is composed primarily of beta2-microglobulin and the condition is almost exclusively seen in ESRD patients on dialysis. The incidence of DRA is now much lower than had been reported previously due to the increased use of high-flux biocompatible dialyzers with enhanced clearance of beta2-microglobulin.

3. d. As a rule, live vaccines are contraindicated in CKD, whereas inactivated and subunit vaccines can be given. However, MMR and varicella vaccines are attenuated viral vaccines and can be given in CKD unless the patient is on concomitant immunosuppressive therapy All CKD patients should receive annual vaccinations with inactivated influenza vaccine.

4. c. Hepcidin blocks mobilization of iron from the reticuloendothelial system. Hepcidin also decreases the influx of iron from the intestinal cells by decreasing the levels of intestinal iron transporter ferroportin. The average RBC life span is reduced by 50% in advanced uraemia. Erythropoietin is a survival factor for erythroblasts, the primary function being to prevent apoptosis of RBC precursors.

5. c. A tendency to phosphate retention, beginning early in CKD due to a decrease in the filtered phosphate load, is thought to play a central role in the development of secondary hyperparathyroidism and the associated CKD-MBD. Hyperphosphataemia is also partially responsible for low serum calcium in these patients.

8

Nephrotic Syndrome

Pankaj Hari and Surjit Tarafdar

Summary

Minimal Change Disease and Focal Segmental Glomerulosclerosis

- Minimal change disease (MCD) is characterized by diffuse foot process effacement on electron microscopy (EM) in the absence of any findings on light microscopy or immunofluorescence (IF)
- About 90% of nephrotic syndrome in children is caused by MCD, whilst it is seen in only 10–15% of adults with nephrotic syndrome
- Focal segmental glomerulosclerosis (FSGS) is a histological pattern of glomerular injury characterized by sclerosis in parts (segmental) of some (focal) glomeruli and is the commonest cause of nephrotic syndrome in adults of African origin
- Both MCD and FSGS are associated with diffuse foot process effacement; due to the focal nature of FSGS, it may be mistaken for MCD if not enough glomeruli are visualized in biopsy
- MCD shows good response to treatment with corticosteroids, with children showing better response than adults
- FSGS may be primary or secondary to genetic mutations in podocyte proteins, viral infections, drug toxicity, maladaptive response to reduced number of functioning nephrons, and increased haemodynamic stress on initially normal renal mass
- 40–60% of primary FSGS cases achieve partial or complete remission with corticosteroids
- About 30% of FSGS recurs in the transplanted kidney

Membranous Nephropathy and Membranoproliferative Glomerulonephritis

- Membranous nephropathy (MN) is characterized by typical subepithelial electron-dense deposits on EM (with absence of endothelial or mesangial changes) which stain for immunoglobulin G and complement components on IF
- MN is the commonest cause of nephrotic syndrome in the Caucasian adult population
- Whilst up to two-thirds of cases of MN are idiopathic, the condition may be associated with infections, drugs, autoimmune conditions or malignancies
- 70% of cases of idiopathic MN have circulating autoantibodies against phospholipase A2 receptor 1 (PLA2R1) located on the surface of podocytes
- Membranoproliferative glomerulonephritis (MPGN), which is also called mesangiocapillary glomerulonephritis, is characterized by increased mesangial and endocapillary hypercellularity (proliferative lesions), with thickening of the glomerular basement membrane (GBM) often leading to a double-contoured appearance
- MPGN is classified as immune complex–mediated or complement-mediated, with the former having a strong association with hepatitis C
- MPGN may present as microscopic haematuria and non-nephrotic proteinuria (35%), as nephrotic syndrome with minimally depressed renal function (35%), as chronically progressive glomerulonephritis (20%) or as rapidly progressive glomerulonephritis (10%)

Lecture Notes Nephrology: A Comprehensive Guide to Renal Medicine, First Edition. Edited by Surjit Tarafdar.
© 2020 John Wiley & Sons Ltd. Published 2020 by John Wiley & Sons Ltd.

Nephrotic syndrome is a constellation of clinical and biochemical features, including heavy proteinuria (>3.5 g/day), hypoalbuminaemia (<25 g/l), and oedema. Patients suffering from nephrotic syndrome are more prone to hyperlipidaemia and accelerated atherosclerosis, thromboembolism, and malnutrition, and have an increased susceptibility to infections. Urine in nephrotic syndrome characteristically does not have casts or dysmorphic red blood cells.

The following conditions can lead to presentation with nephrotic syndrome.

Primarily glomerular pathology:

- Mininal change disease (MCD)
- Focal segmental glomerulosclerosis (FSGS)
- Membranous nephropathy (MN)
- Membranoproliferative glomerulonephritis (MPGN)/ mesangiocapillary glomerulonephritis (MCGN)

Systemic diseases:

- Diabetes mellitus
- Amyloidosis

In adults, FSGS is the commonest cause of nephrotic syndrome worldwide and especially in those of African origin, whilst MN is the commonest in Caucasian males. On the other hand, MCD is responsible for up to 90% of nephrotic syndrome in children younger than 10 years of age, 50–70% of older children, and 10–15% of adults.

It is important to remember that acute kidney injury (AKI) is not very common in nephrotic syndrome. When patients with nephrotic syndrome present with AKI, it is usually due to one of the following factors:

- Hypovolaemia due to aggressive diuresis
- Interstitial nephritis from diuretics
- Angiotensin-converting enzyme (ACE) inhibitor or angiotensin II receptor blocker (ARB) induced AKI
- Intrarenal oedema leading to compression of tubules
- Rarely, bilateral renal vein thrombosis
- Other superimposed renal pathology

Amongst these causes of nephrotic syndrome, childhood MCD has the lowest risk of progression to chronic kidney disease (CKD).

Pathogenesis of the Components of Nephrotic Syndrome

Proteinuria

Defect in the glomerular filtration barrier leads to the leakage of serum proteins into urine. Normal urine formation involves filtration across the following three layers (Figure 8.1):

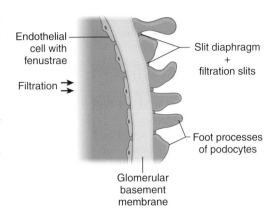

Figure 8.1 Glomerular filtration barrier.

- Endothelium – lined on the luminal side by the negatively charged protein podocalyxin, has pores which are 50–100 nm in diameter.
- Glomerular basement membrane (GBM) – which is rich in type IV collagen, laminin 11, and the negatively charged heparin sulphate.
- 30–40 nm filtration slits (gaps between podocytes) bridged by the negatively charged nephrin-rich slit diaphragms with 8 nm pores.

Albumin molecule with a diameter of 7.2 nm would have been totally filtered by the above barrier (with the smallest pores, i.e. slit diaphragms being 8 nm sized) were it not for the fact that the negative charges on all the three layers in this barrier repel the negatively charged albumin. Glomerular proteinuria can be caused by the lack of negative charges on the filtration barrier (Figure 8.1), as well as disease processes causing abnormal physical widening of the filtration pore.

Hypoalbuminaemia and Hyperlipidaemia

Whilst the liver increases the synthesis of albumin to compensate for hypoalbuminaemia, the urinary losses are usually more than the hepatic increase in albumin production. Hypoalbuminaemia causes the liver to increase lipoprotein synthesis in an attempt to correct the low plasma oncotic pressure, leading to the development of hyperlipidaemia.

Oedema

Traditionally, oedema in nephrotic syndrome has been postulated to be due to the movement of fluid from vascular space to the interstitium due to low plasma oncotic pressure. However, now we know that it is the transcapillary oncotic pressure gradient (plasma minus interstitium), rather than just the plasma oncotic pressure, that determines the movement of fluid. In nephrotic syndrome hypoalbuminaemia leads to less albumin leaking out of the vascular space, causing the interstitial oncotic pressure to fall. The parallel fall in both the plasma oncotic pressure and interstitial oncotic pressure minimizes the change in the transcapillary oncotic pressure gradient, and therefore minimizes fluid movement out of the vascular space. Thus, other factors are involved in the pathogenesis of oedema in nephrotic syndrome. The following two mechanisms are believed to coexist and lead to oedema in these patients:

- *Underfill theory*: fluid movement from the intravascular to the extravascular space as a consequence of low plasma oncotic pressure in the early phase of nephrotic syndrome (when the interstitial oncotic pressure is still normal) leads to decrease in intravascular volume. The resultant stimulation of the renin–angiotensin system (RAS) leads to aldosterone-induced sodium retention in the distal tubule. Water is passively reabsorbed along with sodium in the tubules. This makes more water available in the intravascular space to leak out to the interstitium.
- *Overfill theory*: many patients with nephrotic syndrome are unable to excrete sodium efficiently due to increased sodium reabsorption in the distal tubule, secondary to excessive stimulation of the epithelial sodium channel (ENAC) by filtered proteolytic enzymes (which enter the tubular lumen due to glomerular filtration). This in turn leads to increased intravascular volume and suppression of both the RAS and anti-diuretic hormone production. Elevated intravascular volume in the presence of low plasma oncotic pressure leads to transudation of fluid from the intravascular space to the interstitium. These patients are more prone to hypertension.

If the underfill theory was the only or predominant mechanism leading to oedema, diuretics would lead to AKI by worsening the already low intravascular volume. However, most of these patients tolerate diuretic therapy well, indicating a major role for the overfill theory in the pathogenesis of oedema.

Hypercoagulability

The incidence of both venous and arterial thrombosis is almost eight times higher in patients with nephrotic syndrome compared to the general population [1, 2].

Risk of thrombosis is highest in MN. Whilst the exact mechanism leading to the increased predisposition to hypercoagulability is not very well understood, decreased levels of antithrombin and plasminogen (due to urinary losses) and increased hepatic synthesis of procoagulant proteins are postulated to play roles.

Increased Infections

Increased urinary loss of opsonizing factors is postulated to lead to increased risk of infections in this patient group [3]. In addition, ascites and pleural effusions provide a good culture medium for the bacteria to grow easily.

Minimal Change Disease

MCD is defined by characteristic foot process fusion of podocytes seen on electron microscopy (EM), with normal-looking glomeruli on light microscopy (LM) and absence of findings on immunofluorescence (IF) microscopy. Since both MCD and primary FSGS are associated with diffuse foot process effacement in the absence of immune deposits on IF, there is a debate as to whether the two diseases are two ends of the spectrum of a same disease process, or whether they represent separate pathogenic entities [4]. However, as explained later, whilst MCD is associated with increased CD80 expression in podocytes, elevated circulating soluble urokinase-type plasminogen activator receptor (suPAR) levels seem to play the major pathogenic role in primary FSGS. Also, FSGS is generally less steroid sensitive than MCD.

MCD mostly presents with sudden onset over days to weeks, in contrast to the other causes of nephrotic syndrome where the presentation is generally much more gradual.

Aetiology and Pathogenesis

Whilst most cases of MCD are idiopathic, some known associations include:

- *Drugs*: non-steroidal anti-inflammatory drugs (NSAIDs), Interferon-alpha, antibiotics (ampicillin, rifampicin, cephalosporin), pamidronate, lithium, D-penicillamine, and sulfasalazine.
- *Neoplasm*: Hodgkin lymphoma and less commonly non-Hodgkin lymphoma (NHL) and leukaemia.
- *Allergy*: atopy/asthma/eczema history in up to 30% [5].

Multiple studies have established that podocyte dysfunction is the key factor in the pathogenesis of

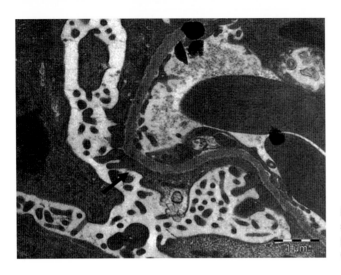

Figure 8.2 Electron microscopy picture showing extensive glomerular foot process effacement in minimal change disease.

both MCD and FSGS, hence these diseases are also referred to as podocytopathies.

Although the exact underlying cause of MCD is unclear, it is now accepted that injury to the slit diaphragm of podocytes is the key event leading to proteinuria. It is postulated that activated T-helper 2 cells (Th2) secrete excess interleukin-13 (IL-13). IL-13 (which is also associated with allergic states) in turn induces excess CD80 expression in podocytes. CD80 is presumed to lead to:

- Decreased expression of the negatively charged protein nephrin found on the slit diaphragm; loss of negative charge on the slit diaphragm allows the negatively charged albumin to leak out of glomerular capillaries.
- Foot process fusion (characteristically seen in MCD).

Whilst urinary CD80 is increased in patients with MCD, it is rarely detected in the urine of patients with other causes of nephrotic syndrome [6].

Pathology

MCD is characterized by normal-appearing glomeruli on LM and IF examination. The only positive findings are seen in EM, which characteristically shows marked foot process effacement of podocytes (Figure 8.2).

Focal Segmental Glomerulosclerosis

FSGS is a histological pattern of glomerular injury characterized by sclerosis in parts (segmental) of some (focal) glomeruli. It is the commonest cause of nephrotic syndrome in adult population of African origin.

Whilst the disease is focal and segmental at the outset, uncontrolled FSGS usually leads to global glomerular sclerosis. Differentiating between primary and secondary FSGS is important, as primary FSGS is potentially treatable with immunosuppression in up to 50% of patients, whereas in secondary FSGS prognosis is linked to treatment of the underlying disorder.

Patients with primary FSGS are more likely to present with acute to subacute nephrotic syndrome, whilst those with secondary FSGS often present in a more chronic pattern, with sub-nephrotic (<3.5 g/day) proteinuria or nephrotic-range proteinuria and a normal serum albumin concentration with or without oedema (i.e. without full-blown nephrotic syndrome). Histologically podocyte effacement is generally more global in primary FSGS (>80%), whilst it is generally more segmental in secondary FSGS (<80%).

Many of the non-sclerotic glomeruli in FSGS show uniform foot process effacement similar to MCD and hence there is the debate as to whether FSGS and MCD represent the same disease process. This argument is also strengthened by the fact that by virtue of being focal, FSGS may be misdiagnosed as MCD on biopsy if the non-sclerosed glomeruli are examined. However, pathogenetically the two diseases appear to be distinct, as MCD is characteristically associated with an increased CD80 level in the urine, whilst, as will be discussed later, primary FSGS is associated with a raised plasma level of soluble urokinase-type plasminogen activator receptor (suPAR).

Aetiology and Pathogenesis

FSGS may be primary (idiopathic) or secondary to various conditions such as genetic mutations in podocyte proteins, viral infections, drug toxicity, maladaptive response to reduced number of functioning nephrons and increased haemodynamic stress on initially normal renal mass (Table 8.1).

Table 8.1 Aetiology of focal segmental glomerulosclerosis (FSGS)

Idiopathic (primary) FSGS

Familial FSGS

Due to mutations

Nephrin (NPHS1)

Podocin (NPHS2)

CD2-associated protein (CD2AP)

Transient-receptor potential ion channel 6 (TRCP6)

Alpha-actinin-4 (ACTN4)

Infections

Parvovirus B19

HIV

Drugs

Lithium

Interferon-alpha

Heroin

Pamidronate

Sirolimus

Adaptive (secondary) FSGS

Reduced renal mass

Unilateral renal agenesis/nephrectomy

Reflux nephropathy

Very low birthweight

Renal dysplasia

Transplant glomerulopathy

Any advanced renal disease with reduction in functioning nephrons, e.g. diabetic nephropathy, lupus or vasculitis

Initially normal renal mass

Hypertension

Obesity

Increased lean body mass, e.g. body builders

Anabolic steroids

Cyanotic congenital heart disease

Sickle cell anaemia

Primary Focal Segmental Glomerulosclerosis

Injury to the podocyte because of a circulating factor or factors seems to be the primary defect in primary FSGS. Plasma level of suPAR, which is implicated in the induction of FSGS, is found to be raised in upto two-third of patients with primary FSGS. Circulating suPAR activates podocyte beta(3) integrin in both native and grafted kidneys in mice, causing foot process effacement, proteinuria, and FSGS-like glomerulopathy [7].

FSGS recurs in approximately 30% of transplanted kidneys and may lead to graft loss [8]. Increased serum levels of suPAR before renal transplantation are associated with an increased risk of recurrent disease in the allograft. Plasmapheresis after transplantation in recurrent FSGS leads to decreased suPAR and improvement in proteinuria.

Expression of a specific microRNA called miR-193a can also produce FSGS in mice [9]. Mechanistically miR-193a inhibits the expression of a variety of genes that are important for podocyte function, including production of the negatively charged podocyte protein nephrin. Expression of miR-193a in podocytes was not found in mouse models of suPAR-induced FSGS, suggesting that they are distinct mechanisms leading to FSGS.

Secondary Focal Segmental Glomerulosclerosis

The primary site of injury in secondary FSGS, as in primary FSGS, is the podocyte. Glomerulosclerosis of secondary FSGS usually results from:

- Adaptive response to glomerular hypertrophy/hyperfiltration, e.g. diabetic nephropathy.
- Scarring due to previous injury, e.g. lupus nephritis.
- Reduced renal mass, e.g. reflux nephropathy, surgical ablation.
- Direct toxic injury to podocytes, e.g. drugs like heroin, interferon, etc.

Polymorphisms in the apolipoprotein L1 (APOL1) gene on chromosome 22 has been shown to be associated with the development of FSGS in people of African origin. Polymorphisms in APOL1 appear to be expressed exclusively in individuals of African descent and have not been identified in any individuals from Europe, Japan or China [10]. APOL1 provides innate immunity against trypanosomiasis.

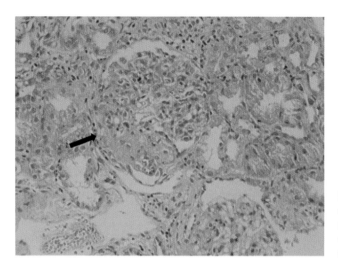

Figure 8.3 Light microscopy picture showing focal sclerosis (arrow pointing at accumulation of extracellular matrix with obliteration of capillary lumen) in focal segmental glomerulosclerosis (FSGS).

Pathology

FSGS is characterized by focal (involving some but not all) and segmental (involving a portion of the glomerular tuft) sclerosis of glomeruli. The sclerosed segment shows collapse of the capillary tuft and increase in matrix deposition, whilst the uninvolved area of the glomerulus is essentially normal on LM (Figure 8.3).

On EM, primary FSGS is associated with comparatively more diffuse foot process fusion than in the secondary forms.

Based on LM findings, both primary and secondary FSGS are classified into the following histological variants:

- *Classic FSGS, also called FSGS NOS (not otherwise specified)*: this is the commonest variant of FSGS and requires the exclusion of the other four more specific subtypes. On LM, classic FSGS is characterized by segmental areas of mesangial collapse and sclerosis in some, but not all, glomeruli.
- *Collapsing variant of FSGS*: in collapsing FSGS at least one glomerulus displays segmental or global obliteration of the glomerular capillary lumen by implosive wrinkling and collapse of the GBM, along with podocyte hypertrophy and hyperplasia. It is most often seen in association with HIV infection, when it is called HIV nephropathy. It can be seen in primary or non-HIV-associated FSGS as well [11]. Patients with the collapsing variant usually have poor prognosis.
- *Tip variant*: the tip variant is characterized by segmental sclerosis involving the tip domain; that is, the outer 25% of the tuft next to the origin of the proximal tubule. The tip lesion may identify patients who are more likely to present abruptly and are also more likely to respond to glucocorticoid therapy than patients with the other FSGS variants (suggesting a resemblance to MCD).
- *Perihilar variant*: the perihilar variant consists of perihilar sclerosis and hyalinosis in more than 50% of segmentally sclerotic glomeruli. It is more likely to be seen in secondary FSGS associated with increased glomerular capillary pressure, such as renal agenesis or diabetic nephropathy.
- *Cellular variant*: the cellular variant is characterized by the presence of at least one glomerulus with segmental endocapillary hypercellularity that occludes the capillary lumen. Other glomeruli may exhibit findings consistent with classic FSGS.

Whilst these histological subtypes of FSGS have no therapeutic implication, it is usually accepted that the tip variant has the best prognosis, whilst the collapsing variant has the worst [12]. Tip variant also shows better steroid responsiveness than the other subtypes.

Membranous Nephropathy

MN is the commonest glomerular cause of nephrotic syndrome in the adult Caucasian population and is rarely seen in children. MN is characterized by typical subepithelial electron-dense deposits on EM (with absence of subendothelial deposits), which stain for immunoglobulin (IgG) and complement components on IF. LM reveals thickening of the GBM with a characteristic absence of mesangial or endocapillary hypercellularity.

Although traditional teaching often mentions that one-third each of patients with MN have spontaneous remission, develop CKD (but not end-stage renal disease, ESRD) or develop ESRD, one must understand that chance of remission is inversely related to the amount of proteinuria. As discussed in the treatment section, whilst only 8% of those with proteinuria of <4 g are likely to develop CKD, up to 75% of those with proteinuria of >8 g develop CKD.

Aetiology and Pathogenesis

Up to two-thirds of cases of MN are primary or idiopathic. The following conditions and agents are associated with MN (Table 8.2):

- *Autoimmune disorders*: systemic lupus erythematosus (common), rheumatoid arthritis, Sjögren's syndrome, Grave's disease, dermatomyositis, mixed connective tissue disorder, systemic sclerosis
- *Infections*: hepatitis B (common), hepatitis C, schistosomiasis, malaria, leprosy, filiariasis
- *Drugs*: gold, penicillamine, NSAIDs, captopril and anti-TNF agents (adalimumab, etanercept and infliximab)
- *Malignancy*: solid organ tumours, e.g. prostate, lung or colon; less commonly haematological malignancies like chronic lymphocytic leukaemia (CLL)
- *Others*: renal transplant, sickle cell disease, sarcoidosis

In regions endemic for hepatitis B infection, up to 40% of children with nephrotic syndrome may have hepatitis B–related MN [13].

Experimental models of MN suggest that the subepithelial immune deposits develop because of movement of IgG across the GBM to bind with antigens on the foot processes of podocytes. These antigens might be endogenous or they may be small, positively charged molecules which by virtue of size and charge manage to cross the negatively charged GBM. The rat model of Heymann nephritis closely resembles the human disease both histologically and clinically [14]. In Heymann nephritis, circulating antibodies target the glycoprotein megalin (gp330) on podocyte foot processes, leading to the development of MN.

In humans, IgG is postulated to cross the GBM to bind to antigens on the podocyte foot processes. This antigen–antibody interaction leads to the activation of complement and subsequent formation of C5b-9 that enters into the podocytes. Although the C5b-9 level inside the podocytes is not enough to cause cell death, this sublytic level of C5b-9 causes the podocytes to release proteases and oxidants that damage the underlying GBM.

The antigen–antibody complexes are shed to form subepithelial deposits between the podocytes and the GBM.

Upregulation of the podocyte production of transforming growth factor B2 (TGFB2) as well as an increase in the number of receptors for TGFB2 (under the influence of C5b-9) leads to overproduction of extracellular matrix molecules that accumulate between and around the immune deposits, leading to the characteristic 'spike and dome' and thickening of GBM.

Phospholipase A2 receptor (PLA2R) is postulated to be a podocyte antigen which can lead to primary MN. Antibody to PLA2R is seen in up to 70% of

Table 8.2 Secondry causes of membranous nephropathy (MN)

Autoimmune diseases	Systemic lupus erythematosus (SLE)
	Rheumatoid arthritis
	Dermatomyositis
	Mixed connective tissue disorder
	Sjögren's syndrome
	Systemic sclerosis
	Hashimoto's disease
	Grave's disease
Infections	Hepatitis B
	Hepatitis C
	Schistosomiasis
	Malaria
	Leprosy
	Filariasis
Drugs	Gold
	Penicillamine
	Non-steroidal anti-inflammatory drugs
	Captopril
Malignancy	Solid organ tumours, e.g. prostate, lung or colon
	Less frequently haematological malignancy, e.g. chronic lymphocytic leukaemia
Others	Renal transplant
	Sickle cell disease
	Sarcoidosis

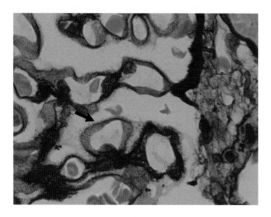

Figure 8.4 Light microscopy picture showing subepithelial spikes along the glomerular basement membrane on silver methenamine stain in membranous nephropathy.

patients with primary MN, but not in secondary MN. Thrombospondin type-1 domain-containing 7A (THSD7A) may be the responsible antigen in approximately 10% of patients with idiopathic MN who are negative for anti-PLA2R antibodies.

It must be mentioned here that although the characteristic IgG subclass seen in primary MN is IgG4, amongst the four subclasses of IgG this is the least likely to activate complement. So, that raises the question as to whether there is a yet undiscovered mechanism or mechanisms involved in the crucial step of complement activation in primary MN.

Lupus-induced MN is usually associated with IgG1 or IgG3 along with IgA, IgM, and C1q. The IgG pattern seen with malignancy-associated MN is usually IgG1 or IgG2.

Pathology

The characteristic abnormality on LM is diffuse global capillary wall thickening due to subepithelial immune complex deposition. The newly formed GBM around the unstained immune complex deposit is stained black and appears as 'spikes' in silver methenamine stain (Figure 8.4). Eventually, the spikes extend all around the deposits to give a dome-like appearance. Over time, the GBM is overtly thickened and spikes become less apparent. The mesangial matrix and cellularity are characteristically normal and the capillary loops are patent. Granular capillary wall staining for IgG and C3 is the characteristic finding seen on IF. EM reveals subepithelial electron-dense immune deposits.

Membranoproliferative Glomerulonephritis (MPGN) or Mesangiocapillary Glomerulonephritis (MCGN)

MPGN, or MCGN, is characterized by increased mesangial and endocapillary hypercellularity (proliferative lesions), with thickening of the GBM often leading to a double-contoured appearance. MPGN accounts for approximately 7–10% of all cases of nephrotic syndrome undergoing renal biopsy and is an important cause of ESRD. MPGN may present as microscopic haematuria and non-nephrotic proteinuria (35%), as nephrotic syndrome with minimally depressed renal function (35%), as chronically progressive GN (20%) or as rapidly progressive glomerulonephritis i.e. RPGN (10%). MPGN may be idiopathic or secondary to chronic infections, cryoglobulinaemia or systemic autoimmune disorders – all these conditions result in aberrant immune complex formation. Cryoglobulinaemia and hepatitis C are the commonest associations seen with MPGN.

Initially MCGN was classified into three types based on EM:

- *Type 1*: characterized by immune complex deposition in the subendothelial space (causing capillary wall thickening) and the mesangium.
- *Type II*: also called 'dense deposit disease', characterized by dense deposits within the mesangium and also the basement membranes of glomeruli, tubules, and Bowman's capsule.
- *Type III*: probably a variant of type I and characterized by extensive subendothelial as well as subepithelial deposits.

However, a better understanding of the pathogenesis of MPGN has led to the following classification based on IF [9]:

- *Immune complex-mediated MPGN*: caused by complement activation via the classic pathway and associated with normal or mildly decreased serum C3 concentration and a low serum C4 concentration.
- *Complement-mediated MPGN*: caused by activation of the alternate pathway leading to low serum C3 and normal C4 levels [13].

Table 8.3 Causes of immune complex membranoproliferative glomerulonephritis (MPGN)

Infections	Hepatitis C (>70% cases), hepatitis B, HIV
	Endocarditis, shunt nephritis, malaria, schistosomiasis
Autoimmune diseases	Systemic lupus erythematosus
	Mixed cryoglobulinemia
	Sjögren's syndrome
	Scleroderma
Monoclonal immunoglobulins Paraproteinemia	Monoclonal gammopathy of undetermined significance (MGUS)
	Myeloma
	Leukaemia
	Lymphoma
Others	Cirrhosis
	Sarcoidosis
	Drugs

Aetiology and Pathogenesis

Immune Complex–Mediated Membranoproliferative Glomerulonephritis

Immune complex-mediated MPGN results from the deposition of immune complexes in the glomeruli owing to persistent antigenaemia, as may be seen in chronic hepatitis or autoimmune diseases (Table 8.3). The immune complexes trigger activation of the classic complement and kidney biopsy typically shows both immunoglobulin and complement deposition on IF.

Causes of immune complex–mediated MPGN:

- Hepatitis C (70–90% of all patients), cryoglobulinemia
- Other infections (hepatitis B, infective endocarditis, HIV, malaria)
- SLE, Sjögren's syndrome
- Myeloma, monoclonal gammopathy of undetermined significance (MGUS), CLL, NHL

Complement-Mediated Membranoproliferative Glomerulonephritis (Dense Deposit Disease and C3 Glomerulonephritis)

Complement activation occurs through classic, lectin or alternative pathways, all of which converge to form C3 convertase, which cleaves C3 into C3a and C3b. In the alternative pathway, circulating autoactivated C3b, in the presence of factor B and factor D, becomes the alternative pathway C3 convertase (Figure 8.5) [10, 11]. Factor H has an inhibitory effect on the alternative complement pathway by inhibiting the continued activation of C3 convertase [11, 12]. Complement-mediated MPGN—that is, either dense deposit disease (DDD) or C3 glomerulonephritis (C3GN)—may result from antibodies to C3 convertase (called C3 nephritic factor, C3Nef) that stabilize the C3 convertase by preventing its degradation by factor H, or by genetic mutation in factor H [11, 14]. Kidney biopsy typically shows complement deposition in the absence of immunoglobulins on IF.

Causes of complement-mediated MPGN (Table 8.4):

- Associated with C3Nef (with/without partial lipodystrophy/retinal defects)
- Inherited mutation of factor H or antibodies to factor H
- Monoclonal gammopathies (commoner in adults)

Pathology

Characteristic finding in both immune complex and complement-mediated MPGN is increased mesangial and endocapillary cellularity (proliferative lesions), with thickened GBM often leading to a double-contour appearance of glomerular capillary walls (Figure 8.6). DDD is typically characterized by linear-appearing dense deposits in the mesangium, GBM, and basement membranes of the tubules and Bowman's capsules.

Typical findings seen on IF in immune complex-mediated MPGN are:

- Hepatitis C–positive cases show granular deposition of IgM, C3, and both kappa and lambda light chains, with C1q typically being negative.

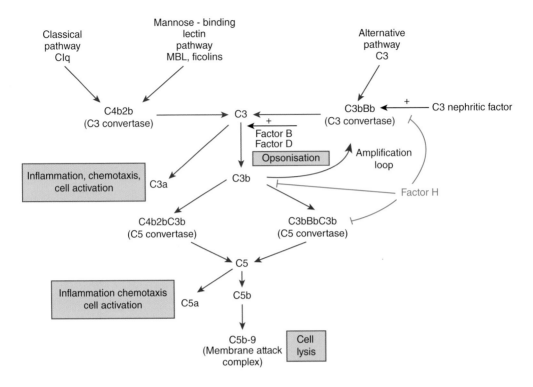

Figure 8.5 Complement pathways: C3 nephritic factor stabilizes alternative pathway C3 convertase, whilst factor H inhibits it.

Table 8.4 Causes of complement-mediated membranoproliferative glomerulonephritis (MPGN)	
Associated with C3 nephritic factor	With or without partial lipodystrophy and retinal abnormalities
Associated with factor H defect	Inherited mutations of factor H (deficiency) or antibodies to factor H
Plasma cell disorder	Mostly seen in adult population, unlike other two causes

- With MGUS/myeloma either kappa or lambda light chains (not both) seen.
- With SLE, 'full-house' pattern of Ig deposition seen: IgG, IgM, IgA, C1q, C3, and both kappa and lambda light chains.

Complement-mediated MPGN (both DDD and C3GN) is characterized by C3 deposition in the absence of Ig deposition.

Treatment

General Principles of Treatment in Nephrotic Syndrome

The following principles apply to the treatment of all patients with nephrotic syndrome.

Oedema

Diuretics and dietary sodium restriction form the cornerstone of treatment for oedema. Patients should be carefully monitored for diuresis-induced hypovolaemia with regular measurement of serum creatinine.

Note: All the major diuretics are highly protein bound. The degree of protein binding is reduced with hypoalbuminaemia, resulting in a larger extravascular space of distribution and a slower rate of delivery to the kidney. This probably explains the larger dose of diuretics needed to treat oedema in patients with nephrotic syndrome compared to heart failure [15].

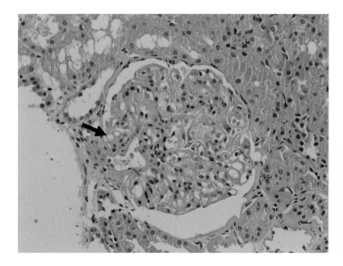

Figure 8.6 Light microscopy picture showing membranoproliferative glomerulonephritis (MPGN) pattern of glomerular injury: the glomerular basement membrane may appear double counted and is always thickened (arrow), whilst the capillaries are barely visible due to their obliteration by the increased mesangial and endocapillary cellularity.

Angiotensin Inhibition

Almost all patients are put on an ACE inhibitor or an ARB to slow down proteinuria. An additional benefit of slowing down proteinuria is the resultant increase in serum albumin, which in turn improves diuretic sensitivity.

Prophylactic Anti-coagulation

In patients with nephrotic syndrome who do not have a contraindication to anti-coagulation, prophylactic anti-coagulation is suggested in the following settings:

- *In any cause of nephrotic syndrome*: patients with atrial fibrillation, genetic thrombophilia, certain surgical procedures (abdominal, gynaecological or orthopaedic), severe heart failure, prolonged immobilization, morbid obesity or a prior idiopathic thromboembolic event.
- *In patients with MN*: in those with a serum albumin less than 20 g/l, irrespective of the presence or absence of the above mentioned co-morbidities [16].

Many patients with nephrotic syndrome are found to be hypertensive and need treatment with second-line anti-hypertensive drugs in addition to ACE inhibitors or ARBs. Patients should also be on therapy to control hyperlipidaemia.

Minimal Change Disease

Glucocorticoid leads to a complete remission of proteinuria in over 85–90% of cases of MCD in both children and adults [17]. Children tend to remit rapidly,

with 50% responding within two weeks and almost all within eight weeks. Adults respond more slowly, with more than 25% of responders taking four months or longer to achieve complete remission. Approximately 50–75% of glucocorticoid-responsive adults have a relapse, and steroid dependence is seen in 25–30%.

Patients who relapse after the cessation of glucocorticoid therapy are offered reinstitution of the same therapy. Those who relapse whilst on prednisolone are treated with cyclophosphamide, cyclosporine or rituximab.

Focal Segmental Glomerulosclerosis

Primary FSGS

- Up to 40–60% achieve complete or partial remission with prednisolone, which may be needed for six months to more than a year. Usually started at a dose of 1 mg/kg/day, with dose reduction by 8–12 weeks.
- In patients at increased risk for glucocorticoid-associated toxicity (e.g. obesity, diabetes mellitus or severe osteoporosis), the calcineurin inhibitors cyclosporine or tacrolimus with or without low-dose prednisolone are an alternative.
- FSGS can recur in up to 30% of patients with primary FSGS.

Secondary FSGS

There is not much evidence for the use of immunosuppressive therapy in secondary FSGS. Management relies on the use of ACE inhibitors or ARBs to reduce proteinuria, and treatment of the underlying pathology where possible.

Membranous Nephropathy

In view of the potential toxicity of immunosuppressive medicines and the fact that those without significant proteinuria may show complete or partial resolution, one should be very careful when deciding on the course of treatment offered to patients with MN. Treatment and prognosis of MN are guided by categorizing patients into the following three subsets:

- *Low risk*: proteinuria <4 g/day and normal creatinine over six months—less than 8% develop CKD. These patients are treated conservatively with ACE inhibitors or ARBs.
- *Moderate risk*: proteinuria between 4 and 8 g/day for >6 months with normal or near normal creatinine—50% progress to CKD. If proteinuria <4 g/day after six months of conservative management, then no immunosuppression offered. If proteinuria >4–6 g/day after six months of conservative treatment, then patients are offered immunosuppression.
- *High risk*: proteinuria >8 g/day and persists for three months and/or renal function that is either below normal or decreases—CKD is seen in 75%. Treated with immunosuppressive regimens.

First-line immunosuppressive therapy usually consists of glucocorticoids and cyclophosphamide. Calcineurin inhibitor (CNI), cyclosporine or tacrolimus is used if cyclophosphamide is contraindicated [18]. Rituximab is used in patients who fail both the cyclophosphamide or CNI-based therapy. Along with monitoring for relapse or worsening of proteinuria, serum PLA2R antibody levels are useful for monitoring treatment in primary MN.

Treatment of secondary MN often depends on the aetiology. Corticosteroids and immunosuppressive agents are effective in controlling proteinuria in lupus MN (discussed in Chapter 10).

Membranoproliferative Glomerulonephritis

Resolution of MPGN usually occurs after successful treatment of the associated underlying disease, for instance initiation of anti-viral therapy in MPGN due to hepatitis C or B virus. Immunosuppressive therapy is not indicated and may be deleterious in patients with hepatitis. MPGN shows at least partial remission with treatment of other underlying conditions like myeloma or autoimmune disorders.

Idiopathic immune complex MPGN that does not respond to ACE inhibitors or ARBs may be offered immunosuppressive therapy e.g. prednisolone and cyclophosphamide or rituximab.

Therapy with corticosteroids has been largely unsatisfactory in complement-mediated MPGN, with the majority of patients progressing to ESRD. Patients with mutations resulting in deficiency of complement factors should receive plasma infusion every two to three weeks. Those with antibodies against complement factor proteins require an initial 7–10 plasma exchanges followed by immunosuppression with corticosteroids and mycophenolate or rituximab.

Depending on the type, median renal survival in MPGN has been reported at between 10 and 20 years. Patients undergoing renal transplant have a high risk of recurrence from graft failure, ranging from 50% in all MPGN to almost 100% in MPGN due to DDD. Though not universally accepted, there is a growing interest in the use of eculizumab, a humanized monoclonal antibody to complement component C5 that prevents the generation of the membrane attack complex, in patients with complement-mediated MPGN [19].

References

1. Anderson, F.A. Jr., Wheeler, H.B., Goldberg, R.J. et al. (1991). A population-based perspective of the hospital incidence and case-fatality rates of deep vein thrombosis and pulmonary embolism. The Worcester DVT study. *Arch. Intern. Med.* 151 (5): 933.
2. Thom, T.J., Kannel, W.B., Silbershatz, H. et al. (1998). Incidence, prevalence and mortality of cardiovascular diseases in the United States. In: *Hurst's the Heart*, 9e (eds. R.W. Alexander, R.C. Schlant and V. Fuster), 3. New York: McGraw-Hill.
3. Ballow, M., Kennedy, T.L. 3rd, Gaudio, K.M. et al. (1982). Serum hemolytic factor D values in children with steroid-responsive idiopathic nephrotic syndrome. *J. Pediatr.* 100 (2): 192–196.
4. Meyrier, A. and Niaudet, P. (2005). Minimal changes and focal-segmental glomerulosclerosis. In: *Oxford Textbook of Clinical Nephrology*, 3e, vol. 1 (eds. A.M. Davison, J.S. Cameron, E. Grünfeld, et al.), 439. Oxford: Oxford University Press.
5. Abdel-Hafez, M., Shimada, M., Lee, P.Y. et al. (2009). Idiopathic nephrotic syndrome and atopy: is there a common link? *Am. J. Kidney Dis.* 54 (5): 945–953.
6. Ishimoto, T., Shimada, M., Araya, C.E. et al. (2011). Minimal change disease: a CD80 podocytopathy? *Semin. Nephrol.* 31 (4): 320–325.

7. Wei, C., El Hindi, S., Li, J. et al. (2011). Circulating urokinase receptor as a cause of focal segmental glomerulosclerosis. *Nat. Med.* 17 (8): 952.

8. Straatmann, C., Kallash, M., Killackey, M. et al. (2014). Success with plasmapheresis treatment for recurrent focal segmental glomerulosclerosis in pediatric renal transplant recipients. *Pediatr. Transplant.* 18 (1): 29–34. https://doi.org/10.1111/petr.12185.

9. Gebeshuber, C.A., Kornauth, C., Dong, L. et al. (2013). Focal segmental glomerulosclerosis is induced by microRNA-193a and its downregulation of WT1. *Nat. Med.* 19 (4): 481–487.

10. Genovese, G., Friedman, D.J., Ross, M.D. et al. (2010). Association of trypanolytic ApoL1 variants with kidney disease in African Americans. *Science* 329 (5993): 841.

11. Mohammadi Torbati, P. (2012). Focal segmental glomerulosclerosis; collapsing variant. *J. Nephropathol.* 1 (2): 87–90. https://doi.org/10.5812/nephropathol.7515.

12. Thomas, D.B., Franceschini, N., Hogan, S.L. et al. (2006). Clinical and pathologic characteristics of focal segmental glomerulosclerosis pathologic variants. *Kidney Int.* 69 (5): 920.

13. Smith, R.J., Alexander, J., Barlow, P.N. et al. (2007). Dense deposit disease focus group. New approaches to the treatment of dense deposit disease. *J. Am. Soc. Nephrol.* 18 (9): 2447.

14. Farquhar, M.G., Saito, A., Kerjaschki, D., and Orlando, R.A. (1995). The Heymann nephritis antigenic complex: megalin (gp330) and RAP. *J. Am. Soc. Nephrol.* 6 (1): 35.

15. Smith, D.E., Hyneck, M.L., Berardi, R.R., and Port, F.K. (1985). Urinary protein binding, kinetics, and dynamics of furosemide in nephrotic patients. *J. Pharm. Sci.* 74 (6): 603.

16. Glassock, R.J. (2007). Prophylactic anticoagulation in nephrotic syndrome: a clinical conundrum. *J. Am. Soc. Nephrol.* 18 (8): 2221–2225. https://doi.org/10.1681/ASN.2006111300.

17. Mak, S.K., Short, C.D., and Mallick, N.P. (1996). Long-term outcome of adult-onset minimal-change nephropathy. *Nephrol. Dial. Transplant.* 11 (11): 2192.

18. Alexopoulos, E., Papagianni, A., Tsamelashvili, M. et al. (2006). Induction and long-term treatment with cyclosporine in membranous nephropathy with the nephrotic syndrome. *Nephrol. Dial. Transplant.* 21 (11): 3127.

19. Bomback, A.S. (2014). Eculizumab in the treatment of membranoproliferative glomerulonephritis. *Nephron. Clin. Pract.* 128: 270–276. https://doi.org/10.1159/000368592.

Questions and Answers

Questions

1. Which of the following is/are true about FSGS in adults?
   a. Collapsing GN is the commonest pathological variant
   b. Obesity is a cause of secondary FSGS
   c. Cyclosporine is an alternative treatment for steroid-resistant FSGS
   d. It can be differentiated from minimal change disease by presence of diffuse foot process effacement

2. Which of the following is/are true about MCD?
   a. 90% of nephrotic syndrome in adults is due to MCD
   b. The disease takes longer to respond to corticosteroids in adults than in children
   c. It can occur in association with Hodgkin disease
   d. It is associated with increased CD80 levels in urine

3. Which of the following is/are true about FSGS?
   a. Its pathogenesis could involve a cytokine soluble mediator
   b. There may be mutation in the genes encoding for the proteins of the podocyte cytoskeleton
   c. Immunofluorescence (IF) of the renal biopsy has characteristic immune complex deposition
   d. Postrenal transplant recurrence occurs in 30–40% of cases with primary FSGS

4. Which of the following is/are true about complement mediated MPGN?
   a. Responds well to oral corticosteroids
   b. Is diagnosed based on characteristic findings on light microscopic examination of renal biopsy
   c. A significant proportion of cases is due to mutation in the genes encoding for the complement regulatory proteins
   d. IF characteristically shows isolated complement deposits in the absence of immunoglobulins

5. Which of the following is/are true about membranous nephropathy?
   a. It is common cause of nephrotic syndrome and ESRF in children
   b. It is caused by autoantibodies to C3 convertase called C3 nephritic factor
   c. The characteristic biopsy finding is the presence of 'spikes' in the GBM on silver methenamine stain
   d. Immunosuppressive treatment is not recommended in those with persistent sub-nephrotic range proteinuria

6. Which of the following statements about FSGS is true?
   a. Primary FSGS is associated with suPAR
   b. Secondary FSGS may result from heroin abuse
   c. Polymorphisms in the apolipoprotein L1 (APOL1) gene can lead to the development of FSGS in people of African origin
   d. a, b, and c are correct

Answers

1. b, c. Obesity is an important cause of secondary FSGS. Classic FSGS (not otherwise specified) is the commonest histologic variant. Both FSGS and MCD are associated with diffuse foot process effacement. Calcineurin inhibitors such as cyclosporine induce remission in significantly higher proportion of patients with steroid-resistant FSGS than prednisolone alone.

2. b, c, d. While majority of nephrotic syndrome in children is due to MCD, 10–15% of cases in adults are caused by MCD. Most children with MCD achieve remission within four weeks of therapy with corticosteroids but adults take longer to respond. MCD has been reported to be associated with Hodgkin's disease. CD80 expression is increased in podocytes in MCD and is reflected by increased levels of CD80 in urine.

3. a, b, d. The pathogenesis of FSGS is believed to involve circulating soluble cytokine mediator such as IL-13 and suPAR (soluble urokinase plasminogen activator receptor). The genetic forms of FSGS are due to mutations in the genes encoding for the podocyte cytoskeleton. There is no immune complex deposition in primary FSGS. There is a high risk of recurrence following renal transplant in those with primary FSGS (up to 30%).

4. c, d. A significant proportion of cases of complement-mediated MPGN is due to mutation in the genes encoding for the complement regulatory proteins. It is differentiated from immune-complex mediated by the presence of isolated C3 deposition on IF and not by findings on light microscopy.

5. c. Idiopathic MN is common in Caucasian males and quite uncommon in children. C3 nephritic factor is involved in the pathogenesis of MPGN. More than 70% of idiopathic MN have circulating autoantibodies against phospholipase A2 receptor (PLA2R) located on the surface of podocytes. The characteristic abnormality on light microscopy is diffuse glomerular capillary wall thickening while "spikes" of glomerular basement membrane extending between the immune deposits may be seen with silver methenamine stain. Patients with sub-nephrotic range proteinuria are treated with ACEI or ARB alone and immunosuppressive therapy is only indicated in those with persistent high-grade proteinuria >4 g/daily despite the use of ACEI or ARB.

6. d. Up to two-third of patients with primary FSGS have increased plasma level of suPAR. Drugs causing secondary FSGS include heroin, interferon, lithium, sirolimus, and pamidronate. Polymorphisms in the apolipoprotein L1 (APOL1) gene which are protective against trypanosomiasis are believed to lead to the development of FSGS in people of African origin.

9

Glomerulonephritis

Surjit Tarafdar

Summary

- Glomerulonephritis (GN), which presents as nephritic syndrome, is characterized by haematuria with dysmorphic red blood cells and red cell casts, variable degree of proteinuria usually in the non-nephrotic range and often hypertension, renal insufficiency and oedema (secondary to sodium retention)

Immunoglobulin A Nephropathy
- Immunoglobulin (Ig) A nephropathy is the commonest glomerular disease, particularly in developed countries where infective GN is less common
- Young adults in their second or third decade present with episodes of macroscopic haematuria within 24–48 hours of upper respiratory tract infections or with asymptomatic haematuria and proteinuria
- Characterized by mesangial deposition of IgA with mesangial proliferation in the absence of any changes in the endothelium, glomerular basement membrane (GBM) or podocytes
- Many patients progress to end-stage renal disease (20% at 20 years and 30% at 30 years)

Infection-Related Glomerulonephritis
- The incidence of poststreptococcal glomerulonephritis (PSGN) has decreased quite dramatically in developed countries, with an increase in staphylococcus-associated GN
- Unlike PSGN, where there is a time lag of one to two weeks between infection and the onset of GN, in staphylococcus-associated GN the clinical presentation of GN accompanies active infection
- Serum complement levels (especially C3, suggesting activation of the alternate complement pathway predominantly) are usually low in infection-related GN
- The most characteristic histological finding in infection-related GN is the presence of dome-shaped subepithelial electron-dense deposits with a hump-like appearance
- Glomerular cellular proliferation with polymorphonuclear calls seen
- Prognosis is worse in staphylococcus-associated GN in comparison to PSGN

Rapidly Progressive Glomerulonephritis
- Rapidly progressive glomerulonephritis (RPGN) is a nephritic syndrome with rapid deterioration in kidney function over days to weeks, along with characteristic finding of crescents on biopsy
- Cellular glomerular crescents are defined as two or more layers of proliferating parietal epithelial cells in Bowman's space (which normally has single layers of parietal and visceral epithelial cells)
- May be due to anti-GBM antibody disease (Goodpasture's disease), immune complex-mediated GN (lupus, IgAN, infectious GN or mesangio-capillary GN) or pauci-immune GN (anti-neutrophil cytoplasmic autoantibody or ANCA-positive GN)
- Initial therapy consists of pulse methylprednisolone for three days followed by daily oral prednisone and oral or intravenous cyclophosphamide or rituximab
- Plasmapheresis is offered if patient has haemoptysis, which may be seen in RPGN associated with anti-GBM disease or ANCA vasculitis

Lecture Notes Nephrology: A Comprehensive Guide to Renal Medicine, First Edition. Edited by Surjit Tarafdar.
© 2020 John Wiley & Sons Ltd. Published 2020 by John Wiley & Sons Ltd.

Anti-Glomerular Basement Membrane Antibody Disease and Goodpasture's Disease

- Goodpasture's disease is due to antibodies against the NC1 domain of the alpha-3 chain of type IV collagen found in the glomerular and alveolar basement membranes
- Patients are positive for anti-GBM antibodies in their plasma
- Renal biopsy shows characteristic immuno-fluorescence finding of IgG deposition in a linear pattern along the GBM

- Typically presents as acute or subacute kidney injury caused by RPGN, often accompanied by pulmonary haemorrhage that may be life threatening
- 10–40% of anti-GBM antibody-positive patients may also be positive for myeloperoxidase (MPO) ANCA and these patients usually have more aggressive disease
- Treatment consists of plasmapheresis in conjunction with prednisolone and cyclophosphamide

Whilst nephrotic syndrome is characterized by increased permeability of the glomerular capillary walls to protein and the resultant nephrotic-range proteinuria (in the absence of active inflammation), glomerulonephritis (GN) which presents as nephritic syndrome is characterized by glomerular inflammation leading to a reduction in glomerular filtration rate (GFR), haematuria with dysmorphic red blood cells (RBCs) and red cell casts, non-nephrotic proteinuria, and hypertension, often with oedema (secondary to sodium retention).

Mechanical damage caused by passage of RBCs through the glomerular basement membrane (GBM) followed by osmotic injury sustained during passage through the hypotonic tubular segment leads to the formation of abnormal-appearing RBCs (dysmorphic RBCs). Quantitatively, dysmorphic RBCs need to be more than 5% of total urinary RBCs to indicate GN.

Note that microscopic haematuria is ≥2 RBCs per high-power field in spun urine.

RBC casts are RBCs embedded in Tamm–Horsfall protein, which is a physiological protein secreted by the thick ascending limb of the loop of Henle cells.

Figure 9.1 is a classification of the various types of GN based on immunofluorescence (IF) findings on renal biopsy.

Anti-neutrophil cytoplasmic autoantibody (ANCA)-positive GN is discussed in Chapter 10, whilst membranoproliferative/mesangiocapillary GN (MPGN/MCGN) is discussed in Chapter 8.

Immunoglobulin A Nephropathy

Immunoglobulin (Ig) A nephropathy (IgAN) is generally considered the commonest cause of primary GN worldwide, especially in developed countries with a low prevalence of infectious diseases [1]. The clinical presentation spans a spectrum from asymptomatic haematuria, to visible haematuria within 24–48 hours of upper respiratory tract infection, to rapidly progressive glomerulonephritis (RPGN). Previously thought to be a benign disease, now we know that upto half of these patients may progress to end-stage renal disease (ESRD). IgAN is most frequently diagnosed in young adults in the second and third decades of life and there is a male predominance.

The condition is characterized by deposition of IgA in the mesangium with mesangial proliferation. It is typically not associated with changes in the GBM, endothelial cells or podocytes, as seen in many of the other GNs. Renal biopsies done on autopsy cases and both living and cadaveric donors suggest that the incidence of IgAN may be as high as 5–16% in the general population [2, 3].

Pathogenesis

Although IgA is predominantly associated with immune function in mucous membranes, it is found in both serum and mucous membranes. IgA exists as two isotypes, namely IgA1 and IgA2, with the latter being more concentrated in the mucous membranes. IgA can also be classified based upon the location: monomeric serum IgA in the blood versus polymeric secretory IgA in the mucous membranes. In its secretory form, two monomers of IgA are joined by a joining chain (J chain), with the big protein 'secretory component' wrapped around them. The secretory component protects IgA from degradation by the gastric acids and enzymes of the digestive system.

IgA1 but not IgA2 has a hinge region that binds O-linked sugars, thus making IgA1 galactosylated.

Most of the circulating IgA is bone marrow derived and is monomeric IgA1 (mIgA1). The IgA found in

GN Classification

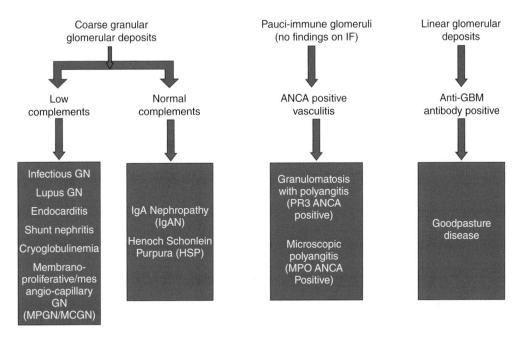

Figure 9.1 Classification of the various types of glomerulonephritis (GN) based on immunofluorescence findings on renal biopsy. ANCA, anti-neutrophil cytoplasmic autoantibody; GBM, glomerular basement membrane; IF, immunofluorescence; Ig, immunoglobulin.

mucous membranes is made by the plasma cells in the mucosa-associated lymphoid tissue on mucosal exposure to antigens. The J chains bind two monomers of IgA and this polymeric IgA (pIgA) is transferred into the intestinal epithelial cells and released into the intestinal secretions, after coupling to the secretory component to make the polymeric secretory IgA.

The mesangial deposit in IgAN is predominantly pIgA1. Because of the fact that pIgA is derived from the mucous membranes and there is an association in many cases of IgAN with respiratory tract infections, the initial belief was that IgAN was the result of exaggerated mucosal immunity. However, it has been shown that in IgAN, pIgA production is down-regulated in the mucosa, whereas pIgA levels are increased in the blood after systemic immunization with antigens such as tetanus toxoid. Theoretically, impaired IgA production in the mucous membranes might cause antigens to reach the systemic circulation and trigger IgA production.

Although serum IgA levels are raised in up to one-third of patients with IgAN, the mesangial deposition of IgA is not dependent on raised serum levels of IgA, as evidenced by the fact that patients with IgA myeloma do not have an increased chance of

developing IgAN. The IgA in patients with IgAN shows less galactose content than healthy controls [4, 5]. It is thought that this poor galactosylation of pIgA1 may contribute to the development of IgAN by the following mechanisms:

- The galactose-deficient IgA are targets for IgG autoantibodies [4, 5]. The resultant immune complex can precipitate in the mesangium, leading to mesangial proliferation.
- Poorly galactosylated IgA1 also tend to self-aggregate and deposit in the mesangium.
- IgA is normally cleared by the liver. Poor galactosylation reduces hepatic clearance of IgA by interfering with its attachment to hepatic cells.

The characteristic immunofluorescence (IF) microscopic finding of mesangial deposition of IgA and C3 in the absence of C1q or C4 suggests that the disease is the result of mesangial deposition of immune complexes, leading to activation of the complement system by the alternate pathway. The resultant inflammation leads to increased local production of platelet-derived growth factor (PDGF) and transforming growth factor B (TGF-B), which in turn are believed to lead to the mesangial proliferative changes.

Pathology

Light Microscopy

Light microscopy (LM) may be completely normal or show diffusely increased mesangial matrix and hypercellularity (Figure 9.2), focal segmental changes or, rarely, aggressive GN with crescents. Focal segmental or global glomerular sclerosis suggests that the disease has been going on for some time.

Electron Microscopy

The characteristic finding on electron microscopy (EM) is mesangial expansion due to both mesangial hypercellularity and mesangial dense deposits, which co-relate with the IgA deposits on IF (Figure 9.3).

Immunofluorescence

IF in IgAN is characterized by mesangial staining for IgA and C3. There may be some IgG and IgM, but C1q is characteristically absent, differentiating from lupus nephritis (Figure 9.4).

The following four histological parameters were found to be independently predictive of clinical outcome in IgAN [6]:

- Mesangial hypercellularity
- Endocapillary hypercellularity
- Segmental glomerulosclerosis
- Tubular atrophy/interstitial fibrosis

This led to the formulation of the Oxford-MEST scoring system for IgAN. Whilst M1, S1 or T1/T2 are associated with worsening kidney function and

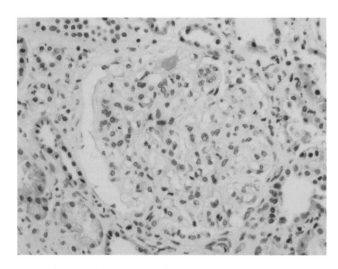

Figure 9.2 H and E stain 20× magnification showing increased mesangial matrix and hypercellularity in immunoglobulin A nephropathy (IgAN) on light microscopy.

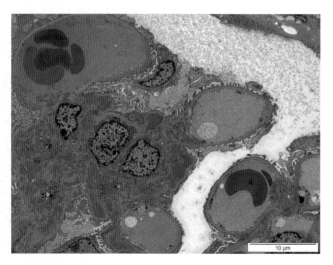

Figure 9.3 Electron micrograph showing increased mesangial matrix in immunoglobulin A nephropathy (IgAN).

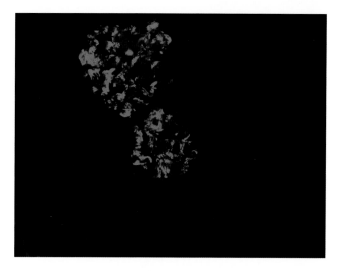

Figure 9.4 Immunofluorescence showing heavy mesangial deposit of immunoglobulin (Ig) A in IgA nephropathy (IgAN).

Table 9.1 MEST criteria for Oxford classification of immunoglobulin (Ig) A nephropathy

Histological variable	Definition	Score
Mesangial hypercellularity (M)	>4 mesangial cells in any mesangial area of glomerulus	M0 (if <50% glomeruli affected) M1 (if >50% glomeruli affected)
Endocapillary hypercellularity (E)	Hypercellularity within glomerular capillary lumens causing narrowing/obliteration of the lumens	E0 (no hypercellularity) E1 (any glomeruli showing hypercellularity)
Segmental glomerulosclerosis (S)	Sclerosis of glomerular tuft	S0 (no glomerular sclerosis) S1 (any part of the glomerular tuft involved in sclerosis)
Tubular atrophy/ interstitial fibrosis (T)	Percentage of the cortical area involved by tubular atrophy or interstitial fibrosis	T0 <25% T1 26–50% T2 >50%

development of ESRD, E1 suggests a better response to immunosuppressive therapy (Table 9.1).

Crescents has been recently added as a fifth variable to the above:

- Crescents: this feature is defined as the presence of cellular and/or fibrocellular crescents in at least one glomerulus (C1) or at least 25% of glomeruli (C2).

Clinical Presentation

In 40–50% of cases, the presentation is with episodic macroscopic haematuria, especially in the second or third decade of life [7]. The haematuria often follows within 24–48 hours of an upper respiratory tract infection. This is in contrast to the 10–14 days gap between infection and subsequent haematuria in those with poststreptococcal glomerulonephritis (PSGN).

Between 30 and 40% of cases are identified on the basis of follow-up for asymptomatic microscopic haematuria identified on urinary dipstick testing [7]. These patients may or may not have proteinuria, and when present, the proteinuria is usually less than 1 g/day.

Less than 5% of patients present with nephrotic-range proteinuria along with haematuria. They usually have widespread proliferative GN or coexistent IgAN and minimal change disease.

Acute kidney injury (AKI) is an uncommon mode of presentation in IgAN. AKI may develop in these patients due to severe necrotizing GN with crescent formation, i.e. RPGN or tubular blockade secondary to heavy glomerular haematuria.

Rarely, patients with IgAN present with malignant hypertension. It is thought that these patients had longstanding IgAN not diagnosed previously.

Although IgAN is defined by abnormalities in the kidney only, there is an association with the following conditions:

- *Rheumatic and autoimmune diseases*: ankylosing spondylitis and reactive arthritis
- *Gastrointestinal tract*: coeliac disease
- *Liver*: alcoholic liver disease and non-alcoholic cirrhosis
- *Lung*: sarcoidosis
- *Infection*: HIV

Natural History and Transplantation

IgAN was initially thought to be a benign condition, but now we know that slow progression to ESRD can occur in up to half of these patients [8]. Besides the prognostic use of the Oxford-MEST scoring system already discussed, the following are considered predictors of poorer renal outcome:

- Elevated serum creatinine concentration
- Hypertension (>140/90 mmHg)
- Persistent (for more than six months) proteinuria above 1 g/day

Although transplantation outcome is not inferior if the primary renal disease is IgAN, mesangial deposit of IgA can be seen in the transplanted kidney in up to 58% of these patients [9]. The following are considered to be possible risk factors for recurrence:

- Use of living-related-donor kidney
- Specific human leukocyte antigen (HLA) alleles in recipient, including HLA-B35, HLA-DR4, HLA-B8, HLA-DR3
- Good HLA match between donor and recipient
- High serum IgA concentration

Treatment

Patients without significant proteinuria, hypertension or low GFR do not need any active treatment, but six-monthly follow-up to monitor for these factors. Angiotensin-converting enzyme (ACE) inhibitors or angiotensin II receptor blockers (ARB) are used for blood pressure control and controlling proteinuria. As per the Kidney Disease: Improving Global Outcomes (KDIGO) guidelines, patients with persistent proteinuria >1 g/day despite three to six months of optimized supportive care (including ACE inhibitors or ARBs and blood pressure control) and GFR >50 ml/min per 1.73 m^2 should receive a six-month course of corticosteroid therapy. KDIGO also suggests fish oil in the treatment of IgAN with persistent proteinuria >1 g/day despite three to six months of optimized supportive care. There is no evidence of benefit in combining other immunosuppressive therapy with corticosteroids in treating IgAN, except in those with severe crescentic disease and RPGN.

Patients with chronically low estimated GFR or substantial glomerulosclerosis and tubulointerstitial atrophy or fibrosis on renal biopsy are not likely to benefit from steroid therapy.

Studies in Japan have suggested a role for tonsillectomy in the treatment of IgAN [10], whilst other studies have not been supportive [11].

Infection-Related Glomerulonephritis

In the past, most cases of infection-related GN occurred in children following streptococcal upper respiratory tract or skin infections and were called PSGN. Now the majority of infection-related GN in developed countries are seen in adults, particularly in the elderly or those with debilitating conditions like diabetes, malignancy, alcoholism or acquired immunodeficiency syndrome (AIDS). Whilst the overall incidence of infection-related GN has been falling in developed countries, the incidence of PSGN has decreased quite dramatically in developed countries [12]. In adults, staphylococcus infections are as common as streptococcus infections and three times more common in the elderly as the cause of GN. Whilst streptococcal and staphylococcal infections cause up to half of all infection-associated GNs, other causes include non-streptococcal bacteria (*salmonella, Escherichia coli, Neisseria*, etc.), virus (hepatitis A, B, and C, HIV, cytomegalovirus, etc.), helminths (schistomiasis, filariasis, etc.), and protozoa (*Falciparum malariae*, toxoplasma and trypanosoma). Table 9.2 lists the main differences between PSGN and staphylococcus-associated GN.

Because staphylococcal and other non-streptococcal infections are usually present at the same time as the GN, the term infection-related GN is now preferred to post-infectious GN, while PSGN is classically seen in streptococcal infections.

Poststreptococcal Glomerulonephritis

The annual burden of PSGN in developing countries ranges from 9.5 to 28.5 cases per 100 000 people [13], whilst it ranges from 0.4 to 0.9 cases per 100 000 in

Table 9.2 Chief differences between poststreptococcal glomerulonephritis (PSGN) and staphylococcus-associated glomerulonephritis (GN)

Staphylococcus-associated GN	Post-streptococcal GN
GN simultaneously with infection	GN up to two weeks after infection
More common in In elderly and especially diabetics/alcoholics/malignancy/AIDS	Commoner in children between 2 and 14 years of age
Associated infections: skin (38%), lung (22%), endocarditis (10%), deep abscess (3%), and urinary tract infection (3%)	Follows throat or skin infections
On Immunofluorescence often immunoglobulin (Ig) A dominance or co-dominance	On immunofluorescence C3 dominance with some IgG as well
Up to half develop chronic kidney disease or end-stage renal disease	Renal recovery in >90%, especially children

developed countries [14]. PSGN mostly affects children between the ages of 2 and 14 years or the elderly. Traditionally, only certain nephritogenic strains of group A *Streptococcus pyogenes* was known to lead to GN. However, PSGN has now been identified following infection with group C streptococcus as well [15].

Pathogenesis

PSGN is an immune complex-mediated glomerular disease with the two leading candidates for the putative streptococcal antigen(s) responsible being:

- Nephritis-associated plasmin receptor (NAPlr), a glycolytic enzyme, which has glyceraldehyde-3-phosphate dehydrogenase (GAPDH) activity. Anti-NAPlr antibody levels are found in 92% of the sera from patients with PSGN [16]. Though NAPlr does not bind immunoglobulins or complements, its nephritogenic role is thought to be related to its plasmin-binding capacity, which facilitates immune complex deposition and inflammation.
- Streptococcal pyrogenic exotoxin B (SPEB), a cationic cysteine proteinase which has been localized in subepithelial electron-dense deposits (humps) that are characteristic of PSGN [17]. SPEB co-localizes with IgG and complements in the glomeruli.

PSGN is thought to occur when persistent streptococcal antigenaemia leads to the development of circulating immune complexes that deposit at the subendothelial and mesangial locations and initiate an inflammatory cascade there. Subepithelial deposits (humps) form because of the presence of the cationic protein SPEB mentioned earlier, or the dissociation of subendothelial complexes with transition and reformation on the outer aspect of the GBM.

Pathology
Light Microscopy

Diffuse endocapillary GN with proliferation of both mesangial and endothelial cells along with numerous neutrophils is the most common finding (Figure 9.5). Trichrome stain may show small subepithelial hump-shaped deposits and uncommonly crescent formation may be seen.

Over a period of weeks, the endocapillary hypercellularity is lost, resulting in a predominantly mesangial proliferative GN.

Electron Microscopy

The most characteristic finding is the hump-shaped subepithelial electron-dense deposits (Figure 9.6).

Immunofluorescence

In the early phase of the disease (the initial two to three weeks), the glomeruli show finely granular deposits of C3 (100% of cases) and usually IgG as well in the capillary walls and mesangial areas, in a 'starry sky' pattern. Later, with resorption of many of the capillary wall deposits, there is a predominantly mesangial pattern of staining. Some cases show a coarse granular to confluent granular staining along the glomerular capillary walls (termed the 'garland' pattern; Figure 9.7).

Clinical Presentation

The typical clinical presentation is of acute nephritic syndrome, whilst up to 20% of adult patients have nephrotic-range proteinuria as well. The latent period between upper respiratory infection and nephritis is

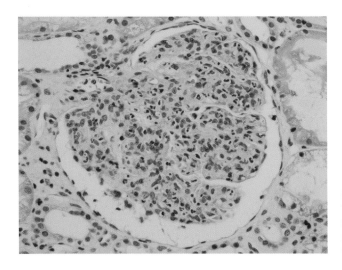

Figure 9.5 H and E stain 20× magnification showing mesangial and endothelial proliferation with occasional neutrophils in poststreptococcal glomerulonephritis (PSGN).

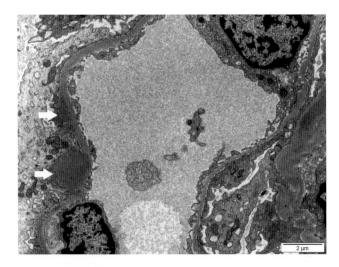

Figure 9.6 Electron micrograph of poststreptococcal glomerulonephritis (PSGN) with subepithelial humps (white arrows).

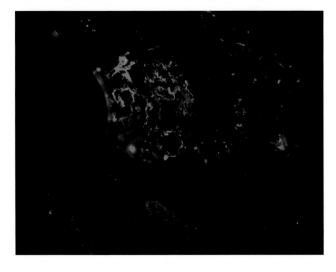

Figure 9.7 Immunofluorescence showing garland pattern of C3 deposition in poststreptococcal glomerulonephritis (PSGN).

7–10 days, whilst nephritis appears 2–4 weeks following skin infection.

In a typical case of PSGN, improvement is observed after two to seven days, with resolution of oedema and improving urine output. Serum complement levels (especially C3, suggesting activation of alternate complement pathway predominantly) are low within the first two weeks in 90% of cases and return to normal in four to eight weeks.

RPGN associated with crescents on biopsy is seen in less than 1% of cases.

Positive cultures for streptococcus are obtained in 10–70% of cases during epidemics and in about 25% of sporadic cases.

The streptozyme test, which measures five different streptococcal antibodies, is positive in more than 95% of patients who develop PSGN due to pharyngitis and 80% of those with skin infections [18]. It includes the following antibodies:

- Anti-streptolysin (ASO)
- Anti-hyaluronidase (AHase)
- Anti-streptokinase (ASKase)
- Anti-nicotinamide-adenine dinucleotidase (anti-NAD)
- Anti-DNase B antibodies

Treatment

If the streptococcal infection is still present at the time of diagnosis, patients should be treated with penicillin (erythromycin in case of penicillin allergy).

Treatment is supportive, as in all nephritic syndromes, with fluid and salt restriction, use of loop diuretics, and anti-hypertensives as needed. Patients with PSGN have variable reductions in renal function, and some patients require dialysis temporarily for severe AKI, life-threatening fluid overload and hyperkalaemia refractory to medical management.

Staphylococcal-Associated Glomerulonephritis

Unlike PSGN where there is a time lag of days to weeks between infection and the onset of GN, in staphylococcus-associated GN the clinical presentation of GN accompanies active infection. In adults and specially the older population, staphylococcus-associated GN is commoner than PSGN.

Pathogenesis

Staphylococcus-associated GN is an immune complex-mediated disease with the antigen derived from the infectious agent. Staphylococcus-associated GN requires continued antigen production, and therefore active and ongoing infection, to perpetuate the renal inflammation. Therefore if the infection is treated successfully, the GN *might* resolve.

Pathology

The renal biopsy findings on LM and EM are similar to those seen in PSGN. Crescents may be seen in as many as 50% of cases associated with infective endocarditis [19]. On IF, many patients have IgA co-deposits along with C3 (unlike the predominance of IgG with C3 in PSGN).

Clinical Presentation

As already mentioned, adults with staphylococcus-associated GN present with haematuria, proteinuria of varying degrees, a rising serum creatinine and/or oedema, with concurrent active infection. Whilst the site of infection can be variable (e.g. cellulitis, osteomyelitis, infective endocarditis, indwelling catheter, etc.), upper respiratory tract infection is very uncommon (unlike in PSGN). Cutaneous vasculitis imitating Henoch–Schönlein purpura (HSP)/IgAN or ANCA vasculitis may be seen in staphylococcus-associated GN. Renal prognosis is usually much worse than for PSGN.

Treatment

Apart from general measures for treatment of nephritis, which include fluid and salt restriction, use of loop diuretics, and anti-hypertensives as needed, staphylococcal infection should be eradicated with appropriate antibiotics and, if needed, surgery, for example for abscess or infective endocarditis.

Rapidly Progressive Glomerulonephritis

RPGN refers to the clinical syndrome of nephritic syndrome along with rapid deterioration in kidney function over days to weeks. Histologically RPGN is characterized by the finding of crescent in the glomeruli (crescentic GN).

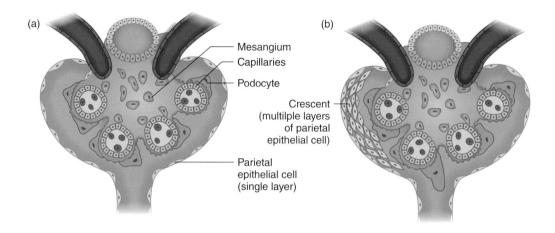

Figure 9.8 (a) Normal glomeruli with single layer of parietal epithelium; (b) glomeruli with multiple layers of parietal epithelial cells forming crescent.

Normally Bowman's space has single layers of parietal and visceral epithelial cells. Cellular glomerular crescents are defined as two or more layers of proliferating parietal epithelial cells in Bowman's space (Figure 9.8). Crescents are a hallmark of severe inflammatory GN. Usually RPGN results when >50% of the glomeruli exhibit crescents, though at times severe GN may lead to rapid AKI with a lower number of crescents.

Pathogenesis

Crescent formation is a non-specific inflammatory response to severe glomerular injury [20]. Rents in the glomerular capillary wall lead to leakage of plasma products, including fibrinogen, into Bowman's space with subsequent fibrin formation. This is followed by the influx of macrophages and T cells and the release of proinflammatory cytokines.

Types of Crescentic Glomerulonephritis

Crescentic GN leading to RPGN is classified into three types:

- *Anti-GBM antibody disease–associated RPGN*: characterized by the presence of anti-GBM antibodies and linear staining of the GBM on IF; this leads to 20% of all RPGN.
- *Immune complex-mediated RPGN*: IF characteristically shows the presence of coarse immune deposits in the glomeruli; about 25% of all RPGN is immune complex mediated and may be due to lupus, IgAN, infectious GN or MCGN.
- *Pauci-immune RPGN*: causing more than 50% of all RPGN, this group is due to ANCA-associated

vasculitis such as granulomatosis with polyangiitis, microscopic polyangiitis or, rarely, eosinophilic granulomatosis with polyangiitis (Churg–Strauss).

Treatment

Initial therapy for biopsy-proven crescentic GN presenting clinically as RPGN consists of pulse methylprednisolone for three days followed by daily oral prednisone and oral or intravenous cyclophosphamide or rituximab. Plasmapheresis is offered if the patient has haemoptysis, which may be seen in RPGN associated with anti-GBM disease or ANCA vasculitis. Sometimes, empirical therapy with pulse methylprednisolone and cyclophosphamide is started when the clinical suspicion of RPGN is very high and there is a delay in renal biopsy or interpretation of the biopsy.

This is accompanied by specific therapy for the renal pathology causing RPGN.

The presence of circumferential crescents in >80% glomeruli is associated with a very poor response to therapy.

Anti-Glomerular Basement Membrane Antibody Disease and Goodpasture's Disease

Anti-GBM disease is characterized by circulating antibodies against an antigen intrinsic to the type IV collagen chain found in GBM. The condition typically

Table 9.3 Causes of lung haemorrhage with rapidly progressive glomerulonephritis (Goodpasture's syndrome)	
Goodpasture's disease: associated with anti-GBM disease (20–40% of cases)	**Not associated with anti-GBM antibodies (60–80% of cases)** • Granulomatosis with polyangiitis (commonest) • Microscopic polyangiitis • Churg–Strauss syndrome • Systemic lupus erythematosus • Henoch–Schonlein purpura • Bechet's syndrome • Cryoglobulinemic vasculitis • Rheumatoid vasculitis • Drugs: penicillamine, propylthiouracil, hydralazine

GBM, glomerular basement membrane.

presents as AKI caused by RPGN, often accompanied by pulmonary haemorrhage that may be life threatening [21].

It must be borne in mind that Goodpasture's *syndrome* refers to the coexistence of RPGN with lung haemorrhage due to any cause (e.g. systemic lupus erythematosus, granulomatosis with polyangiitis or microscopic polyangiitis), whilst Goodpasture's *disease* specifically refers to the combination of renal failure, lung haemorrhage, and anti-GBM antibodies detected in the patient's sera.

Only 20–40% of Goodpasture's syndrome is caused by Goodpasture's disease, with the rest being caused by the other diseases mentioned in Table 9.3.

Pathogenesis

Collagen consists of three polypeptides called alpha-chains (about 1400 amino acids long) wrapped around each other in a triple helical rope-like structure. Of the four types of collagen, type IV is found exclusively in basement membranes. The three alpha-chains in type IV collagen can be of six types, designated types 1–6 alpha-chains, and the combinations of these alpha-chains can give rise to the following three distinct types of type IV collagen:

• Alpha1–alpha1–alpha2: found in all basement membranes.
• Alpha3–alpha4–alpha5: exclusively in GBM, alveolar membranes in lungs, eye, and cochlea.
• Alpha5–alpha5–alpha6: skin, distal tubular basement membrane (*but not GBM*).

Collagen has a C-terminal non-collagenous domain (NC1) of 230 amino acids and a smaller N-terminal non-collagenous domain of 20 amino acids. Anti-GBM disease is due to antibodies against the NC1 domain of the alpha-3 chain of type IV collagen [22].

Whilst the collagen in GBM is always exposed to blood due to the gaps between the glomerular endothelial cells, the tightly aligned endothelial cells in lungs prevent the collagen in the alveolar basement membrane from being exposed to circulating blood. Pulmonary insults due to smoking, infection, cocaine inhalation, fluid overload or hydrocarbon exposure cause gaps between the pulmonary endothelial cells and predispose to the development of pulmonary haemorrhage in patients with circulating anti-GBM antibody. This explains why pulmonary haemorrhage is observed in only 40–60% of patients with anti-GBM disease, whilst renal insult is seen almost universally in these patients.

Pathology

LM and EM show typical appearances of diffuse proliferative GN, often with crescent formation. IF shows characteristic IgG deposition in a linear pattern along the GBM.

Clinical Presentation

Pulmonary haemorrhage may present with overt haemoptysis, shortness of breath, cough, pulmonary infiltrates on chest X-ray or an increased carbon monoxide diffusing capacity (DLCO) due to the presence of haemoglobin in the alveoli. The pulmonary symptoms often precede the renal failure and may have been present for days to weeks and at times for months. Renal involvement in the form of RPGN usually proceeds quite rapidly.

Diagnosis is based on the presence of anti-GBM antibody in sera along with typical IF findings on renal biopsy.

Between 10 and 40% of anti-GBM antibody-positive patients may also be positive for myeloperoxidase (MPO) ANCA [23]. These patients tend to have a more aggressive disease and also have more frequent relapses.

Treatment

Early diagnosis is vital for response to therapy and prognosis. Delay in treatment can lead to death or dialysis dependence in up to 90% of patients.

Most patients are treated with plasmapheresis in conjunction with prednisolone and cyclophosphamide. Plasmapheresis removes circulating anti-GBM antibodies, whilst the immunosuppressive agents minimize new antibody formation.

Plasmapheresis for 14 days or until the anti-GBM antibody levels are suppressed is an absolute indication in patients with pulmonary haemorrhage independent of the severity of renal involvement. Plasmapheresis is not useful in those who are dialysis dependent on presentation or have >85% crescents on renal biopsy in the absence of pulmonary haemorrhage. Patients who are double positive for anti-GBM and ANCA antibody are offered plasmapheresis irrespective of the presence or absence of pulmonary haemorrhage.

Crescents seen on renal biopsy mandate treatment as for RPGN already discussed, with pulse methylprednisolone for three days followed by oral prednisolone along with oral or intravenous cyclophosphamide.

Prednisolone is started at 1 mg/kg orally and reduced weekly to one-sixth of the dose at eight weeks, with the aim of tapering down the dose and usually stopping by three to four months. Cyclophosphamide is normally used orally at a dose of 2 mg/kg/day for up to three months [24]. Maintenance therapy is not advised by the KDIGO 2012 guidelines, although local practices vary, with many offering maintenance therapy for up to nine months.

Relapses are uncommon except in those who are double positive for anti-GBM and ANCA antibodies, with most patients relapsing with the ANCA vasculitis rather than Goodpasture's disease [25].

References

1. Donadio, J.V. and Grande, J.P. (2002). IgA nephropathy. *N. Engl. J. Med.* 347: 738–748. https://doi.org/10.1056/NEJMra020109.

2. Suzuki, K., Honda, K., Tanabe, K. et al. (2003). Incidence of latent mesangial IgA deposition in renal allograft donors in Japan. *Kidney Int.* 63 (6): 2286.

3. Waldherr, R., Rambausek, M., Duncker, W.D., and Ritz, E. (1989). Frequency of mesangial IgA deposits in a non-selected autopsy series. *Nephrol. Dial. Transplant.* 4 (11): 943.

4. Suzuki, H., Kiryluk, K., Novak, J. et al. (2011). The pathophysiology of IgA nephropathy. *J. Am. Soc. Nephrol.* 22 (10): 1795–1803. https://doi.org/10.1681/ASN.2011050464.

5. Boyd, J.K., Cheung, C.K., Molyneux, K. et al. (2012). An update on the pathogenesis and treatment of IgA nephropathy. *Kidney Int.* 81 (9): 833–843.

6. Working Group of the International IgA Nephropathy Network and the Renal Pathology Society, Cattran, D.C., Coppo, R. et al. (2009). The Oxford classification of IgA nephropathy: rationale, clinicopathological correlations, and classification. *Kidney Int.* 76 (5): 534.

7. Galla, J.H. (1995). IgA nephropathy. *Kidney Int.* 47 (2): 377.

8. Moriyama, T., Tanaka, K., Iwasaki, C. et al. (2014). Prognosis in IgA nephropathy: 30 year analysis of 1012 patients at a single Centre in Japan. *PLoS One* 9 (3): e91756. https://doi.org/10.1371/journal.pone.0091756.

9. Odum, J., Peh, C.A., Clarkson, A.R. et al. (1994). Recurrent mesangial IgA nephritis following renal transplantation. *Nephrol. Dial. Transplant.* 9 (3): 309.

10. Komatsu, H., Fujimoto, S., Hara, S. et al. (2008). Effect of tonsillectomy plus steroid pulse therapy on clinical remission of IgA nephropathy: a controlled study. *Clin. J. Am. Soc. Nephrol.* 3 (5): 1301.

11. Kawamura, T., Yoshimura, M., Miyazaki, Y. et al. (2014). A multicenter randomized controlled trial of tonsillectomy combined with steroid pulse therapy in patients with immunoglobulin a nephropathy. *Nephrol. Dial. Transplant.* 29 (8): 1546–1553. Epub 2014 Mar.

12. Nasr, S.H., Radhakrishnan, J., and D'Agati, V.D. (2013). Bacterial infection-related glomerulonephritis in adults. *Kidney Int.* 83 (5): 792–803. https://doi.org/10.1038/ki.2012.407.

13. Carapetis, J.R., Steer, A.C., Mulholland, E.K., and Weber, M. (2005). The global burden of group a streptococcal diseases. *Lancet Infect. Dis.* 5 (11): 685–694.

14. Nasr, S.H., Fidler, M.E., Valeri, A.M. et al. (2011). Postinfectious glomerulonephritis in the elderly. *J. Am. Soc. Nephrol.* 22 (1): 187–195. https://doi.org/10.1681/ASN.2010060611.

15. Rodriguez-Iturbe, B. and Haas, M. Post-strepto-coccal glomerulonephritis. In: *Streptococcus Pyogenes: Basic Biology to Clinical Manifestations* (eds. J.J. Ferretti, D.L. Stevens and V.A. Fischetti). Oklahoma City, OK: University of Oklahoma Health Sciences Center https://www.ncbi.nlm.nih.gov/books/NBK333429.

16. Yoshizawa, N., Yamakami, K., Fujino, M. et al. (2004). Nephritis-associated plasmin receptor and acute poststreptococcal glomerulonephritis: characterization of the antigen and associated immune response. *J.Am. Soc. Nephrol.* 15 (7): 1785–1793.

17. Batsford, S.R., Mezzano, S., Mihatsch, M. et al. (2005). Is the nephritogenic antigen in post-streptococcal glomerulonephritis pyrogenic exo-toxin B (SPEB) or GAPDH? *Kidney Int.* 68 (3): 1120–1129.

18. Kaplan, E.L., Anthony, B.F., Chapman, S.S. et al. (1970). The influence of the site of infection on the immune response to group a streptococci. *J. Clin. Invest.* 49 (7): 1405.

19. Boils, C.L., Nasr, S.H., Walker, P.D. et al. (2015). Update on endocarditis-associated glomerulone-phritis. *Kidney Int.* 87 (6): 1241–1249. Epub 2015 Jan 21.

20. Greenhall, G.H.B. and Salama, A.D. (2015). What is new in the management of rapidly progressive glomerulonephritis? *Clin. Kidney J.* 8 (2): 143–150. https://doi.org/10.1093/ckj/sfv008.

21. Greco, A., Rizzo, M.I., De Virgilio, A. et al. (2015). Goodpasture's syndrome: a clinical update. *Autoimmun. Rev.* 14 (3): 246–253. https://doi.org/10.1016/j.autrev.2014.11.006. Epub 2014 Nov 15.

22. Pedchenko, V., Vanacore, R., and Hudson, B. (2011). Goodpasture's disease: molecular archi-tecture of the autoantigen provides clues to etiol-ogy and pathogenesis. *Curr. Opin. Nephrol. Hypertens.* 20 (3): 290–296. https://doi.org/10.1097/MNH.0b013e328344ff20.

23. Hellmark, T., Niles, J.L., Collins, A.B. et al. (1997). Comparison of anti-GBM antibodies in sera with or without ANCA. *J. Am. Soc. Nephrol.* 8 (3): 376.

24. (2012). Chapter 14: Anti-glomerular basement membrane antibody glomerulonephritis. *Kidney Int. Suppl* 2: 240–242. https://doi.org/10.1038/kisup.2012.27.

25. Jayne, D.R., Marshall, P.D., Jones, S.J., and Lockwood, C.M. (1990). Autoantibodies to GBM and neutrophil cytoplasm in rapidly progressive glomerulonephritis. *Kidney Int.* 37 (3): 965.

Questions and Answers

Questions

1. Glomerulonephritis associated with low complement levels is seen in:
   a. IgA nephropathy
   b. Goodpasture's disease
   c. Lupus nephritis
   d. ANCA positive vasculitis

2. Mesangial deposits of IgA are characteristically seen in:
   a. Lupus nephritis
   b. Anti-GBM disease
   c. Post-streptococcal GN
   d. HSP

3. True about IgA nephropathy:
   a. Is common in the age group of 50–60 years
   b. Half the patients present in rapidly progressive GN
   c. Half the patients present with asymptomatic episodic haematuria
   d. AKI is the mode of initial presentation in >30% patients

4. A 35 year-old man with no known previous medical history is referred by GP for new renal failure. His creatinine is 220 µmol/l and dipstick reveals ++++hematuria and + proteinuria. USG rules out an obstructive cause for the renal failure and clinical examination reveals blood pressure of 180/96 mmHg and pedal edema till mid shins. Rest of the routine blood tests including LFT and FBC are normal. Which of the following is unlikely to be the diagnosis for this man?
   a. IgAN
   b. Lupus nephritis
   c. FSGS
   d. Cryoglobulinemia

5. Which of the following is NOT the treatment of choice for rapidly progressive GN?
   a. Pulse methylprednisolone
   b. Intravenous cyclophosphamide
   c. Oral cyclophosphamide
   d. Mycophenolate

Answers

1. c. GN associated with low complements is seen in lupus, infectious GN, infective endocarditis, cryoglobulinemia, and MCGN.
2. d. HSP is a systemic form of IgAN and hence characteristically associated with glomerular IgA deposits on IF.
3. c. In 40–50% of cases with IGAN, the presentation is with episodic macroscopic haematuria especially in the second or third decades of life.

About 30–40% cases are identified on the basis of follow up for asymptomatic microscopic haematuria identified on urinary dipstick testing. AKI is an unusual mode of presentation and likely seen in <10% of cases.

4. c. FSGS presents with nephrotic syndrome and not nephritis.
5. d. There is no evidence for the use of mycophenolate in RPGN. Those who have a contraindication to cyclophosphamide or are unwilling to accept are offered rituximab.

10

Renal Vasculitis and Lupus Nephritis

Anthea Anantharajah, Sanjay Swaminathan, and Surjit Tarafdar

Summary

- Vasculitis is a group of disorders characterized by inflammation of blood vessel walls
- The clinical manifestations are due to either rupture of the inflamed vessel wall or luminal blockage due to inflammation leading to downstream tissue ischaemia and necrosis
- Classified as large, medium or small vessel vasculitis; the latter might lead to glomerulonephritis (GN), which is often rapidly progressive without treatment
- Although prognosis has improved in recent years, patients often experience poor quality of life due to frequent relapses, persisting low-grade disease activity, and the burden of immunosuppression-related toxicity

- Systemic lupus erythematosus (SLE) is a multi-system autoimmune disorder that predominantly affects females, with a female to male ratio of 10:1
- SLE is characterized by the presence of autoantibodies against various nuclear antigens and detection of these antibodies plays an important role in diagnosis.
- 30–50% of patients with SLE have renal involvement in the course of their disease
- Lupus nephritis may present as either GN or nephrotic syndrome which is usually due to membranous nephropathy
- Lupus-associated proliferative GN needs treatment with immunosuppression

Vasculitis

Vasculitis is a group of disorders characterized by inflammation of the vessel wall. The clinical manifestations of vasculitis are largely due to the following two effects:

- An inflamed and thinned vessel wall may protrude out as an aneurysm that may rupture and bleed.
- Luminal obstruction due to inflammation may lead to downstream ischaemia and/or necrosis.

Systemic vasculitis is often serious and sometimes fatal. Despite a poor understanding of the aetiology of specific vasculitides, there has been a significant reduction in mortality in the last few decades [1]. However, many treated patients experience poor quality of life due to frequent relapses, persisting low-grade disease activity, and the burden of immunosuppression-related toxicity.

Vasculitis can be classified as large vessel, medium vessel, and small vessel vasculitis. The small vessel vasculitides can be further subdivided as immune complex mediated or pauci-immune mediated. The

Lecture Notes Nephrology: A Comprehensive Guide to Renal Medicine, First Edition. Edited by Surjit Tarafdar.
© 2020 John Wiley & Sons Ltd. Published 2020 by John Wiley & Sons Ltd.

organs most commonly involved in vasculitis are the skin, musculoskeletal system, peripheral nerves, gastrointestinal tract, respiratory tract, and the kidneys.

Large Vessel Vasculitis

- Takayasu arteritis
- Giant cell arteritis (GCA)

Medium Vessel Vasculitis

- Polyarteritis nodosa (PAN)
- Kawasaki disease (seen in children)

Small Vessel Vasculitis

Pauci-immune, Antineutrophil Cytoplasmic Antibody (ANCA) Associated

- Granulomatosis with polyangiitis (GPA, formerly Wegener's granulomatosis)
- Microscopic polyangiitis
- Eosinophilic granulomatosis with polyangiitis (EGPA, formerly Churg–Strauss syndrome)

Immune Complex Mediated

- Cryoglobulinemic vasculitis
- Anti-glomerular basement membrane (anti-GBM) disease
- Immunoglobulin (Ig) A nephropathy/Henoch–Schönlein purpura (HSP)

How is the Kidney Affected in Vasculitis?

The nature of kidney involvement and presentation depends on the size of the blood vessel involved by the vasculitis:

- *Large vessel vasculitis*: affects aorta/main renal arteries, leading to renovascular hypertension with presentation similar to renal artery stenosis.
- *Medium vessel vasculitis*: inflammation of the intra-renal medium-sized arteries, causing thrombosis or rupture and leading to foci of renal infarction (and resultant hypertension due to activation of the renin–angiotensin–aldosterone system) or haemorrhage, respectively.
- *Small vessel vasculitis*: involvement of the small glomerular vessels leads to glomerulonephritis (GN) and often acute kidney injury (AKI).

Note that only small vessel vasculitis, which involves the small glomerular capillaries, leads to GN.

Large Vessel Arteritis

Takayasu Arteritis

Takayasu arteritis primarily affects the aorta and its main branches, with the subclavian artery being more commonly affected in the early stages of the disease. Women in their second and third decades are at the greatest risk, and the disease is more common in Asian populations. Primarily characterized by granulomatous inflammation, the abdominal aorta is eventually involved in up to 50% patients. The vessels may be either dilated and aneurysmal due to destruction of the muscular media, or stenotic due to scarring and intimal proliferation (Figure 10.1).

Systemic symptoms such as fatigue, weight loss, and low-grade fever are common. Most patients have diminished or absent pulses in the arm, and blood-pressure discrepancies between the right and left arms due to subclavian stenosis [2]. Stenotic lesions proximal to the origin of the vertebral artery can cause neurological symptoms or syncope due to subclavian steal syndrome (Figure 10.1) [3]. Involvement of the renal arteries leading to renovascular hypertension is the major manifestation of renal involvement and may be seen in up to 50% of patients.

Histological confirmation is often not possible given the location of the lesions and diagnosis frequently rests on the combination of clinical scenario, raised inflammatory markers—such as C-reactive protein (CRP) and erythrocyte sedimentation rate (ESR)—and radiographic evidence of smoothly tapered stenotic arterial lesions on magnetic resonance imaging (MRI), computed tomography (CT) or angiography. Fluorodeoxyglucose-positron emission tomography (FDG-PET) is also frequently used to identify inflammatory lesions in large blood vessels.

Whilst the mainstay of treatment is corticosteroids, up to half of patients will require steroid-sparing agents such as methotrexate or azathioprine. Angioplasty or bypass grafts may be needed for large aneurysms or irreversible arterial stenosis causing significant ischaemic symptoms [4].

Giant Cell Arteritis

Although pathologically both Takayasu arteritis and GCA are characterized by granulomatous vasculitis involving the large-sized arteries, there are significant

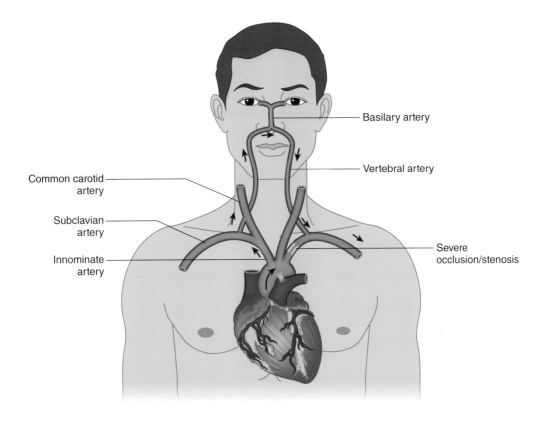

Figure 10.1 Takayasu arteritis affecting subclavian artery proximal to origin of vertebral artery can lead to the subclavian steal syndrome.

differences in the type of artery predominantly involved and the age of presentation. Unlike Takayasu arteritis, which has a predilection for major arteries supplying the upper limbs, GCA tends to affect the cranial branches of the arteries originating from the aortic arch (particularly the extra-cranial branches of the carotid artery). Takayasu arteritis is more common in Asians and usually presents before the age of 40 years, whilst GCA is frequently seen in people of northern European ancestry and presents after the age of 50 years [5, 6].

According to the American College of Rheumatology, three positive criteria (out of five) help to diagnose GCA [7]:

- Age greater than or equal to 50 years at time of disease onset.
- Localized headache of new onset.
- Tenderness or decreased pulse of the temporal artery.
- ESR greater than 50 mm/hour.
- Biopsy revealing a necrotizing arteritis with a predominance of mononuclear cells or a granulomatous process with multinucleated giant cells.

Clinically significant renal disease is rare in GCA. Polymyalgia rheumatica, which is usually characterized by aching and morning stiffness about the shoulder and hip girdles, may be seen in 40–50% of patients with GCA.

Treatment of GCA consists of corticosteroids and long-term prognosis is usually good.

Medium Vessel Arteritis

Polyarteritis Nodosa

PAN is a systemic necrotizing vasculitis that typically affects medium-sized muscular arteries. The characteristic absence of involvement of veins and smaller arteries or capillaries, and ANCA negativity, helps to differentiate PAN from some of the other vasculitis conditions. The aetiology and pathogenesis of PAN are unknown, but there is a strong association with hepatitis B, suggesting that circulating immune complexes might localize on vessel walls, causing the condition. Whilst up to one-third of patients with PAN

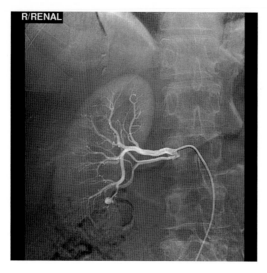

Figure 10.2 Computed tomography angiogram showing multiple aneurysms and irregular constrictions in the medium-sized renal blood vessels suggestive of polyarteritis nodosa (PAN).

Table 10.1 Clinical presentation of polyarteritis nodosa (PAN)

Systemic features – fever/malaise	80%
Peripheral neuropathy	75%
Arthralgia/myalgia	60%
Skin – livedo reticularis, purpura	50%
Kidney – infarction or haemorrhage	50%
Gastrointestinal – abdominal pain, blood in stool	40%
Hypertension	35%
Orchitis	20%
Stroke	20%
Cardiac – cardiomyopathy, pericarditis	10%

may be hepatitis B positive [8], the association is probably stronger in areas where hepatitis B is endemic. Histologically, PAN is characterized by segmental transmural fibrinoid necrosis of arteries accompanied by infiltrating leucocytes and lack of granulomas. Recessive loss of function mutations of the gene encoding adenosine deaminase 2 (ADA2), a growth factor that is the major extracellular adenosine deaminase, is thought to be associated with childhood presentation of PAN.

More than 80% of patients have non-specific systemic complaints such as fever and weight loss. Peripheral neuropathy, typically in the form of mononeuritis multiplex, is seen in up to three-quarters of patients. Almost half of patients have gastrointestinal involvement presenting as abdominal pain or blood in the stool. Kidney involvement may lead to infarction or haemorrhage, which may present with flank pain and haematuria. Up to one-third of patients develop hypertension, whilst 20% of patients may present with testicular pain due to orchitis (Table 10.1).

There is no single diagnostic test for PAN. Acute-phase reactants like ESR and CRP are often elevated and up to one-third of patients are hepatitis B positive. Whilst a tissue biopsy should be done where possible, a mesenteric or renal angiogram in the setting of a suggestive history and clinical presentation is often diagnostic. The angiogram characteristically shows multiple aneurysms and irregular constrictions in the larger vessels, with occlusion of smaller penetrating arteries (Figure 10.2).

Remember, in PAN:

- No GN
- No lung involvement
- No ANCA
- No involvement of arterioles/capillaries/veins
- No granuloma on biopsy

The treatment of PAN depends on the degree of disease severity and presence or absence of hepatitis:

- *Mild disease*: arthritis, anaemia, and skin lesions without renal, cardiac, gastrointestinal or neurological involvement are treated with prednisolone.
- *Moderate to severe disease*: involvement of the above or life-threatening complications warrant treatment with prednisolone and a second immunosuppressive agent, typically cyclophosphamide.
- *Hepatitis B positive*: anti-viral therapy rather than immunosuppression is the mainstay of treatment. However, if PAN is severe, short-term treatment with glucocorticoids and plasma exchange is advised until anti-viral therapy becomes effective [9].

Kawasaki Disease

Kawasaki disease is rare in adults and mostly seen below the age of 5 years. Termed mucocutaneous lymph node (MCLN) syndrome, it is self-limited and associated with fever, conjunctivitis, erythaema of the lips and oral mucosa, desquamation of the extremities, rash, and cervical lymphadenopathy. Coronary artery aneurysms or ectasia develop in approximately 15–25% of untreated children and may lead to ischaemic heart disease or sudden death [10]. Renal involvement is uncommon. Treatment consists of intravenous immunoglobulin and aspirin to decrease the risk of coronary artery aneurysms [11]. Steroids are of no benefit in this condition.

Small Vessel Arteritis

Immune complex-mediated small vessel vasculitis, namely anti-GBM disease and immunoglobulin A nephropathy are discussed in Chapter 9.

Pauci-immune Vasculitis

Pauci-immune vasculitis—characterised lack of immunoglobulin and or complements seen on immunofluorescence (IF) microscopy includes granulomatosis with polyangiitis (GPA, formerly called Wegener's granulomatosis), microscopic polyangiitis (MPA), and eosinophilic granulomatosis with polyangiitis (EGPA, formerly termed Churg–Strauss syndrome). These conditions have a strong association with ANCA, which are autoantibodies directed against cytoplasmic antigens of neutrophils and monocytes.

The two main types of ANCA are:

- *Cytoplasmic or c-ANCA:* on IF, the staining is diffuse throughout the cytoplasm and the main antigen is proteinase 3 (PR3).
- *Perinuclear or p-ANCA:* a perinuclear pattern of staining is actually an artefact of ethanol fixation. With ethanol fixation of neutrophils, the positively charged cytoplasmic antigens arrange themselves around the negatively charged nuclear membrane, leading to perinuclear fluorescence [12]. The chief antigen is myeloperoxidase (MPO).

The two types of ANCA assays generally used are indirect IF, to detect the ANCA pattern, and enzyme-linked immunosorbent assay (ELISA), to quantify the MPO or PR3 positivity. Whilst the former is more sensitive, ELISA is more specific. Usually indirect IF is the first test performed for screening. If positive, the more specific and quantitative ELISA is performed as a confirmatory test.

False positive immunofluorescence results for p-ANCA could be due to antibodies reacting to other cytoplasmic antigens such as lactoferrin, elastase, cathepsin G, bactericidal permeability inhibitor, and catalase (Table 10.2).

Whilst there is a degree of overlap in the mode of presentation of the three types of pauci-immune small vessel vasculitis, there are sufficient differences to warrant individual description. All patients typically develop constitutional symptoms that may include fever, malaise, anorexia, arthralgia, myalgia, and weight loss.

Granulomatosis with Polyangiitis

GPA (previously called Wegner's granulomatosis) is characterized by granulomatous inflammation affecting the upper and lower respiratory tracts, in addition to renal involvement leading to GN [13]:

- Lung involvement in 90%: pulmonary haemorrhage and nodular or cavitating lesions seen radiologically.
- Ear, nose, and throat (ENT) involvement in 90%: sinusitis, rhinitis, subglottic stenosis, ocular inflammation, septal perforation, and/or saddle nose deformity.
- Kidney involvement in 80%: GN with/without proteinuria and renal failure, rapidly progressive GN (RPGN).
- Cutaneous manifestations in 40%: leukocytoclastic angiitis causing purpura, ulceration, and necrosis.
- Gastrointestinal (GI) involvement in 50% and neurological in 30%.
- ANCA positive in up to 90%: usually PR3 positive.

Microscopic Polyangiitis

MPA is characterized by non-granulomatous inflammation of the kidneys, leading to GN with absence of asthma or eosinophilia:

- Kidney involvement in 80%: GN with/without proteinuria and AKI, RPGN.
- Skin involvement in 40%, lung involvement in 40%, GI involvement in 40%, ENT involvement in 35%, and neurological system involvement in 30%.
- ANCA positive in more than 80%: usually MPO-ANCA.

Eosinophilic Granulomatosis with Polyangiitis

EGPA (previously called Churg–Strauss syndrome) is characterized by asthma, eosinophilia, and granulomatous changes on histology [14]:

- Asthma and eosinophilia with vasculitis affecting multiple organs and extravascular granulomas.
- Kidney involvement in 50% and less severe than GPA and MPA.
- ANCA positive in up to 50%: MPO slightly more common than PR3 antibodies.
- Develops in the following sequential phases with overlap at times:
  - *Prodromal phase:* in second to third decades with atopic disease/asthma.
  - *Eosinophilic phase:* pulmonary opacities, asthma, and peripheral eosinophilia with eosinophilic infiltration of lungs and GI tract.

Table 10.2 Antineutrophil cytoplasmic antibody (ANCA)-associated small vessel vasculitis

Disease or associations	Frequency of ANCA positivity	Type of ANCA
Granulomatosis with polyangiitis	90%	Mostly PR3
Microscopic polyangiitis	70%	Mostly MPO
Eosinophilic granulomatosis with polyangiitis	50%	MPO slightly >PR3
Anti-GBM antibody disease	10–40%	Mostly MPO
Drugs: anti-thyroid drugs (propylthiouracil and methimazole), hydralazine, penicillamine, cocaine contaminated with levamisole		MPO≫PR3

GBM, glomerular basement membrane; MPO, myeloperoxidase; PR3, proteinase 3.

Table 10.3 Chief differences between granulomatosis with polyangiitis (GPA), microscopic polyangiitis (MPA), and eosinophilic granulomatosis with polyangiitis (EGPA)

GPA	MPA	EGPA
Granulomatous inflammation affecting the upper and lower respiratory tracts, with glomerulonephritis but without eosinophilia	Necrotizing inflammation causing glomerulonephritis but without asthma/eosinophilia/granulomas	Asthma, eosinophilia, and necrotizing granulomatous inflammation involving the respiratory tract; renal involvement is less common and usually less severe than in GPA or MPA

○ *Vasculitic phase*: in third to fourth decades, with vascular/extravascular granulomatosis and fever, weight loss, malaise, and lassitude.

Asthma usually precedes the vasculitis by up to 10 years and is often poorly controlled with inhaled corticosteroids. For this reason, patients are often on oral corticosteroids, which in turn probably helps to keep the disease suppressed in the initial stage and explains the time difference between the prodromal and the vasculitic phases (Table 10.3).

Renal biopsy in all three conditions shows segmental necrotizing GN, often with crescents, and IF is characteristically negative. Granulomas are very infrequently seen on renal biopsy specimens in patients with GPA or EGPA, although they may be seen in biopsy from other sites such as nasal mucosa or lungs.

Treatment

The treatment of small vessel pauci-immune vasculitis consists of induction and maintenance phases, as follows [15].

Induction Phase

Intravenous methylprednisolone for three days followed by oral prednisolone at 1 g/kg and cyclophosphamide (intravenous or oral) for induction: 3–6 months is effective in 80–90% of cases. The RAVE and RITUXIVAS trials have shown the non-inferiority of using rituximab as an effective induction strategy in achieving remission [16, 17].

Plasmapheresis is offered in patients with:

- Severe renal disease; that is, those with a serum creatinine of 354 umol/l or needing dialysis
- Concurrent anti-GBM autoantibody disease
- Pulmonary haemorrhage

Patients with EGPA generally have less severe renal disease and are unlikely to need plasmapheresis.

Maintenance Phase

Azathioprine or methotrexate and low-dose prednisolone are usually given for 12–24 months. There is evidence for the use of rituximab for up to 18 months as maintenance therapy with good outcomes, as per the

Maintenance of Remission Using Rituximab in Systemic ANCA-Associated Vasculitis (MAINRITSAN) trial [18]. Methotrexate should be avoided in those with glomerular filtration rate (GFR)<50 ml/min, whilst rituximab should be avoided in those who are positive for hepatitis B surface antigen (HBsAg) or have antibodies to the hepatitis B core antigen (anti-HBc), due to the elevated risk of reactivation and potentially fatal hepatitis.

Prior to the use of this treatment, the small vessel pauci-immune vasculitis was universally fatal. Ten-year survival rates for treated patients now approach 90% for EGPA [19] and 60–80% for GPA and MPA [20, 21].

Systemic Lupus Erythematosus and the Kidneys

Systemic lupus erythematosus (SLE) is a multisystem autoimmune disorder that predominantly affects females, with a female to male ratio of 10 : 1. There is an increased prevalence of SLE in certain ethnic populations (such as those from Africa, Indo-Chinese populations, and people from South East Asia), strongly suggesting a genetic component to susceptibility. To illustrate this, the prevalence varies from approximately 40 per 100 000 people in North European populations to >200 per 100 000 persons in patients of African heritage [22]. With current therapeutic tools, the life expectancy of patients with SLE has significantly improved, with 4-year survivals of around 50% reported in the 1950s and 15-year survival rates of ~80% in more recent times [23].

SLE is characterized by the presence of autoantibodies against various nuclear components, suggesting an autoimmune disorder, though recent work has shown that numerous other immune pathways may be also involved [24]. It is a spectrum disorder, with a variety of clinical presentations (discussed below), which can vary from mild to life threatening in severity. This can make the recognition, diagnosis, and management of SLE challenging, with a tailored approach necessary for each patient. Not uncommonly, SLE may be diagnosed in the context of renal impairment, with a suggestive renal biopsy and the presence of characteristic autoantibodies. It is therefore an important condition to have in the differential diagnosis of renal disorders.

Aetiological Factors

With a variety of antibodies directed against self-antigens, there is little doubt that autoimmunity is a major player in both clinical manifestations and disease progression in SLE. However, the factors that drive the autoimmune process remain poorly understood. Given the much higher incidence of SLE in women, hormonal influences have been postulated to play an important role. Hormonal changes may also explain the high incidence of SLE in postpubertal individuals and flares during pregnancy or the menstrual cycle [25].

There is a 25% concordance of SLE between monozygotic twins (and 2% in dizygotic twins). This suggest that though genetic factors are important [26], they are not sufficient by themselves to definitively cause the disease, thereby indicating that environmental factors are at play. Apart from deficiencies in early complement components such as C1q, C2 or C4 (which strongly predict lupus nephritis) [27], genome-wide association studies (GWAS) have identified other loci such as CD44, STAT4, TNFAIP3, ITGAM, FcRγ, and PRDM1-ATG5 [28]. Many of the loci identified via GWAS implicate immune system-related proteins.

Along with genetic factors, a viral aetiology has also been postulated in disease pathogenesis, with Epstein–Barr virus (EBV) being touted as being a leading contender [29]. Interestingly, other autoimmune diseases have also been linked to EBV (notably multiple sclerosis).

Certain drugs have also been associated with the development of SLE (drug-induced lupus). These drugs include hydralazine, procainamide (the two most likely drugs to induce lupus), quinidine, penicillamine, and anti-tumour necrosis factor-alpha agents such as infliximab and etanercept. In fact, there are more than 50 drugs that are known to potentially induce autoimmunity in general [30]. Drug-induced lupus is associated with the presence of anti-histone antibodies, whilst anti-dsDNA and anti-Smith antibodies are usually absent [31].

Pathogenesis of Lupus and Autoantibodies

Before we discuss the pathogenesis of SLE, we need to understand the following terms:

- *Chromatin*: a complex found only in eukaryotic cells consisting of DNA, RNA, and supporting proteins called histones. The main roles of chromatin are to package the DNA into a smaller volume to fit into the cell, prevent DNA from being damaged and also control DNA replication.
- *Histone*: these are the chief protein components of chromatin, acting as a spool around which DNA

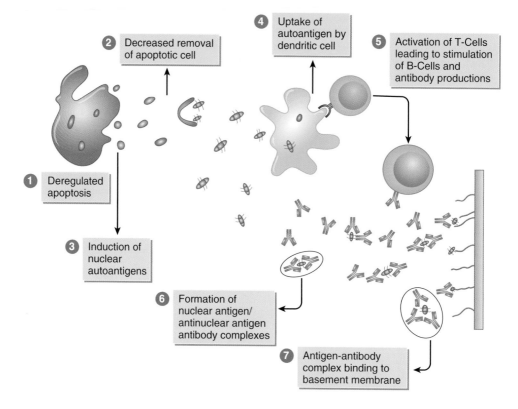

Figure 10.3 Pathogenesis of lupus.

winds. Without histones, the unwound DNA in chromosomes would be very long (a length to width ratio of more than 10 million: 1 in human DNA).

- *Nucleosome*: this is the basic unit of DNA packaging and consists of a segment of DNA wound around eight histone protein cores. The nucleosome core particle represents the first level of chromatin organization.

The defining feature of SLE is the presence of autoantibodies directed against a relatively limited range of nuclear antigens. These nuclear antigens include DNA, histone, chromatin, and nucleosome.

Exposure to these autoantibody-stimulating nuclear antigens may occur as a consequence of aberrant cellular apoptosis and their release into the systemic circulation (Figure 10.3). There are thought to be defects in the clearance of immune complexes and persistence of debris of apoptotic cells in these patients. Some of the nuclear antigens are also

postulated to trigger immunogenic response through interaction with Toll-like receptors [32]. These autoantibodies may be present for many years prior to disease manifestation.

The antigen–autoantibody complexes are carried by blood vessels to different organs, where they stimulate inflammation and complement activation.

Although the detection of antinuclear antibodies (ANA) in serum facilitates the diagnosis of patients with SLE, it must be borne in mind that up to 5% of these patients might be negative for ANA. The following autoantibodies are commonly found in patients with SLE:

1. DNA: anti-double-stranded DNA antibodies are highly specific for lupus; they are present in 70% of patients with lupus, but in less than 0.5% of healthy people or patients with other autoimmune diseases such as rheumatoid arthritis. Although they generally tend to reflect disease activity, sometimes they may precede the disease manifestation by years.

Table 10.4 Specificity and sensitivity of antibodies to extractable nuclear antigens for the diagnosis of systemic lupus erythematosus (SLE)

Antibody (tested using enzyme-linked immunosorbent assay, ELISA)	Sensitivity (%) for SLE	Specificity (%) for SLE
Anti-Ro (SS-A)	61	80–93
Anti-La (SS-B)	27–35	88–97
Anti-Sm	34–45	88–100
Anti-RNP (ribonuclear protein)	39–64	84–97

2. Nucleosome: anti-nucleosome antibodies are found in up to 75% of patients with SLE and may be a useful marker for diagnosis and activity assessment of anti-dsDNA negative SLE [33].
3. The following antigens commonly come under the umbrella term 'extractable nuclear antigens' (ENA) (Table 10.4). These antigens are associated with RNA:
   - Smith (Sm) antigens: Sm antigens are part of small nuclear RNAs. Anti-Smith antibody levels are elevated in 34–45% of SLE cases and 8% of those with mixed connective tissue disease (MCTD). Although they have low sensitivity, they are highly specific for lupus nephritis.
   - RNP: Also called U1RNP, this is a small ribonuclear protein. Anti-RNP antibodies are seen in up to 50% of SLE cases.
   - SS-A (Ro), a ribonucleoprotein complex, and SS-B (La), an RNA-binding protein: the presence of anti-Ro antibodies (SS-A/Ro), anti-La antibodies (SS-B/La) or both in pregnancy confers a 1–2% risk of foetal heart block. Ro antigens are exposed on foetal (but not maternal) cardiac myocytes and maternal anti-Ro antibodies that cross the placenta interact with these antigens. The maternal autoantibodies damage the conducting tissues of the foetal heart, leading to heart block.
4. Histone: whilst anti-histone antibodies are present in 50–70% of patients with SLE, they are seen in more than 95% of patients with drug-induced lupus.
5. N-methyl-D-aspartate (NMDA) receptor: NMDA is an excitatory amino acid released by neurons. Anti-NMDA-receptor antibodies are present in up to 50% of patients with cerebral lupus [34].
6. C1q: anti-C1q antibody is more common in patients of Asian background. Anti-C1q in combination with anti-dsDNA and low complements has the strongest serological association with renal lupus [35].
7. Phospholipids: antiphospholipid (aPL) antibodies are found in approximately 30–40% of patients with SLE, but only about 10% of these patients have antiphospholipid syndrome [36].

There is growing evidence that a persistently active B cell response leading to antibody production in lupus may be partly driven by excess activity of the B cell activating factor (BAFF) [37].

Clinical Features of Lupus

SLE can affect virtually any organ in the body. The disease course is usually characterized by episodes of disease flares followed by periods of remission. Constitutional symptoms such as fatigue, fever, and weight loss are present in most patients at some point during the disease. Table 10.5 lists the American College of Rheumatology criteria for the diagnosis of lupus; the presence of four or more criteria has 96% sensitivity and specificity for the diagnosis. It is important to highlight that patients do not necessarily have to meet four criteria to have lupus, particularly if they have characteristic laboratory or biopsy findings.

From 30 to 50% of patients have clinically evident renal disease at presentation (discussed later).

The most common presenting complaints in acute-onset drug-induced lupus are skin and joint manifestations, with renal, haematological, and neurological features seen uncommonly (Table 10.6).

Laboratory Tests for Lupus

Laboratory tests for SLE can be divided into those that are useful for diagnosis and those that have utility in prognosis. The presence of moderate to high titres of

Table 10.5 American College of Rheumatology Criteria for the diagnosis of lupus – presence of four or more criteria diagnoses lupus

1	Malar rash
2	Discoid rash
3	Photosensitivity
4	Oral ulcers
5	Non-erosive arthritis
6	Pleuro-pericarditis
7	Renal disease (proteinuria and/or RBC casts)
8	Neurologic disorder (unexplained seizures or psychosis)
9	Hematologic disorder (hemolytic anemia/leukopenia/lymphopenia/thrombocytopenia)
10	High ANA titers
11	Immunologic disorder: positive anti-dsDNA, anti-Sm, antiphospholipid antibodies, and low complements

ANA, antinuclear antibodies; RBC, red blood cells; Sm, Smith.

ANA is an important screening test that may suggest the presence of SLE. There are many staining patterns seen with a positive ANA, including speckled, homogeneous, and nucleolar patterns that may give an indication of the nuclear components that are targeted by the positive autoantibodies. For example, the presence of high titres of a homogeneous ANA often correlates with the presence of raised anti-DsDNA antibodies and anti-histone antibodies seen in lupus.

There are two speckled patterns: fine and coarse. The fine speckled pattern is associated with anti-Ro and anti-La antibodies, whilst the coarse speckled pattern is caused by anti-U1-RNP and anti-Sm antibodies. The nucleolar staining pattern is associated with antibodies against Scl-70 (seen in scleroderma). The ANA test is measured using indirect immunofluorescence; that is, a patient's serum is added to slides coated with human cells and a fluorescently labelled antibody targeting immunoglobulins is added. If there is fluorescence seen under a microscope, the serum is diluted to see the lowest dilution that still leads to fluorescence under the microscope. A titre is given as the reciprocal of the dilution. For example, if positive fluorescence is seen with a dilution of 1/640, the ANA titre is given as 1:640.

Measuring the autoantibodies is useful in both the diagnosis and measuring activity of SLE. In addition, their levels can help in monitoring disease activity or guiding response to therapy. The various antibodies are discussed in the section on pathogenesis.

Testing for ENA is also a valuable additional test in the diagnosis of SLE.

The complement proteins C3 and C4 are often reduced in immune complex disease (for example in lupus nephritis), with activation/consumption of complement pathways due to antigen–antibody interactions. Other useful markers for disease activity include CRP and ESR. Patients with SLE may also present with immune-mediated thrombocytopenia and leukopenia, particularly lymphopenia.

Patients with SLE should be tested for the presence of antiphospholipid antibodies. These tests include lupus anticoagulant, beta2 glycoprotein I antibodies, and cardiolipin antibodies (both IgG and IgM isotypes should be measured). These antibodies are associated with a pro-thrombotic tendency. To qualify as having the antiphospholipid antibody syndrome, a patient needs to have a significant thrombotic event (or pregnancy-related complication such as recurrent first trimester miscarriage) in the setting of two positive tests for antiphospholipid antibodies, with the tests being done at least 12 weeks apart.

Table 10.6 Features of spontaneous versus drug-induced lupus

Clinical feature	Idiopathic systemic lupus erythematosus (SLE)	Drug-induced lupus
Sex predisposition (female : male)	9 : 1	1 : 1
Symptom onset	Gradual	Abrupt
Usual age	20–40 years	Drug dependent, tends to be older population (>50 years)
Fever/malaise	40–85%	40–50%
Arthralgias/arthritis	75–95%	80–95%
Rash (all)	50–70%	10–30%
Rash (malar/acute cutaneous)	42%	2%
Pleuritis/pleural effusion	16–60%	10–50% (procainamide)
Pulmonary infiltrates	0–10%	5–40% (procainamide)
Pericarditis	6–45%	2–18%
Hepatomegaly/splenomegaly	10–45%	5–25%
Renal involvement	30–50%	0–5%
Central nervous system/neurological involvement	25–70%	0–2%
Haematological	Common	Unusual
Laboratory feature	**Idiopathic SLE**	**Drug-induced lupus**
Antinuclear antibodies	95–98%	95–100%
Anti-dsDNA	50–80%	<5% (rare)
Anti-Smith	20–30%	<5% (rare)
Anti-RNP (ribonuclear protein)	40–50%	20%
Anti-Ro/SS-A	30–40%	Uncertain
Anti-histone	60–80%	90–95%
Low complement levels	40–65%	Rare
Anaemia	30–90%	0–46%
Leukopenia	35–66%	2–33%

Lupus Nephritis

Renal disease is a common manifestation of SLE. The kidneys receive a significant proportion of total cardiac output, therefore the deposition of circulating immune complexes in the renal microcirculation appears to be a foreseeable consequence of renal haemodynamics. Other factors such as autoantibody cross reactivity with kidney-specific antigens (such as type IV collagen, laminin, and heparin sulphate) may also explain the propensity for kidney injury in SLE [38]. Up to 75% of patients have abnormal urinalyses during the course of their disease trajectory and 30–50% of patients have clinically overt disease [39].

Prior to the advent of immunosuppressive therapies, the mortality associated with lupus nephritis approached 70% [40]. At present, although a proportion of patients may still progress to end-stage renal disease (ESRD) and require renal replacement therapy, a significant morbidity of lupus nephritis is related to treatment toxicity. Consequently, a major research focus has been to delineate pathogenesis and develop targeted therapies that are able to ameliorate renal inflammation whilst minimizing 'collateral damage' to other tissues. Some of these novel therapeutic strategies will be discussed later in this chapter.

Pathogenesis

Glomerular injury in SLE is primarily due to the deposition of immune complexes. The clinical presentation as in nephritic versus nephrotic syndrome depends on whether the deposits are predominantly in the mesangium and subendothelial space versus the subepithelial space [41]. Deposits in the mesangium and subendothelial space are proximal to the GBM and in communication with the vascular space. As a result, complement activation (via the classic pathway) with the generation of the chemo-attractants C3a and C5a results in the influx of neutrophils and mononuclear cells. The presentation is often with active urine sediment (red cell casts and dysmorphic red blood cells), proteinuria, and an acute decline in renal function. Histologically, this clinical presentation is often associated with mesangial or focal or diffuse proliferative GN.

Deposits in the subepithelial space are separated from the glomerular capillary circulation by the GBM, and hence less likely to lead to complement activation and influx of inflammatory cells. The injury here is limited to the glomerular epithelial cells with a membranous nephropathy-like picture and patients present with proteinuria, which often progresses to the nephrotic range.

Clinical Manifestations

Lupus nephritis may develop at any time point from the diagnosis of SLE, although manifestations most commonly occur within five years of diagnosis. The spectrum of renal presentations includes asymptomatic abnormalities in urinalysis, including proteinuria and haematuria, to overt clinical disease with nephritic or nephrotic syndromes and progressive renal impairment. Renal disease may be accompanied by extra-renal manifestations of disease flare.

Diagnosis

Due to the prevalence of renal involvement in SLE, patients should be monitored routinely for this complication with the performance of urinalysis and quantitation of proteinuria (spot urine or 24-hour collection). However, the gold standard for the diagnosis of lupus nephritis is renal biopsy. Non-invasive strategies such as monitoring serology (dsDNA, ESR, C3, C4) provide useful adjunctive information but do not replace histopathological examination. Patients with isolated low-level proteinuria (<500 mg/day) can be monitored at the clinician's discretion without biopsy, but the presence of active urinary sediment or decreasing GFR mandates renal biopsy.

Lupus nephritis is classified based on consensus criteria published in 2004 by the International Society of Nephrology/Renal Pathology Society (ISN/RPS), as listed in Table 10.7.

The utility of this classification is in identifying lesions that will respond to immunosuppressive therapy and determining the intensity of treatment required. For example, class IV-A lupus nephritis describes active inflammation affecting most glomeruli, hence aggressive immunosuppressive treatment is warranted. In contrast, in class VI disease, the glomerular injury is chronic and irreversible, therefore immunosuppressive therapy would be futile. These lesions may be indistinguishable clinically, which highlights the key role of renal biopsy in the assessment and management of lupus nephritis. In addition to standard light microscopy techniques, this classification utilizes direct IF to identify immune deposits (identification of a 'full house' of IgG, IgA, IgM, C3, and C1q is highly suggestive of lupus nephritis) and electron microscopy to define glomerular ultrastructure and localize immune deposits. A strong staining for C1q is highly suggestive of lupus nephritis (Figures 10.4 and 10.5).

Management of Lupus Nephritis

Treatment of lupus nephritis is guided by the ISN/RPS class.

Non-proliferative Renal Lesions

Class I, II, V, and VI lesions typically do not involve significant active inflammatory processes; therefore treatment focuses on general renoprotective measures such as control of proteinuria and hypertension with angiotensin converting enzyme inhibitors and

Table 10.7 Histological classification of lupus nephritis by the International Society of Nephrology and the Renal Pathology Society, 2004

Class I: Minimal mesangial lupus nephritis

Normal glomeruli by LM, but mesangial immune deposits by IF

Class II: Mesangial proliferative lupus nephritis

Purely mesangial hypercellularity of any degree or mesangial expansion by LM, with mesangial immune deposits

May be a few isolated subepithelial or subendothelial deposits visible by IF or EM, but not by LM

Class III: Focal lupus nephritis

Active or inactive focal, segmental or global endo- or extracapillary GN involving <50% of all glomeruli, typically with focal subendothelial immune deposits, with or without mesangial alterations

Class III (A): Active lesions: focal proliferative lupus nephritis

Class III (A/C): Active and chronic lesions: focal proliferative and sclerosing lupus nephritis

Class III (C): Chronic inactive lesions with glomerular scars: focal sclerosing lupus nephritis

Class IV: Diffuse lupus nephritis

Active or inactive diffuse, segmental or global endo- or extracapillary GN involving ≥50% of all glomeruli, typically with diffuse subendothelial immune deposits, with or without mesangial alterations. This class is divided in diffuse segmental (IV-S) when ≤50% of the involved glomeruli have segmental lesions, and diffuse global (IV-G) when ≥50% of the involved glomeruli have global lesions. Segmental is defined as a lesion that involves less than half of the glomerular tuft. This class includes cases with diffuse wire loop deposits but with little or no glomerular proliferation.

Class IV-S (A): Active lesions: diffuse segmental proliferative lupus nephritis

Class IV-G (A): Active lesions: diffuse global proliferative lupus nephritis

Class IV-S (A/C): Active and chronic lesions: diffuse segmental proliferative and sclerosing lupus nephritis

Class IV-G (A/C): Active and chronic lesions: diffuse global proliferative and sclerosing lupus nephritis

Class IV-S (C): Chronic inactive lesions with scars: diffuse segmental sclerosing lupus nephritis

Class IV-G (C): Chronic inactive lesions with scars: diffuse global sclerosing lupus nephritis

Class V: Membranous lupus nephritis

Global or segmental subepithelial immune deposits or their morphological sequelae by LM and by IF or EM, with or without mesangial alterations

Class V lupus nephritis may occur in combination with class III or IV, in which case both will be diagnosed

Class V can have any degree of mesangial hypercellularity and can show advanced sclerosis

Class VI: Advanced sclerosing lupus nephritis

≥90% of glomeruli globally sclerosed without residual activity

EM, electron microscopy; GN, glomerulonephritis; IF, immunofluorescence; LM, light microscopy.

angiotensin 2 receptor blockers. Another important measure is minimizing the use of nephrotoxins (such as non-steroidal anti-inflammatory drugs) used routinely in the management of SLE. Patients with class V (membranous) disease may have additional complications related to the nephrotic syndrome; in this group anticoagulation and management of hyperlipidaemia are warranted [42].

Although there are no randomized trials comparing immunosuppressive therapy in addition to non-immunosuppressive therapy with non-immunosuppressive therapy alone in patients with class V lupus

nephritis, most renal physicians advocate the use of immunosuppressive drugs in these patients in the following scenarios:

- Persistent proteinuria >3.5 g/day despite maximum non-immunosuppressive therapy.
- Progressively rising serum creatinine.
- Mixed membranous and proliferative lesions on biopsy (i.e. class V plus either class III or IV lupus nephritis), which may be present at diagnosis or develop later, or the presence of superimposed crescentic disease.

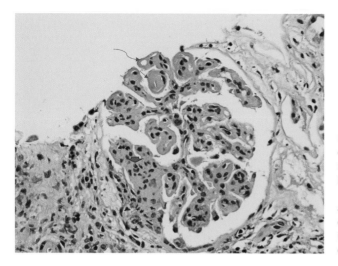

Figure 10.4 Light microscopy image of class IV lupus nephritis showing increased mesangial hypercellularity (thick arrow-head), hyaline thrombi (straight arrow), 'wire loop' lesion which is homogeneous and 'rigid' thickening of peripheral capillary loops due to subendothelial immune deposits (curved arrow) and endocapillary proliferation.

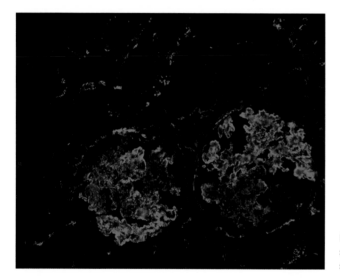

Figure 10.5 Direct immunofluorescence showing strong mesangiocapillary staining with C1q in lupus nephritis.

Proliferative Renal Lesions

Immunosuppression is the cornerstone of management of proliferative lupus nephritis (classes III–IV). The treatment strategy consists of *induction* and *maintenance phases*. The principle of induction therapy is to provide potent initial immunosuppression to achieve disease remission; the aim of maintenance therapy is to maintain remission with a lower degree of immunosuppression. In the absence of maintenance therapy up to 50% of patients will develop recurrent disease [43]. Corticosteroids are used in both the induction and maintenance phases.

Induction Therapy

Until recently, the sole agent available for the induction of remission was cyclophosphamide, a cytotoxic alkylating agent used in the treatment of solid organ and haematological malignancies. Cyclophosphamide induction is highly effective in achieving remission [44]. The major disadvantages of cyclophosphamide, however, are the short-term and cumulative toxicities. Acute toxicities include alopecia and leukopenia, the latter predisposing to opportunistic infection. Long-term toxicities include ovarian failure, haemorrhagic cystitis, and bladder cancer. A low-dose cyclophosphamide protocol (the Euro-Lupus protocol) has also been used in patients with lupus nephritis, with the risk of ovarian failure greatly reduced compared to higher dosing regimens [45]. Mesna is recommended along with cyclophosphamide to minimize bladder toxicity.

As the majority of patients with lupus nephritis are women of childbearing age, a major consideration for the patient and clinician is preservation of fertility. Egg or sperm storage should be discussed if high-dose cyclophosphamide is being considered. Both azathioprine and hydroxychloroquine are considered relatively safe in lupus patients in pregnancy [46].

Mycophenolate, an antimetabolite used in organ transplantation, has recently emerged as an equally effective agent for the induction of remission in lupus nephritis [25]. Although there is a similar propensity towards leukopenia and opportunistic infections, there are no detrimental effects on fertility and hence mycophenolate is a more attractive option in many patients. Mycophenolate may be more effective than cyclophosphamide in certain ethnic groups (African American and Hispanic) [47].

Maintenance Therapy

The two agents most commonly used in the maintenance of remission are mycophenolate and azathioprine. Mycophenolate is generally favoured over azathioprine due to initial evidence pointing at greater tolerability and efficacy. However, long-term data now suggest that these drugs are equally efficacious [48]. Azathioprine is favoured by patients in whom pregnancy is planned (see Box 10.1). Maintenance therapy is usually offered for 12–24 months.

Novel and Emerging Therapies

Although conventional immunosuppressive therapies are highly effective in inducing and maintaining remission in lupus nephritis, these agents exert a 'broad-spectrum' mechanism of action and do not specifically target the underlying pathogenesis of SLE. The challenge in developing targeted therapies in lupus is our incomplete understanding of pathogenic mechanisms. Currently, emerging therapy focuses on B cell depletion and inhibition. The most studied agent is rituximab, a monoclonal antibody directed against CD20 (a pan B cell marker). Although definitive evidence is lacking, rituximab appears to have a role in the treatment of refractory lupus nephritis [49, 50]. Another novel agent is belimumab, a humanized monoclonal antibody targeting BAFF

 Box 10.1 Lupus Nephritis and Pregnancy

Given the demographics affected by lupus nephritis, the issue of pregnancy is highly relevant. The activity of SLE is influenced by the altered immunological milieu of pregnancy, and in turn pregnancy outcomes are affected by the presence of lupus nephritis, particularly if a flare occurs during pregnancy. The aim in obstetric management of patients with lupus nephritis is to ensure optimal disease control prior to conception and to modify medications to prevent teratogenicity. Patients with active disease preconception are more likely to experience significant flares during pregnancy, and this is associated with adverse maternal and foetal outcomes including foetal death, intrauterine growth retardation, and preeclampsia. Other considerations during pregnancy are the presence of specific antibodies such as anti-SS-A and anti-SS-B (associated with neonatal lupus and congenital heart block) and anti-phospholipid antibodies, which are associated with early and late trimester miscarriage.

which may decrease B cell activation and the production of pathogenic antibodies. This agent is currently being studied as a potential adjunctive therapy in induction and maintenance regimens.

References

1. Exley, A.R., Carruthers, D.M., Luqmani, R.A. et al. (1997). Damage occurs early in systemic vasculitis and is an index of outcome. *QJM* 90 (6): 391–399.

2. Weyand, C.M. and Goronzy, J.J. (2003). Medium- and Large-Vessel Vasculitis. *N. Engl. J. Med.* 349: 160–169. https://doi.org/10.1056/NEJMra022694.

3. Peera, M.A., LoCurto, M., and Elfond, M. (2011). A case of Takayasu arteritis causing subclavian steal and presenting as syncope. *J. Emerg. Med.* 40 (2): 158–161. https://doi.org/10.1016/j.jemermed.2007.11.031. Epub 2008 May 12.

4. Rao, S.A., Mandalam, K.R., Rao, V.R. et al. (1993). Takayasu arteritis: initial and long-term follow-up in 16 patients after percutaneous transluminal angioplasty of the descending thoracic and abdominal aorta. *Radiology* 189 (1): 173.

5. Arend, W.P., Michel, B.A., Bloch, D.A. et al. (1990). The American College of Rheumatology 1990 criteria for the classification of Takayasu arteritis. *Arthritis Rheum.* 33 (8): 1129.

6. Goodwin, J.S. (1992). Progress in gerontology: polymyalgia rheumatica and temporal arteritis. *J. Am. Geriatr. Soc.* 40 (5): 515–525.

7. Hunder, G.G., Bloch, D.A., Michel, B.A. et al. (1990). The American College of Rheumatology 1990 criteria for the classification of giant cell arteritis. *Arthritis Rheum.* 33 (8): 1122–1128.

8. Pagnoux, C., Seror, R., Henegar, C. et al. (2010). Clinical features and outcomes in 348 patients with polyarteritis nodosa: a systematic retrospective study of patients diagnosed between 1963 and 2005 and entered into the French Vasculitis study group database. *Arthritis Rheum.* 62 (2): 616.

9. Guillevin, L., Mahr, A., Cohen, P. et al. (2004). Short-term corticosteroids then lamivudine and plasma exchanges to treat hepatitis B virus-related polyarteritis nodosa. *Arthritis Rheum.* 51 (3): 482.

10. Newburger, J.W., Takahashi, M., Gerber, M.A. et al. (2004). Diagnosis, treatment, and long-term management of Kawasaki disease: a statement for health professionals from the committee on rheumatic fever, endocarditis and Kawasaki disease, council on cardiovascular disease in the young, American Heart Association. *Circulation* 110 (17): 2747.

11. Terai, M. and Shulman, S.T. (1997). Prevalence of coronary artery abnormalities in Kawasaki disease is highly dependent on gamma globulin dose but independent of salicylate dose. *J. Pediatr.* 131 (6): 888.

12. Falk, R.J. and Jennette, J.C. (1988). Anti-neutrophil cytoplasmic autoantibodies with specificity for myeloperoxidase in patients with systemic vasculitis and idiopathic necrotizing and crescentic glomerulonephritis. *N. Engl. J. Med.* 318 (25): 1651.

13. Almouhawis, H.A., Leao, J.C., Fedele, S., and Porter, S.R. (2013). Wegener's granulomatosis: a review of clinical features and an update in diagnosis and treatment. *J. Oral Pathol. Med.* 42 (7): 507–516. https://doi.org/10.1111/jop.12030. Epub 2013 Jan 10.

14. Vaglio, A., Buzio, C., and Zwerina, J. (2013). Eosinophilic granulomatosis with polyangitis (Churg–Strauss): state of the art. *Allergy* 68 (3): 261–273. https://doi.org/10.1111/all.12088. Epub 2013 Jan 18.

15. Furuta, S. and Jayne, D.R.W. (2013). Antineutrophil cytoplasm antibody-associated vasculitis: recent developments. *Kidney Int.* 84 (2): 244–249.

16. Stone, J.H., Merkel, P.A., Spiera, R. et al. (2010). Rituximab versus cyclophosphamide for ANCA-associated Vasculitis. *N. Engl. J. Med.* 363: 221–232. https://doi.org/10.1056/NEJMoa0909905.

17. Jones, R.B., Tervaert, J.W.C., Hauser, T. et al. (2010). Rituximab versus cyclophosphamide in ANCA-associated renal Vasculitis. *N. Engl. J. Med.* 363: 211–220. https://doi.org/10.1056/NEJMoa0909169.

18. Guillevin, L., Pagnoux, C., Karras, A. et al. (2014). Rituximab versus azathioprine for maintenance in ANCA-associated vasculitis. *N. Engl. J. Med.* 371 (19): 1771.

19. Moosig, F., Bremer, J.P., Hellmich, B. et al. (2013). A vasculitis centre based management strategy leads to improved outcome in eosinophilic granulomatosis and polyangitis (Churg-Strauss, EGPA): monocentric experiences in 150 patients. *Ann. Rheum. Dis.* 72 (6): 1011.

20. Koldingsnes, W. and Nossent, H. (2002). Predictors of survival and organ damage in Wegener's granulomatosis. *Rheumatology (Oxford)* 41 (5): 572–581.

21. Corral-Gudino, L., Borao-Cengotita-Bengoa, M., Del Pino-Montes, J., and Lerma-Márquez, J.L. (2011). Overall survival, renal survival and relapse in patients with microscopic polyangiitis: a systematic review of current evidence. *Rheumatology (Oxford)* 50 (8): 1414–1423. https://doi.org/10.1093/rheumatology/ker112. Epub 2011 Mar 15.

22. Rahman, A. and Isenberg, D.A. (2008). Systemic lupus erythematosus. *N. Engl. J. Med.* 358 (9): 929–939.

23. Abu-Shakra, M., Urowitz, M.B., Gladman, D.D., and Gough, J. (1995). Mortality studies in systemic lupus erythematosus. Results from a single center. II. Predictor variables for mortality. *J. Rheumatol.* 22 (7): 1265–1270.

24. Lisnevskaia, L., Murphy, G., and Isenberg, D. (2014). Systemic lupus erythematosus. *Lancet* 384 (9957): 1878–1888.

25. Costenbader, K.H., Feskanich, D., Stampfer, M.J., and Karlson, E.W. (2007). Reproductive and menopausal factors and risk of systemic lupus erythematosus in women. *Arthritis Rheum.* 56 (4): 1251–1262.

26. Sullivan, K.E. (2000). Genetics of systemic lupus erythematosus. Clinical implications. *Rheum. Dis. Clin. N. Am.* 26 (2): 229–256. v–vi.

27. Walport, M.J. (2002). Complement and systemic lupus erythematosus. *Arthritis Res.* 4 (Suppl 3): S279–S293.

28. Guerra, S.G., Vyse, T.J., and Cunninghame Graham, D.S. (2012). The genetics of lupus: a functional perspective. *Arthritis Res. Ther.* 14 (3): 211.

29. James, J.A., Neas, B.R., Moser, K.L. et al. (2001). Systemic lupus erythematosus in adults is associated with previous Epstein-Barr virus exposure. *Arthritis Rheum.* 44 (5): 1122–1126.

30. Rubin, R.L. (2015). Drug-induced lupus. *Expert Opin. Drug Saf.* 14 (3): 361–378.

31. Fritzler, M.J. and Tan, E.M. (1978). Antibodies to histones in drug-induced and idiopathic lupus erythematosus. *J. Clin. Invest.* 62 (3): 560–567.

32. Theofilopoulos, A.N., Gonzalez-Quintial, R., Lawson, B.R. et al. (2010). Sensors of the innate immune system: their link to rheumatic diseases. *Nat. Rev. Rheumatol.* 6 (3): 146–156.

33. Min, D.J., Kim, S.J., Park, S.H. et al. (2002). Antinucleosome antibody: significance in lupus patients lacking anti-double-stranded DNA antibody. *Clin. Exp. Rheumatol.* 20 (1): 13–18.

34. Husebye, E.S., Sthoeger, Z.M., Dayan, M., Zinger, H. et al. (2005). Autoantibodies to a NR2A peptide of the glutamate/NMDA receptor in sera of patients with systemic lupus erythematosus. *Ann Rheum. Dis.* 64 (8): 1210–1213.

35. Orbai, A.M., Truedsson, L., Sturfelt, G. et al. (2015). Anti-C1q antibodies in systemic lupus erythematosus. *Lupus* 24 (1): 42–49.

36. Lockshin, M.D. (2008). Update on antiphospholipid syndrome. *Bull. NYU Hosp. Jt. Dis.* 66 (3): 195–197.

37. Vincent, F.B., Morand, E.F., Schneider, P., and Mackay, F. (2014). The BAFF/APRIL system in SLE pathogenesis. *Nat. Rev. Rheumatol.* 10 (6): 365–373.

38. Borchers, A.T., Leibushor, N., Naguwa, S.M. et al. (2012). Lupus nephritis: a critical review. *Autoimmun. Rev.* 12 (2): 174–194.

39. Hanly, J.G., O'Keeffe, A.G., Su, L. et al. (2016). The frequency and outcome of lupus nephritis: results from an international inception cohort study. *Rheumatology (Oxford)* 55 (2): 252–262.

40. Ropes, M.W. (1976). *Systemic Lupus Erythematosus*. Cambridge, MA: Harvard University Press.

41. Weening, J.J., D'Agati, V.D., Schwartz, M.M. et al. (2004). The classification of glomerulonephritis in systemic lupus erythematosus revisited. *Kidney Int.* 65 (2): 521–530.

42. Griffin, B. and Lightstone, L. (2013). Renoprotective strategies in lupus nephritis: beyond immunosuppression. *Lupus* 22 (12): 1267–1273.

43. Illei, G.G., Takada, K., Parkin, D. et al. (2002). Renal flares are common in patients with severe proliferative lupus nephritis treated with pulse immunosuppressive therapy: long-term followup of a cohort of 145 patients participating in randomized controlled studies. *Arthritis Rheum.* 46 (4): 995–1002.

44. Austin, H.A. 3rd, Klippel, J.H., Balow, J.E. et al. (1986). Therapy of lupus nephritis. Controlled trial of prednisone and cytotoxic drugs. *N. Engl. J. Med.* 314 (10): 614–619.

45. Houssiau, F.A., Vasconcelos, C., D'Cruz, D. et al. (2010). The 10-year follow-up data of the Euro-Lupus Nephritis Trial comparing low-dose and high-dose intravenous cyclophosphamide. *Ann. Rheum. Dis.* 69 (1): 61–64.

46. Bramham, K., Soh, M.C., and Nelson-Piercy, C. (2012). Pregnancy and renal outcomes in lupus nephritis: an update and guide to management. *Lupus* 21 (12): 1271–1283.

47. Appel, G.B., Contreras, G., Dooley, M.A. et al. (2009). Mycophenolate mofetil versus cyclophosphamide for induction treatment of lupus nephritis. *J. Am. Soc. Nephrol.* 20 (5): 1103–1112.

48. Tamirou, F., D'Cruz, D., Sangle, S. et al. (2016). Long-term follow-up of the MAINTAIN nephritis trial, comparing azathioprine and mycophenolate mofetil as maintenance therapy of lupus nephritis. *Ann. Rheum. Dis.* 75 (3): 526–531.

49. Davies, R.J., Sangle, S.R., Jordan, N.P. et al. (2013). Rituximab in the treatment of resistant lupus nephritis: therapy failure in rapidly progressive crescentic lupus nephritis. *Lupus* 22 (6): 574–582.

50. Weidenbusch, M., Rommele, C., Schrottle, A., and Anders, H.J. (2013). Beyond the LUNAR trial. Efficacy of rituximab in refractory lupus nephritis. *Nephrol. Dial. Transplant.* 28 (1): 106–111.

Questions and Answers

Questions

1. True about PAN:
   a. Can affect both arteries and veins
   b. Is ANCA positive in 30% cases
   c. Kidney involvement manifests as glomerulonephritis
   d. Characterized by absence of vasculitis in veins
   e. Can affect both large and small blood vessels

2. ANCA positive vasculitis is not seen in
   a. Lupus nephritis
   b. Goodpasture's syndrome
   c. Use of anti-thyroid disease
   d. Microscopic polyangitis
   e. Anti-GBM antibody drugs

3. Which of the following is true about microscopic polyangitis?
   a. There is a strong association with hepatitis B
   b. Histology shows granuloma formation
   c. Usually leads to saddle nose deformity of the nose
   d. Kidney histology often shows crescents
   e. Is associated with eosinophilia

4. The commonest clinical manifestation of PAN is:
   a. Abdominal pain
   b. Testicular pain
   c. Haemoptysis
   d. Hypertension
   e. Peripheral neuropathy

5. Renal involvement is usually the least severe in:
   a. GPA
   b. Microscopic polyangitis
   c. Lupus nephritis class 4
   d. EGPA
   e. Anti-GBM disease

6. Lupus nephritis is a serious complication of SLE that requires intensification of immunosuppression. Which feature on the renal biopsy is **least** suggestive of the diagnosis?
   a. C1q staining in a Mesangiocapillary pattern
   b. C3 staining in the glomerulus
   c. IgG, IgA, and IgM staining in a Mesangiocapillary pattern
   d. Pauci immune glomerular staining
   e. Membranoproliferative change seen on light microscopy

7. Belimumab is the first novel agent specifically approved for the treatment of SLE in 50 years. What is its mechanism of action?
   a. Belimumab targets CD19 on the surface of B cells, dramatically reducing the number of circulating B cells as a result.
   b. This biologic agent targets DNA antibodies and hence modulates disease pathogenesis.
   c. Belimumab directly inhibits intracellular B cell signalling pathways.
   d. Belimumab is humanized monoclonal antibody that targets B cell activation factor (BAFF).
   e. Belimumab removes apoptotic blebs and reduces the chance of an autoinflammatory reaction.

Answers

1. d. PAN is a systemic necrotizing vasculitis that typically affects medium-sized muscular arteries with characteristic absence of involvement of veins, smaller arteries, or capillaries and is ANCA negative. Absence of capillary involvement rules out the possibility of glomerulonephritis which is associated with glomerular capillary involvement.

2. a. ANCA positive vasculitis is associated with the pauci-immune vasculitis, being positive in 90% of GPA, 70% of microscopic polyangitis, and 50% of EGPA. Anti-GBM antibody disease can be associated with ANCA positivity in 10–40% of cases. ANCA positivity can be associated with certain drugs with the most common association being seen with anti-thyroid drugs (propylthiouracil and methimazole).

3. d. While PAN is associated with Hepatitis B positivity, both PAN and microscopic polyangitis do not show granulomas on histology (unlike Takayasu arteritis, GCA, GPA, and EGPA). Severe ENT involvement leading to saddle nose deformity of the nose is sometimes seen with GPA. EGPA is characterized by difficult to control asthma, eosinophilia, and vasculitis. Renal biopsy shows segmental necrotizing glomerulonephritis often with crescents in the pauci-immune vasculitis. Interestingly, granulomas are usually not seen on renal biopsy in both GPA and EGPA.

4. e. While peripheral neuropathy may be seen in up to 75% of cases with PAN, gastrointestinal symptoms with abdominal pain or blood in stool may be seen in up to 40%. Hypertension and orchitis may be seen in 35% and 20% cases, respectively. Pulmonary involvement is uncommon in PAN.

5. d. Amongst the three types of pauci-immune vasculitis, EGPA affects kidney the least frequently and also the severity of renal involvement here is the least. Lupus nephritis class 4 is the most severe form of lupus nephritis. Anti-GBM disease typically presents with the syndrome of glomerulonephritis and pulmonary haemorrhage and has a poor prognosis without treatment.

6. d. IF finding of a 'full house' of IgG, IgA, IgM, C3, and C1q is highly suggestive of lupus nephritis. Pauci immune glomerular staining is seen with ANCA-associated vasculitis.

7. d. Belimumab is humanized monoclonal antibody that targets B cell activation factor (BAFF). Excessive levels of BAFF causes abnormally high antibody production leading to conditions like SLE.

11

Renovascular Hypertension, Pregnancy-Related Hypertension, and Thrombotic Microangiopathies

Amanda Mather and Muh Geot Wong

Summary

Renovascular Hypertension

- Renovascular hypertension (HTN) is an important cause of secondary HTN, with approximately 80% of cases due to atherosclerotic renal artery stenosis (RAS) and 20% due to fibromuscular dysplasia (FMD)
- Duplex Doppler ultrasonography, computed tomography angiography, and/or magnetic resonance angiography are all useful for detection of renovascular HTN
- For patients with atherosclerotic RAS, revascularization procedures have not been shown to confer clinical benefit when compared to medical therapy
- Revascularization should be offered to those with a short duration of blood pressure (BP) elevation, failure or intolerance to medical therapy, recurrent flash pulmonary oedema or otherwise unexplained renal failure
- Revascularization procedures are often considered useful in patients with FMD

Pregnancy-Related Hypertension

- The hypertensive disorders of pregnancy include gestational HTN, preeclampsia (de novo or superimposed on chronic HTN), chronic HTN in pregnancy, and white coat HTN
- Gestational HTN is characterized by the new onset of HTN after 20 weeks of gestation without any maternal or foetal features of preeclampsia, followed by return of BP to normal within three months post-partum
- The likelihood of gestational HTN progressing to preeclampsia is related to the gestational age at which HTN develops and the severity of the HTN
- Antihypertensive agents considered safe for pregnancy include methyldopa, labetalol or oxprenolol, hydralazine, and nifedipine

Lecture Notes Nephrology: A Comprehensive Guide to Renal Medicine, First Edition. Edited by Surjit Tarafdar.
© 2020 John Wiley & Sons Ltd. Published 2020 by John Wiley & Sons Ltd.

- Preeclampsia is a pregnancy-specific, multi-system disorder that occurs in about 5–10% of pregnancies and is a leading cause of maternal and foetal morbidity and mortality
- Preeclampsia is defined as HTN developing after 20 weeks of gestation and the coexistence of either proteinuria or renal insufficiency, abnormal liver transaminases, pulmonary oedema, neurological complications (e.g. new-onset headache or altered mental status, flashing lights or visual scotomata) or platelet count <100 000/microl^3
- Delivery is the only definite treatment of pre-eclampsia

Thrombotic Microangiopathies Including Thrombotic Thrombocytopenic Purpura and Haemolytic Uraemic Syndrome

- Thrombotic microangiopathies (TMA) are characterized by abnormalities in the walls of arterioles and capillaries leading to platelet thrombi
- Clinically, TMA presents with microangiopathic haemolytic anaemia (MAHA) and thrombocytopenia with variable signs of organ injury due to platelet thrombosis in the microcirculation
- Whilst disseminated intravascular coagulation (DIC) seen in infections or malignancies can also present with MAHA and thrombocytopenia, the thrombi in DIC are composed of red blood cells and not platelets
- The two main categories of primary TMA are haemolytic uraemic syndrome (HUS) and thrombotic thrombocytopenic purpura (TTP)
- HUS is characterized by acute kidney injury (AKI) with minimal or no neurological manifestations
- Whilst Shiga toxin-producing *Escherichia coli* (STEC) HUS accounts for over 90% of cases of HUS, complement-mediated HUS, which is also called atypical HUS (aHUS), is seen more commonly in adults
- STEC HUS usually resolves spontaneously with supportive management of anaemia, thrombocytopenia, HTN, electrolyte disorders, and AKI
- Treatment of aHUS consists of eculizumab and plasma exchange
- TTP is characteristically associated with neurological findings with usually minimal abnormalities of kidney function, despite microthrombi observed on renal biopsy
- TTP is caused by severely reduced activity of the von Willebrand factor-cleaving protease ADAMTS13
- The mainstay of treatment for TTP is plasma exchange therapy with fresh frozen plasma

About 10% of all hypertensive patients have hypertension (HTN) secondary to a defined pathology in a specific organ, although a higher percentage has been reported in referral centres focused on the investigation of hypertension. Table 11.1 lists the common causes of secondary HTN. Screening for secondary HTN should be considered in the following scenarios:

- Severe or resistant HTN: persistent HTN despite adequate doses of three antihypertensive agents from different classes including a diuretic.
- Malignant HTN: severe HTN with signs of end-organ damage such as retinal haemorrhages/papilloedema, heart failure, neurological disturbance or acute kidney injury (AKI).
- Acute rise in blood pressure (BP) in a patient with previously stable values.
- Severe HTN in a patient with an unexplained atrophic kidney or asymmetry in renal sizes of >1.5 cm.
- Hypokalaemia and/or metabolic alkalosis in a hypertensive patient.
- Adrenal incidentaloma in a hypertensive patient (should lead to screening for endocrine causes of

Table 11.1 Aetiology of secondary hypertension (the first two causes are the commonest ones)

- **Renovascular hypertension**
- **Primary aldosteronism**
- Cushing syndrome
- Pheochromocytoma
- Drugs, e.g. oral contraceptive pills, prednisolone, non-steroidal anti-inflammatory drugs, cyclosporine, tacrolimus, erythropoietin, amphetamines and cocaine
- Primary renal disease e.g. glomerulonephritis
- Coarctation of aorta
- Polyarteritis nodosa
- Conditions other than primary aldosteronism leading to hypertension with metabolic alkalosis and hypokalaemia:
  - Liddle syndrome
  - Chronic liquorice ingestion
  - Apparent mineralocorticoid excess
  - Glucocorticoid remediable hypertension

HTN, i.e. primary hyperaldosteronism, Cushing syndrome, and pheochromocytoma).
- Age less than 30 years in non-obese, non-black patients with a negative family history.

The first part of this chapter will focus on renovascular HTN (a renal cause of secondary HTN), whilst primary aldosteronism, which is the other common cause of secondary HTN, is discussed in Chapter 3.

The second and third parts of this chapter will cover pregnancy-related HTN (gestational HTN, preeclampsia, and eclampsia) and thrombotic microangiopathies causing microangiopathic haemolytic anaemia (MAHA) and thrombocytopenia; thrombotic thrombocytopenic purpura (TTP) and haemolytic uraemic syndrome (HUS).

Renovascular Hypertension

Renovascular HTN is considered one of the most common causes of secondary HTN. Its prevalence amongst hypertensive patients has been mentioned to be from 4 to 53% in different studies, with increased prevalence in the older population [1]. The condition reflects the causal relation between anatomically evident arterial occlusion of renal arteries and BP. To cause HTN, the renal artery occlusive lesion should obstruct more than 70–75% of the lumen.

There are two common clinical variants of renovascular HTN: atherosclerotic renal artery stenosis (RAS) and fibromuscular dysplasia (FMD). About 80% of renovascular HTN cases are due to atherosclerotic disease and 20% are related to FMD. Other rarer causes include emboli, trauma, accidental ligation of renal artery during surgery and extrinsic compression of the renal pedicle by tumours.

HTN appearing in younger individuals (i.e. children or young adults) is suggestive of FMD, whilst atherosclerotic RAS should be suspected in recent onset of HTN in previously normotensive individuals above the age of 55 years [2]. Other situations where renovascular HTN is suspected are resistant or malignant HTN, more than 1.5 cm discrepancy in kidney sizes, episodes of unexplained flash pulmonary oedema and a rise in serum creatinine of more than 30% after initiating an angiotensin-converting enzyme (ACE) inhibitor or angiotensin-receptor blocker (ARB).

Fibromuscular Dysplasia

In contrast to the more common atherosclerotic RAS, FMD is a non-atherosclerotic and non-inflammatory disorder that generally affects medium-sized arteries, leading to arterial stenosis, occlusion, aneurysm, and dissection. The condition affects nearly every arterial bed, but the most frequently affected arteries are renal and internal carotid (affected in 75% of cases), followed by the vertebral, visceral, and external iliac arteries [3]. Therefore, the most common presentations are either with HTN due to renal artery involvement or stroke/transient ischaemic attack due to involvement of the carotid or vertebral arteries.

FMD most often affects women under the age of 50 years and typically involves the mid to distal part of the main renal artery beyond the first 2 cm from the aorta [4]. Most patients have renal artery aneurysms along with stenosis, and at times this 'string of beads' appearance of the renal arteries can mimic radiological appearances seen in polyarteritis nodosa (PAN). Unlike FMD, however, PAN is a vasculitis and patients are usually systemically unwell with evidence of skin, musculoskeletal or peripheral nervous system involvement.

Atherosclerotic Renovascular Disease (Renal Artery Stenosis)

Atherosclerosis primarily affects older patients (more than 50 years of age), who usually have coexistent cardiovascular risk factors. Unlike FMD, atherosclerotic RAS commonly involves the aortic orifice or the first 2–3 cm of the main renal artery. It can manifest as part of a diffuse atherosclerotic disease, but can involve the renal artery alone, being bilateral in 20–40% of patients. The incidence of atherosclerotic RAS is increasing and possibly reflects the fact that more people are living to older age, enabling the atherosclerotic arterial narrowing to reach critical levels.

Pathogenesis of Renovascular Hypertension

The pathogenesis of HTN differs in unilateral versus bilateral RAS [5]. In unilateral RAS, low blood flow to the kidney leads to increased renin release from the affected side, leading in turn to increased angiotensin II and aldosterone production; that is, activation of the renin–angiotensin–aldosterone system (RAAS). The non-stenotic kidney compensates by pressure natriuresis with excretion of extra sodium and water; perfusion to the stenotic kidney remains reduced.

Thus, the RAAS stays chronically activated in unilateral RAS leading to HTN.

In contrast, in bilateral RAS, there is no compensatory natriuresis as both the kidneys are hypoperfused. HTN in this case is due to the volume expansion and RAAS is actually inhibited due to the chronically expanded fluid volume. The mechanisms producing HTN in unilateral and bilateral RAS were first demonstrated in animals by Harry Goldblatt in 1934 by clipping one or both renal arteries. Some patients with bilateral RAS present with recurrent episodes of flash pulmonary oedema due to the volume expansion.

Diagnosis

Advances in contrast imaging have led to an increase in 'incidental finding' of RAS. Therefore, the diagnosis of RAS should only be considered in patients with clinical suspicion (Table 11.2). Also, testing for RAS is only indicated if a corrective procedure would be performed if clinically significant renovascular disease were detected.

Whilst renal artery angiography remains the gold standard for the diagnosis of RAS, it is not recommended for screening because of the risks associated with the procedure. Non-invasive screening tests including duplex Doppler ultrasonography, computed tomography angiography (CTA) and magnetic resonance angiography (MRA) are reasonably safe alternatives for initial testing (Figure 11.1). Whilst the advantage of Doppler ultrasound is that it is relatively inexpensive and does not involve administration of contrast, it is highly operator dependent and not very useful in the distal lesions seen in FMD. Whilst both MRA and CTA have the drawback of needing some sort of contrast, CTA is more sensitive for identification of the distal lesions seen in FMD.

With Doppler ultrasonography, an increased peak systolic velocity above 300 cm/sec, and with CTA or MRA, a stenosis greater than 75% in one or both renal arteries, especially associated with post-stenotic dilatation, is indicative of a haemodynamically significant RAS. Other non-invasive tests, such as peripheral plasma renin activity and captopril scintigraphy, are no longer considered suitable for initial testing because of their poor sensitivity and specificity. However, a captopril renogram may help to assess the haemodynamic significance of a stenotic lesion and determine the relative function of each kidney.

Management

The first-line management of RAS is most often medical, whilst FMD patients are often treated with revascularization procedures.

Atherosclerotic Renal Artery Stenosis

Medical therapy should be offered to all patients, with revascularization only offered (in conjunction with medical therapy) in the following group of patients:

- Short duration of BP elevation prior to the diagnosis of renovascular disease
- Failure of optimal medical therapy
- Intolerance to optimal medical therapy
- Recurrent flash pulmonary oedema
- Otherwise unexplained progressive renal insufficiency

Revascularization can be achieved by either percutaneous angioplasty with (Figure 11.1) or without stenting, or surgical revascularization in selected patients (usually in those with complex renal artery anatomy).

As the underlying pathogenesis of unilateral renovascular HTN involves the RAAS system, the initial drug of choice in unilateral RAS is an ACE inhibitor or ARB [6]. Bilateral renovascular disease is characterized by impaired sodium excretion resulting in expansion of the extracellular fluid volume and inhibitory

---

Table 11.2 Clinical clues to the diagnosis of renovascular hypertension

1. Onset of hypertension before age of 30 years or after the age of 55 years
2. Accelerated, resistant or malignant hypertension
   (a) Accelerated hypertension is defined as sudden and persistent worsening of previously well-controlled hypertension
   (b) Resistant hypertension is defined as the failure to achieve goal blood pressure in patients who are adhering to full doses of an appropriate three-drug regimen that includes a diuretic
   (c) Malignant hypertension is defined as hypertension with coexistent evidence of acute end-organ damage, i.e. acute renal failure, acutely decompensated congestive heart failure, new visual or neurological disturbance, and/or advanced (grade III–IV) retinopathy
2. Significant deterioration of renal function in response to angiotensin-converting enzyme inhibitors or angiotensin-receptor blocker
3. Unexplained atrophic kidney or a discrepancy in size between the two kidneys of greater than 1.5 cm
4. Sudden unexplained pulmonary oedema

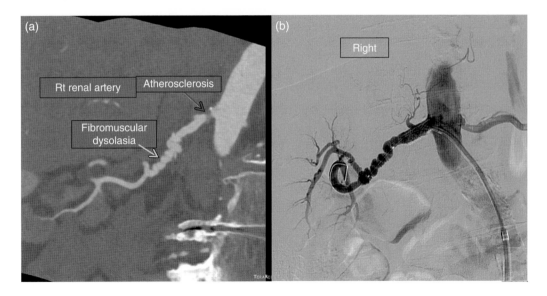

Figure 11.1 (a) Spiral computed tomography image of a right renal artery stenosis due to fibromuscular dysplasia (FMD) as well as atherosclerosis. The atherosclerotic lesion typically involved the proximal third of the renal artery near the orifice, showing near occlusive disease (blue arrow). The FMD, more commonly seen in the distal third of the renal artery, gives the 'string of beads' appearance (yellow arrow). (b) Digital subtraction renal angiography showing revascularization procedure by angioplasty and stenting. Figures Courtesy: Dr. Eisen Liang, intervention radiologist, Sydney Adventist Hospital, NSW.

influence on the RAAS system. Administration of diuretic causes volume depletion with subsequent activation of the RAAS system, and hence combination therapy with a thiazide diuretic and ACE inhibitor (or ARB) may be more useful to control HTN in these patients. Following initiation of ACE inhibitors or ARBs in patients with renovascular disease (or in those where there is clinical suspicion for renovascular disease), serum creatinine and electrolytes should be checked after one week and then at least every six months thereafter. A rise of serum creatinine by more than 30% warrants discontinuation of these drugs.

If target BP is not reached with angiotensin inhibition alone, other antihypertensive drugs (e.g. thiazide diuretic or calcium channel blocker) should be added. Concurrent aggressive control of any cardiovascular risk factor is very important.

Most patients with RAS can be managed with antihypertensive drug therapy, which should be the first line of treatment even for those for whom a revascularization procedure is planned. For atherosclerotic RAS, two large randomized prospective studies, the CORAL and ASTRAL [7] studies, independently reported that revascularization procedure by stenting did not confer a significant benefit over medical management.

Fibromuscular Dysplasia

Although there are no randomized trials comparing revascularization with medical therapy in patients with FMD, a revascularization procedure in FMD is often considered to be curative, or at least can allow BP control with fewer antihypertensive agents [8]. Revascularization trials in patients with atherosclerotic RAS are not applicable to the FMD population because the two disorders have differing pathophysiology and natural history.

Although there is a paucity of prospective data demonstrating the superiority of percutaneous transluminal angioplasty over surgical revascularization, the percutaneous approach has emerged as the mainstay of treatment for patients with FMD. Percutaneous transluminal angioplasty is less expensive, less invasive, and associated with quicker recovery and lower morbidity compared to surgery.

Primary stenting of the renal artery is not recommended for FMD, as these lesions tend to respond well to angioplasty. However, repeated need for angioplasty is not uncommon due to restenosis. Stenting should be reserved for lesions that fail recurrent balloon angioplasty or develop flow-limiting dissection.

Pregnancy-Related Hypertension

The hypertensive disorders of pregnancy include:

- Gestational HTN (commonest cause of HTN in pregnancy)
- De novo preeclampsia and eclampsia
- Preeclampsia superimposed on chronic HTN
- Chronic HTN in pregnancy
- White coat HTN

HTN is the most common medical disorder of pregnancy and is estimated to complicate 1 in 10 pregnancies, accounting for significant morbidity and mortality.

Many physiological changes occurring during pregnancy are relevant to the assessment and management of HTN in pregnancy. In normal pregnancy, mean arterial BP decreases, reaching its lowest point between the 16th and 20th weeks, after which the BP slowly returns to pre-pregnancy levels by the 40th week of gestation. This is accompanied by a parallel rise in cardiac output along with an increase in both stroke volume and heart rate [9]. Given this rise in cardiac output and an accompanying rise in plasma volume, the reduction in arterial BP reflects a profound reduction in vascular tone.

The kidneys also undergo a number of changes during pregnancy that are important to understand, particularly when assessing kidney function in the context of pregnancy. In uncomplicated pregnancies, the kidneys undergo glomerular hyperfiltration, leading in turn to an increase in glomerular filtration rate (GFR) [10]. Glomerular hyperfiltration is also seen in the early stages of chronic kidney disease (CKD), for example in diabetic nephropathy, but unlike in those cases where there is glomerular HTN, the glomerular pressure in pregnancy is always normal. The glomerular hyperfiltration in pregnancy is due to increased blood flow to the kidney, which in turn is secondary to the low vascular resistance and increased cardiac output. Pregnancy-associated glomerular hyperfiltration is therefore characteristically not associated with increased glomerular pressure. The GFR is increased by 40–60% over non-pregnant states, leading to a corresponding reduction in serum creatinine. Therefore, it is important to be aware that creatinine levels at the higher end of the normal range may reflect abnormal renal function during pregnancy.

Gestational Hypertension

Gestational HTN is defined as the new onset of HTN (systolic BP ≥140 mmHg and/or diastolic BP ≥90 mmHg) at ≥20 weeks of gestation on two separate occasions, with measurements at least 4–6 hours apart, in the absence of proteinuria or signs of end-organ damage [11]. It complicates 6% of all pregnancies. Gestational HTN at first presentation may persist through the pregnancy as HTN alone, or in approximately 15–45% of women it is the first sign of evolving preeclampsia. Additionally, women who have not had regular exposure to medical care prior to conception may be labelled with 'gestational HTN' based on elevated BP readings towards the end of pregnancy, but will eventually be classified as chronic HTN when BP readings do not normalize by 12 weeks post-partum. It is therefore not possible to make a definitive diagnosis of gestational HTN until the pregnancy is complete without the development of preeclampsia and the patient's BP has normalized post-partum.

The likelihood of gestational HTN progressing to preeclampsia is related to the gestational age at which HTN develops and the severity of the HTN, with early gestation and severe HTN being associated with a greater chance of progression.

Treatment of Hypertension in Pregnancy

The general strategy is to treat HTN to prevent maternal complications whilst limiting medication toxicity to the foetus and preserving uteroplacental circulation.

Although there is controversy in the literature regarding the level of BP at which antihypertensive therapy should commence, BP ≥ 160/110 mmHg should be treated with antihypertensive drugs to reduce the risk of maternal stroke.

The CHIPS trial confirmed the foetal safety of treating BP to a target diastolic pressure of 85 mmHg but different targets may apply for women with pre-existing organ dysfunction.

The antihypertensive medications usually considered safe for pregnancy are methyldopa, labetalol, oxprenolol, hydralazine, nifedipine, prazosin, and clonidine [12]. ACE inhibitors and ARBs are contraindicated in the second and third trimester of pregnancy due to their teratogenic effects. Patients who are receiving these drugs for antihypertensive treatment alone should be changed to alternative agents prior to pregnancy. Patients receiving these drugs for reno- or cardioprotection will need to consider the risk-benefit ratio of continuing until pregnancy occurs and then changing within the first trimester.

Preeclampsia

Preeclampsia is a pregnancy-specific, multisystem disorder that occurs in about 5% of all pregnancies and is a leading cause of maternal and foetal mortality and morbidity. It is also a leading cause for induction of delivery before 37 weeks. Preeclampsia is defined as HTN developing after 20 weeks of gestation and the coexistence of one or more of the following new-onset conditions [11]:

1. Proteinuria defined by urine protein-creatinine ratio >0.3 mg/mg (30 mg/mmol) $or \geq$ 0.3 g in a 24-hour urine specimen
2. One or more of the following maternal complications (with or without proteinuria):
   - Renal insufficiency (creatinine >97.2 umol/l or 1.1 mg/dL)
   - Liver transaminases at least twice the upper limit of normal concentrations
   - Pulmonary oedema
   - Neurological complications (new-onset headache not responding to analgesics, altered mental status, blurred vision, flashing lights or visual scotomata)
   - Platelet count <100 000/microl^3

Pathophysiology of Preeclampsia

The pathophysiology of preeclampsia involves poor placental implantation leading to placental hypoperfusion. The central role for the placenta in this condition is reinforced by the fact that preeclampsia is always cured within days to weeks after delivery of the placenta. The chain of events appears to be defective trophoblastic invasion of the uterus followed by abnormal spiral artery remodelling. Before we discuss the pathogenesis, let us remind ourselves about spiral arteries, the decidua, and the trophoblast:

- *Spiral arteries*: these highly muscular coiled arteries are terminal branches of the uterine artery that supply blood to the developing foetus/placenta.
- *Decidua*: after ovulation, the maternal uterine endometrium becomes transformed into the secretory lining called decidua in preparation for accepting the embryo.
- *Trophoblast*: the trophoblast is the outer layer of cells that surrounds the blastocyst, which is an early form in the development of the embryo. It plays a vital role in embryo implantation and interaction with the decidualized maternal uterus and eventually forms a large part of the placenta. The trophoblast consists of the inner single-celled layer, called the cytotrophoblast, and the outer multinucleated syncytiotrophoblast, which actively invades the uterine wall and the maternal arteries, thus establishing nutrient circulation between mother and embryo.

- *Abnormal spiral artery remodelling*: in normal pregnancies, the cytotrophoblastic cells of the developing placenta migrate through the decidua and part of the myometrium to invade both the endothelium and highly muscular tunica media of the maternal spiral arteries (Figure 11.2). This, in turn, leads to the transformation of these small and muscular vessels into large-capacitance vessels of low resistance, thus facilitating adequate blood flow to the placenta [13]. In preeclampsia, though the cytotrophoblast infiltrates the decidual part of the spiral arteries, it fails to infiltrate the myometrial portion, causing the spiral arteries to remain narrow, which in turn leads to placental hypoperfusion.
- *Defective trophoblast invasion*: defective differentiation of the trophoblast is postulated to lead to defective trophoblast invasion of the spiral arteries. In normal pregnancy, invading trophoblasts alter their adhesion molecule expression from those that are characteristic of epithelial cells (integrin alpha6/beta1, alphav/beta5, and E-cadherin) to those of endothelial cells (integrin alpha1/beta1, alphav/beta3, and VE-cadherin) [14]. Preeclampsia is characterized by a failure of this differentiation and the trophoblast retains its epithelial character.

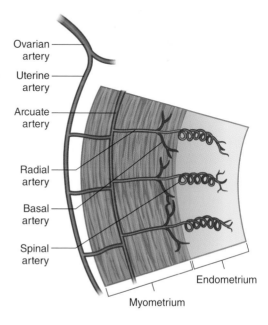

Figure 11.2 Blood supply to the uterus showing the highly coiled spiral arteries in the endometrium.

It is widely accepted that as the placenta becomes progressively dysfunctional, there is a release of pro-inflammatory substances into the maternal circulation that trigger a systemic inflammatory response and maternal endothelial dysfunction, which is postulated to lead to HTN.

There are several clinical risk factors that are associated with an increased likelihood of developing preeclampsia (Table 11.3), but patients can develop preeclampsia in the absence of risk factors.

Table 11.3 Clinical risk factors that are associated with the likelihood of developing preeclampsia

Chronic hypertension

Pre-gestational diabetes

Multiple gestation

African American race

Prior preeclampsia

Nulliparity

Assisted reproductive techniques

Body mass index (BMI) >25

To date, the most promising biomarkers to reflect placental dysfunction are decreased levels of placental growth factor (PlGF) and increased levels of soluble fms-like tyrosine kinase-1 (sFLT-1). We know that sFLT-1 is a potent antagonist to the angiogenic factors vascular endothelial growth factor (VEGF) and PlGF (Figure 11.3). Studies have shown that administration of sFLT-1 to pregnant and non-pregnant rats produces a picture clinically and histologically similar to human preeclampsia. A high plasma sFlt-1: PlGF ratio may identify women at risk of requiring delivery within two weeks because of severe preeclampsia. However, additional studies are required to validate these findings [15].

Prevention of Preeclampsia

Successful prevention of preeclampsia can considerably improve maternal and neonatal morbidity and mortality. According to the National Institute for Health and Care Excellence (NICE) Guideline 107, pregnant women with one high risk factor or more than one moderate risk factor for preeclampsia should be advised to take low dose aspirin (75 to 150 mg daily) from 12 weeks' gestation until the birth of the baby [16]. More recent data has suggested that

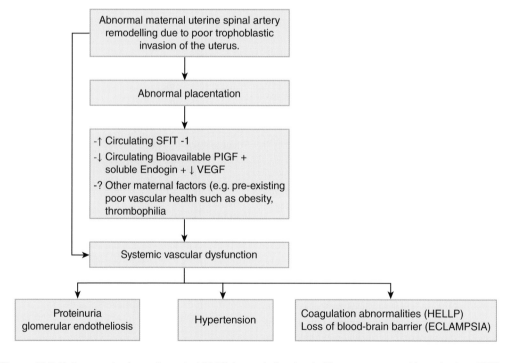

Figure 11.3 Pathogenesis of preeclampsia. HELLP, **h**aemolysis, **e**levated **l**iver enzymes, and **l**ow **p**latelets; PlGF, placental growth factor; sFLT-1, soluble fms-like tyrosine kinase-1; VEGF, vascular endothelial growth factor.

the optimal dose of aspirin for preeclampsia prevention is 150 mg taken at night.

High risk factors for preeclampsia:

- Hypertensive disease during a previous pregnancy
- CKD
- Autoimmune disease such as systemic lupus erythematosus (SLE) or antiphospholipid syndrome (APS)
- Type 1 or type 2 diabetes
- Chronic HTN

Moderate risk factors for preeclampsia:

- First pregnancy
- Age 40 years or older
- Pregnancy interval of more than 10 years
- Body mass index (BMI) of 35 kg/m² or more at first visit
- Family history of preeclampsia
- Multiple pregnancy

Although there was some early interest, available data do not support the use of low molecular weight heparin or nitric oxide donors (glyceryl trinitrate) for the prevention of preeclampsia.

Management of Preeclampsia

The definitive treatment of preeclampsia is delivery to prevent development of both maternal and foetal complications (Table 11.4). Severe preeclampsia (defined by the criteria in Table 11.5) is an indication for urgent delivery regardless of gestational age because of the high risk of serious maternal morbidity.

There is evidence that magnesium sulphate prevents eclampsia in women with severe preeclampsia [17]. However, most of these data have come from developing countries where the risk of eclampsia is high. Developed countries still lack consensus on magnesium prophylaxis, but selective use in women with severe preeclampsia and signs of neurological irritability would seem reasonable.

Complications of Preeclampsia

HELLP Syndrome

HELLP syndrome presents as a variant of preeclampsia characterized by **h**aemolysis, **e**levated **l**iver enzymes and **l**ow **p**latelets. It occurs in about 0.5% of all pregnancies and complicates 10–20% of severe preeclamptic pregnancies. As some patients with HELLP syndrome do not have HTN or proteinuria, some clinicians believe that HELLP is a separate disorder from preeclampsia [18].

HELLP syndrome is associated with significant maternal morbidity and mortality, with life-threatening

Table 11.4 Indications for delivery of women with preeclampsia

- Women with preeclampsia at 37 weeks' gestation should be delivered
- Women with preeclampsia between 34 and 37 weeks can be managed with an expectant conservative approach
- Women with preeclampsia at <34 weeks' gestation should be managed with a conservative (expectant) approach at a centre with maternal and foetal medicine expertise, delivery being necessary when one or more of the following indications emerges:
  (a) Inability to control maternal blood pressure despite antihypertensives
  (b) Maternal pulse oximetry <90% or pulmonary oedema unresponsive to initial diuretics
  (c) Progressive deterioration in liver function, glomerular filtration rate, haemolysis or platelet count
  (d) Ongoing neurological symptoms or eclampsia
  (e) Placental abruption
  (f) Reversed end-diastolic flow in the umbilical artery Doppler velocimetry, a non-reassuring cardiotocography or stillbirth

Of note is that neither the serum uric acid nor the level of proteinuria should be used as an indication for delivery

complications including placental abruption, pulmonary oedema, disseminated intravascular coagulation (DIC), cerebral haemorrhage, septic shock, AKI, and hepatic rupture. As hypertension and proteinuria may not always be present, it is vital to detect symptoms that could suggest HELLP syndrome, including right upper quadrant pain, nausea, vomiting, and general malaise. It is important to differentiate this condition from other conditions seen in pregnancy, such as thrombocytopenia of pregnancy, acute fatty liver of pregnancy, microangiopathic disorders, SLE, viral hepatitis, and cholangitis. Once a diagnosis of HELLP has been established, women should typically be delivered; there is no role for expectant management.

Eclampsia

Eclampsia is the convulsive form of preeclampsia and occurs in 2–3% of women with severe features of preeclampsia not receiving anti-seizure prophylaxis and up to 0.6% of women with preeclampsia without severe features [19]. Eclampsia is defined as the development of convulsions during pregnancy or post-partum in women with symptoms and signs of preeclampsia. However, 25% of patients may not have hypertension and up to 14% may not demonstrate proteinuria,

Table 11.5 Indications of severe preeclampsia. In preeclampsia, the presence of one or more of the following indicates severe preeclampsia

Symptoms of central nervous system dysfunction:

New-onset cerebral or visual disturbance, such as:
- Flashing lights, scotomata, cortical blindness or retinal vasospasm
- Severe headache (i.e. incapacitating, 'the worst headache I've ever had') or headache that persists and progresses despite analgesic therapy
- Altered mental status

Hepatic abnormality:

Severe persistent right upper quadrant or epigastric pain unresponsive to medication and not accounted for by an alternative diagnosis or serum transaminase concentration ≥2 times the upper limit of normal range, or both

Severe blood pressure elevation:

Systolic blood pressure ≥160 mmHg or diastolic blood pressure ≥110 mmHg on two occasions at least four hours apart whilst the patient is on bedrest (antihypertensive therapy may be initiated upon confirmation of severe hypertension, in which case criteria for severe blood pressure elevation can be satisfied without waiting until four hours have elapsed)

Thrombocytopenia:

<100 000 platelets/microl

Renal abnormality:

Progressive renal insufficiency (serum creatinine >1.1 mg/dl [97.2 micromol/l] or a doubling of the serum creatinine concentration in the absence of other renal disease)

Pulmonary oedema

making prediction and diagnosis challenging. Clinical symptoms are important in predicting the development of eclampsia, and the majority of women will have one of the following: persistent occipital or frontal headaches, blurred vision, photophobia, right upper quadrant pain, or altered mental state.

Whilst 60% of eclampsia occurs ante-partum, 20% of cases are intra-partum and 20% occur post-partum [20]. Post-partum presentations most commonly occur within 48 hours, but uncommonly up to as long as three weeks later.

Foetal bradycardia for at least three to five minutes is a common finding during and immediately after the seizure. Transient neurological findings in patients may include memory deficits, increased deep tendon reflexes, visual perception deficits, altered mental status, and cranial nerve deficits [21]. Whilst there is not much literature available regarding electroencephalography (EEG) findings in eclampsia, magnetic resonance imaging (MRI) characteristically shows symmetrical white matter oedema in the posterior cerebral hemispheres, particularly the parieto-occipital regions, similar to posterior reversible encephalopathy syndrome (PRES) discussed in the next section.

The most feared complication is haemorrhagic stroke and management consists of control of BP, administration of magnesium sulphate (both to treat the seizure as well as for preventing further seizures) and urgent delivery.

Posterior Reversible Encephalopathy Syndrome

PRES is a syndrome characterized by typical findings on neuroimaging in combination with neurotoxicity. The neurotoxicity often manifests as visual disturbances such as loss of vision, blurred vision, scotomata, and visual hallucinations, but may also include headache, aphasia, facial numbness, seizure, and ataxia. The diagnostic feature, however, is symmetrical white matter oedema in the posterior cerebral hemispheres, particularly the parieto-occipital regions seen on neuroimaging.

The appearance of PRES is not confined to eclampsia alone, but is also associated with a number of non-pregnancy conditions including acute severe HTN, immunosuppression with cyclosporine or tacrolimus, systemic inflammatory response syndrome and a number of autoimmune conditions such as SLE, PAN, and cryoglobulinaemia. The pathogenesis appears to relate to a breakdown of the blood–brain barrier, causing vasogenic cerebral oedema. Treatment in pregnancy associated PRES consists of gradual control of BP, magesium suphate prophylasxis and delivery.

Thrombotic Microangiopathies Including Thrombotic Thrombocytopenic Purpura and Haemolytic Uraemic Syndrome

Thrombotic microangiopathy (TMA) describes a specific condition in which abnormalities in the vessel wall of arterioles and capillaries lead to microvascular thrombosis. TMA is a histological diagnosis characterized by:

- Platelet microthrombi, typically within small arterioles and capillaries.
- Vessel wall changes characterized by swelling of endothelial cells and the subendothelial space, along with vessel wall thickening.

Clinically, TMA often presents with Micro-angiopathic haemolytic anaemia (MAHA) and thrombocytopenia with variable signs of organ injury due to platelet thrombosis in the microcirculation. Of note is that DIC seen in infections or malignancies can also present with MAHA and thrombocytopenia. However, the thrombi in TMAs are composed primarily of platelets and von Willebrand factor (VWF), whilst in DIC they are composed predominantly of red blood cells (RBCs) and fibrin. Coagulation tests are abnormal in DIC but normal in the TMAs.

MAHA in TMAs is caused by mechanical fragmentation of the RBCs as they traverse platelet-rich thrombi in the microcirculation, leading to the formation of the characteristic schistocytes (helmet-shaped fragmented RBCs) seen on peripheral blood film. The thrombocytopenia is due to the platelet consumption within the mesh of ultra-large molecules of VWF leading to the generation of the platelet-rich thrombi.

Injury to the endothelial cells is the central event leading to the development of TMAs. Many systemic disorders can lead to the clinical presentation of MAHA and thrombocytopenia (Table 11.6). It is important to be able to clinically differentiate primary TMAs from the secondary causes of TMAs because of different therapeutic approaches. The clinical entities seen in the context of primary TMA include [22]:

- HUS, which is characterized by AKI with minimal or no neurological manifestations. Whilst Shiga toxin-producing *Escherichia coli* (STEC) HUS accounts for over 90% of cases of HUS in children, complement-mediated HUS is seen more commonly in adults.
- TTP, which is characteristically associated with neurological findings and usually minimal abnormalities of kidney function despite microthrombi observed throughout the kidney on biopsy. TTP is a TMA caused by severely reduced activity of the VWF-cleaving protease ADAMTS13 (**A d**isintegrin and **m**etalloprotease with a **t**hrombo**s**pondin type 1 motif, member **13**).
- Drug-induced TMA has two distinct categories:

(a) *Immune-mediated*: caused by drug-dependent antibodies that react with platelets, neutrophils or endothelial cells. Quinine is the most widely recognized causative drug, with other drugs implicated being quetiapine, oxaliplatin, and gemcitabine.

(b) *Drug dose-dependent toxicity-related*: presentation might be acute, caused by a toxic dose of an approved or illegal drug, or chronic, when the patient may present after weeks to months of drug exposure. The four classes of drugs which can lead to this presentation are chemotherapeutic agents (such as gemcitabine and mitomycin), immunosuppressive agents (such as cyclosporine and tacrolimus), VEGF inhibitors (such as sirolimus and bevacizumab) and narcotics taken inappropriately or illegal agents (such as oxymorphone and cocaine).

- Metabolism-mediated TMA. Disorders of intracellular vitamin B$_{12}$ (cobalamin) metabolism can cause TMA. These syndromes appear to be exclusively hereditary and are characterized by elevated homocysteine and low methionine levels in plasma, whilst urine often shows methylmalonic aciduria.

The following systemic disorders can cause MAHA and thrombocytopenia:

- *Pregnancy associated*: preeclampsia with severe features and HELLP syndrome (discussed earlier in this chapter).
- *Severe HTN*: severe HTN can cause MAHA and thrombocytopenia with AKI, though at times the renal failure can be absent or mild.
- *Systemic rheumatic disorders*: conditions such as SLE, systemic sclerosis (SSc or scleroderma), and antiphospholipid syndrome (APS).
- *Systemic infections*: associations include bacterial endocarditis, HIV infection, cytomegalovirus (CMV) infection, Rocky Mountain spotted fever, malaria, and systemic aspergillosis.
- *Malignancy*: any systemic malignancy can lead to MAHA and thrombocytopenia by causing microvascular metastases or DIC.
- *Haematopoietic stem cell transplant or organ transplantation*: These patients may develop MAHA and thrombocytopenia from regimens for bone marrow ablation (e.g. total body radiation, high-dose chemotherapy) or immunosuppressive drugs (e.g. calcineurin inhibitors - cyclosporine and tacrolimus).
- *DIC*: whilst both malignancies and severe sepsis can lead to DIC and the resultant MAHA with thrombocytopenia, the characteristically low fibrinogen and high D-dimer help to recognize DIC.

Table 11.6 Differential diagnosis of microangiopathic haemolytic anaemia (MAHA) with thrombocytopenia

Primary thrombotic microangiopathy (TMA) syndromes	Secondary causes of MAHA with thrombocytopenia
Thrombotic thrombocytopenic purpura (TTP)	Pregnancy-associated
	• Preeclampsia with severe features
Haemolytic uraemic syndrome (HUS)	• HELP syndrome (haemolysis, elevated liver enzymes and low platelets
• Shiga toxin-producing *Escherichia coli* haemolytic uraemic syndrome (STEC HUS)	Systemic rheumatic disorders
• Complement-mediated or atypical haemolytic uraemic syndrome (aHUS)	• Systemic lupus erythematosus (SLE)
	• Systemic sclerosis
	• Antiphospholipid syndrome
Drug-induced TMA	Systemic infections
• Immune-mediated (quinine, quetiapine, oxaliplatin, and gemcitabine)	• Bacterial endocarditis
• Drug dose-dependent toxicity-related: chemotherapeutic agents (such as gemcitabine and mitomycin), immunosuppressive agents (such as cyclosporine and tacrolimus), vascular endothelial growth factor (VEGF) inhibitors (such as sirolimus and bevacizumab), and narcotics taken inappropriately or illegal agents (such as oxymorphone and cocaine)	• HIV infection
	• Cytomegalovirus (CMV) infection
	• Rocky Mountain spotted fever
	• Malaria
	• Systemic aspergillosis
Metabolism-mediated TMA (disorders of vitamin B_{12} metabolism)	Malignancy
	Haematopoietic stem cell transplant or organ transplantation
	• Bone marrow ablation (e.g. total body radiation, high-dose chemotherapy)
	• Immunosuppressive drugs (e.g. calcineurin inhibitors)
	Disseminated intravascular coagulation (DIC), characterized by low fibrinogen and high D-dimer, associated with systemic infections and malignancies

Thrombotic Thrombocytopenic Purpura

TTP refers to the primary TMA caused by severe deficiency of ADAMTS13. The ADAMTS13 activity in TTP is typically less than 10%. It is often accompanied by neurological dysfunction, and renal involvement is usually not severe. Endothelial cells synthesize and secrete the ultra-large VWF molecules into plasma, which tend to stick to the luminal surface of the endothelial cells. Normally, ADAMTS13 cleaves these big molecules to the physiologically important smaller VWF fragments. In TTP, a deficiency of ADAMTS13 causes the ultra-large VWF molecules to accumulate on the endothelial cells and this provides a nidus for the trapping of platelets, leading in turn to thrombocytopenia. As the RBCs make their way through these platelet-rich plugs, they are fragmented, leading to the formation of the characteristic schistocytes and the resultant haemolytic anaemia.

The classic clinical pentad of TTP consists of thrombocytopenia, MAHA, neurological abnormalities, fever, and renal dysfunction. The complete pentad is seen in less than 40% of patients, but the majority will have the first three clinical findings. Sometimes differentiation from HELLP can be difficult; TTP should be suspected in pregnant patients with fever and normal liver function in the presence of thrombocytopenia and haemolytic anaemia, especially in those who present at less than 24 weeks of pregnancy or fail to improve upon delivery.

The major cause of severe ADAMTS13 deficiency is an acquired antibody, with genetic mutations accounting for only a small number of cases. Although conditions like sepsis, cardiac surgery, pancreatitis, and liver disease can lead to low ADAMTS13 levels, the levels are usually between 10 and 60%; not low enough to cause TTP.

TTP is a medical emergency and is fatal without prompt treatment. The mainstay of treatment for TTP is plasma exchange therapy with fresh frozen plasma (which has improved the mortality rates from 90% to less than 15%) [23]. Corticosteroids are commonly given to patients with TTP. The use of rituximab along with plasma exchange is shown to be associated with a significantly decreased incidence of relapse in TTP [24]. In patients with a genetic deficiency of ADAMTS13, treatment consists of plasma infusion or plasma exchange (if volume overload is an issue with plasma infusion). Corticosteroids or rituximab do not have a role in hereditary TTP.

Haemolytic Uraemic Syndrome

HUS is clinically defined by the simultaneous occurrence of MAHA, thrombocytopenia, and renal failure. It is much more common in children than adults.

STEC (mostly O157:H7) haemolytic uraemic syndrome (STEC HUS) is the most common cause of paediatric HUS, accounting for 90% of cases. The remaining childhood HUS cases are generally divided into primary HUS, caused by complement dysregulation (termed aHUS), and secondary HUS, caused by pneumococcal infection.

Shigella *dysenteriae* type 1-associated HUS occurs in India, Bangladesh, and southern Africa, and has a more severe presentation with worse mortality figures. In Australia, about 50% of cases of post-diarrhoeal HUS are due to *E. coli* O111 [25]. In *E. Coli*-associated HUS, undercooked meat is the most common culprit, with secondary person-to-person spread also playing an important role [26].

Children with STEC HUS typically have a prodromal illness with abdominal pain, vomiting, and diarrhoea that generally precede the development of HUS by 5–10 days. HUS is diagnosed by the sudden onset of haemolytic anaemia with fragmented RBCs on the peripheral blood film, thrombocytopenia, and AKI. Neurological signs including stroke, seizure or coma may be seen in up to 25% [27]. Pancreatitis may be seen in up to 20%, with occasional patients presenting with severe haemorrhagic colitis (which may be misdiagnosed as ulcerative colitis), bowel necrosis, and perforation.

Diagnosis is usually suspected on the basis of characteristic clinical and laboratory findings; that is, a prodrome of diarrhoea followed by abrupt onset of MAHA, thrombocytopenia, and AKI. Confirmation rests on the detection of offending organisms, which may be demonstrable even several weeks after the event in stool samples.

Antibiotics and antimotility drugs are not helpful in treatment, and there is some evidence that antimotility drugs may increase the risk of central nervous system dysfunction [28]. HUS usually resolves spontaneously in children and supportive management of anaemia, thrombocytopenia, HTN, electrolyte disorders and AKI has improved mortality in the past few decades. Whilst there is no role for plasma exchange in children with HUS, some studies suggest that plasma exchange may be beneficial in adults with STEC HUS in both lowering mortality and risk of end-stage renal disease (ESRD) [29].

The indications for dialysis in HUS are similar to those for dialysis in other causes of AKI.

Whilst mortality rates are less than 5%, another 5% may be left with significant sequelae (e.g. stroke or ESRD) [30].

Complement-mediated or aHUS, which represents 5–10% of all HUS cases, is postulated to arise from dysfunction of the complement system. The various complement pathways converge on the generation of C3 convertases, and the alternative C3 convertase (C3bBb) is tightly regulated by a number of plasma- and membrane-bound factors, including factor H, factor I, membrane cofactor protein, and decay-accelerating factor. In aHUS, mutations in one or more genes encoding these factors are responsible for a lack of control over the alternative C3 convertase, leading to complement-induced lesions of endothelial cells. Pregnancy may activate the onset or relapse of a-HUS. Its diagnosis is therefore suggested by the absence of ADAMTS13 deficiency, and genetic testing is now available for a number of the complement factor gene defects.

Patients with the diagnosis of aHUS should receive eculizumab as the first-line treatment along with plasma exchange [31]. Eculizumab binds to complement factor C5 and blocks its cleavage, thereby preventing production of the terminal complement components C5a and the membrane attack complex C5b-9. Initiating early treatment with eculizumab is associated with significant inhibition of complement-mediated TMA, as measured by an improvement in the platelet count, an absence of thrombotic microangiopathic events and sustained improvement in renal function [32].

References

1. Zoccali, C., Mallamaci, F., and Finocchiaro, P. (2002). Atherosclerotic renal artery stenosis: epidemiology, cardiovascular outcomes, and clinical prediction rules. *J. Am. Soc. Nephrol.* 13: S179–S183.

2. Textor, S.C. (2009). Current approaches to renovascular hypertension. *Med. Clin. North Am.* 93 (3): 717. https://doi.org/10.1016/j.mcna.2009.02.012.

3. Olin, J.W., Froehlich, J., Gu, X. et al. (2012). The United States registry for fibromuscular dysplasia: results in the first 447 patients. *Circulation* 125 (25): 3182.

4. Slovut, D.P. and Olin, J.W. (2004). Fibromuscular dysplasia. *N. Engl. J. Med.* 350: 1862–1871. https://doi.org/10.1056/NEJMra032393.

5. Pickering, T.G. (1989). Renovascular hypertension: etiology and pathophysiology. *Semin. Nucl. Med.* 19 (2): 79–88. https://doi.org/10.1016/S0001-2998(89)80003-0.

6. Tullis, M.J., Caps, M.T., Zierler, R.E. et al. (1999). Blood pressure, antihypertensive medication, and atherosclerotic renal artery stenosis. *Am. J. Kidney Dis.* 33 (4): 675.

7. The ASTRAL Investigators (2009). Revascularization versus medical therapy for renal-artery stenosis. *N. Engl. J. Med.* 361: 1953–1962. https://doi.org/10.1056/NEJMoa0905368.

8. Olin, J.W., Gornik, H.L., Bacharach, J.M. et al. (2014). Fibromuscular dysplasia: state of the science and critical unanswered questions: a scientific statement from the American Heart Association. *Circulation* 129 (9): 1048.

9. Soma-Pillay, P., Catherine, N.-P., Tolppanen, H., and Mebazaa, A. (2016). Physiological changes in pregnancy. *Cardiovasc. J. Afr.* 27 (2): 89–94. https://doi.org/10.5830/CVJA-2016-021.

10. Cheung, K.L. and Lafayette, R.A. (2013). Renal physiology of pregnancy. *Adv. Chronic Kidney Dis.* 20 (3): 209–214. https://doi.org/10.1053/j.ackd.2013.01.012.

11. American College of Obstetricians and Gynecologists, Task Force on Hypertension in Pregnancy (2013). Hypertension in pregnancy. Report of the American College of Obstetricians and Gynecologists' Task Force on Hypertension in Pregnancy. *Obstet. Gynecol.* 122 (5): 1122.

12. Queensland Clinical Guideline (2015). *Hypertensive disorders of pregnancy. MN15.13-V7-R20.* Brisbane: Queensland Health.

13. Uzan, J., Carbonnel, M., Piconne, O. et al. (2011). Pre-eclampsia: pathophysiology, diagnosis, and management. *Vasc. Health Risk Manag.* 7: 467–474. https://doi.org/10.2147/VHRM.S20181.

14. Zhou, Y., Damsky, C.H., and Fisher, S.J. (1997). Preeclampsia is associated with failure of human cytotrophoblasts to mimic a vascular adhesion phenotype. One cause of defective endovascular invasion in this syndrome? *J. Clin. Invest.* 99 (9): 2152.

15. Rana, S., Powe, C.E., Salahuddin, S. et al. (2012). Angiogenic factors and the risk of adverse outcomes in women with suspected preeclampsia. *Circulation* 125 (7): 911.

16. National Institute for Health and Care Excellence (2010). *Hypertension in pregnancy: Diagnosis and management. Clinical guideline CG107.* London: NICE.

17. Roberts, J.M., Villar, J., and Arulkumaran, S. (2002). Preventing and treating eclamptic seizures. *BMJ* 325 (7365): 609–610.

18. Sibai, B.M. (1990). The HELLP syndrome (hemolysis, elevated liver enzymes, and low

platelets): much ado about nothing? *Am. J. Obstet. Gynecol.* 162 (2): 311.

19. Sibai, B.M. (2004). Magnesium sulfate prophylaxis in preeclampsia: lessons learned from recent trials. *Am. J. Obstet. Gynecol.* 190 (6): 1520.

20. Berhan, Y. and Berhan, A. (2015). Should magnesium sulfate be administered to women with mild pre-eclampsia? A systematic review of published reports on eclampsia. *J. Obstet. Gynaecol. Res.* 41 (6): 831.

21. Shah, A.K., Rajamani, K., and Whitty, J.E. (2008). Eclampsia: a neurological perspective. *J. Neurol. Sci.* 271 (1–2): 158.

22. Scully, M., Cataland, S., Coppo, P. et al. (2017). Consensus on the standardization of terminology in thrombotic thrombocytopenic purpura and related thrombotic microangiopathies. *J. Thromb. Haemost.* 15 (2): 312.

23. von Baeyer, H. (2002). Plasmapheresis in thrombotic microangiopathy-associated syndromes: review of outcome data derived from clinical trials and open studies. *Ther. Apher.* 6 (4): 320.

24. Page, E.E., Hovinga, J.A.K., Terrell, D.R. et al. (2016). Rituximab reduces risk for relapse in patients with thrombotic thrombocytopenic purpura. *Blood* 127: 3092–3094. https://doi.org/10.1182/blood-2016-03-703827.

25. Elliott, E.J., Robins-Browne, R.M., O'Loughlin, E.V. et al. (2001). Contributors to the Australian Paediatric Surveillance Unit. Nationwide study of haemolytic uraemic syndrome: clinical, microbiological, and epidemiological features. *Arch. Dis. Child.* 85 (2): 125.

26. Su, C. and Brandt, L.J. (1995). Escherichia coli O157:H7 infection in humans. *Ann. Intern. Med.* 123 (9): 698.

27. Nathanson, S., Kwon, T., Elmaleh, M. et al. (2010). Acute neurological involvement in diarrhea-associated hemolytic uremic syndrome. *Clin. J. Am. Soc. Nephrol.* 5 (7): 1218.

28. Cimolai, N., Morrison, B.J., and Carter, J.E. (1992). Risk factors for the central nervous system manifestations of gastroenteritis-associated hemolytic-uremic syndrome. *Pediatrics* 90 (4): 616.

29. Carter, A.O., Borczyk, A.A., Carlson, J.A. et al. (1987). A severe outbreak of E coli O157:H7 associated hemorrhagic colitis in a nursing home. *NEJM* 317: 1496–1500.

30. Siegler, R.L., Pavia, A.T., Christofferson, R.D., and Milligan, M.K. (1994). A 20-year population-based study of postdiarrheal hemolytic uremic syndrome in Utah. *Pediatrics* 94 (1): 35.

31. Rathbone, J., Kaltenthaler, E., Richards, A. et al. (2013). A systematic review of eculizumab for atypical haemolytic uraemic syndrome (aHUS). *BMJ Open* 3 (11): e003573.

32. Legendre, C.M., Licht, C., Muus, P. et al. (2013). Terminal complement inhibitor eculizumab in atypical hemolytic–uremic syndrome. *N. Engl. J. Med.* 368: 2169–2181. https://doi.org/10.1056/NEJMoa1208981.

Questions and Answers

Questions

1. The pentad of TTP includes all the following except:
   a. Fever
   b. Thrombocytopenia
   c. Raised transaminases
   d. Neurologic dysfunction
   e. Haemolytic anaemia

2. Which of the following intervention helps to reduce the risk of severe preeclampsia in women with risk factors?
   a. Prophylactic beta blockers
   b. Heparinoids
   c. Aspirin
   d. Multivitamins
   e. Folic acid

3. First-line treatment of aHUS consists of:
   a. Haemodialysis
   b. Eculizumab
   c. Rituximab
   d. Antibiotics
   e. Blood transfusion

4. Which of the following statements regarding the treatment of renovascular hypertension is not true:
   a. Revascularization should be offered to patients with fibromuscular dysplasia
   b. Computed tomography angiography (CTA) and magnetic resonance angiography (MRA) are equally useful for diagnosis of FMD
   c. There is no advantage of revascularization over medical therapy in those with renal artery stenosis
   d. FMD does not affect the proximal part of the renal artery
   e. ACE-I are the drugs of choice for unilateral RAS

5. Although DIC can also present with micro-angiopathic haemolytic anaemia (MAHA) and thrombocytopenia, it is not considered as thrombotic microangiopathy (TMA) because:
   a. DIC is usually seen in the context of infection and malignancy
   b. DIC is characterized by haemorrhage rather than thrombosis
   c. The thrombocytopenia in DIC is usually very mild
   d. The thrombi in DIC consist of red blood cells rather than platelets
   e. DIC is not associated with AKI

Answers

1. c. The classic clinical pentad of TTP consisting of thrombocytopenia, microangiopathic haemolytic anaemia, neurological abnormalities, fever, and renal dysfunction is seen in less than 40% of patients. Most patients with TTP have the first three clinical findings. Renal dysfunction is often not present or not very severe in this condition.

2. c. According to the National Institute for Health and Care Excellence (NICE) guideline 107, pregnant women with one high risk factor or more than one moderate risk factor for preeclampsia should be advised to take 150 mg aspirin nightly from 12 weeks until the birth of the baby.

3. b. Patients with the diagnosis of atypical HUS should receive eculizumab as the first-line treatment. Plasma exchange should be used until TTP has been excluded. Shiga toxin-producing

Escherichia coli (STEC) HUS usually resolves spontaneously with supportive management of anaemia, thrombocytopenia, hypertension, electrolyte disorders, and AKI.

4. b. CTA is more sensitive for identification of the distal lesions seen in FMD. Revascularization is offered to patients with FMD

5. d. While TMA often presents with MAHA and thrombocytopenia, it is essentially a histological diagnosis characterized by:

- Platelet microthrombi typically within small arterioles and capillaries
- Vessel wall changes characterized by swelling of endothelial cells and the subendothelial space along with vessel wall thickening

The degree of thrombocytopenia and presence of AKI has no bearing on the diagnosis of TMA. The thrombi in DIC characteristically consist of red blood cells rather than platelets.

12

Hereditary and Familial Renal Diseases

Surjit Tarafdar

Summary

Autosomal-Dominant Polycystic Kidney Disease (ADPKD)

- ADPKD is characterized by enlarged kidneys with multiple and bilateral renal cysts
- Common disorder – seen in 1 in 400 to 1000 births with half the patients remaining undiagnosed
- Clinical manifestations include abdominal pain, haematuria, urinary tract/cyst infection, hypertension, renal stones, urinary-concentrating defect, and end-stage renal disease (ESRD)
- Extra-renal manifestations include cerebral aneurysm, hepatic cysts, pancreatic cysts, seminal vesicle cysts, valvular abnormalities, diverticular disease, and hernia
- Ultrasound is the usual modality for diagnosis
- No specific therapy yet known, but increasing interest in the use of vasopressin receptor antagonists, somatostatin analogues, and mammalian target of rapamycin (mTOR) inhibitors

Autosomal-Recessive Polycystic Kidney Disease (ARPKD)

- Characterized by cystic dilations of the renal collecting ducts (unlike cystic dilatation of any part of nephron in the more common ADPKD) and congenital hepatic fibrosis
- Usually identified in utero or at birth with ultrasonographic evidence of markedly enlarged kidneys

- Severely affected neonates generally present with respiratory distress due to pulmonary insufficiency, whilst others present in early childhood with progressive chronic kidney disease (CKD) and portal hypertension
- Renal transplantation is curative

Alport's Syndrome (AS)

- AS is the commonest form of hereditary nephritis and is often associated with sensorineural deafness and ocular abnormalities
- Mutation in type IV collagen affects the glomerular basement membrane (GBM) and basement membranes in the eye and ear
- X-linked AS (XLAS) in more than 80% of cases, where males are affected more severely
- Usual presentation in the first two decades with microscopic and at times overt haematuria
- ESRD develops in 90% of XLAS males by the age of 40 (compared to 12% in females)
- Renal transplantation is the only definitive therapy, though 5% of patients develop anti-GBM disease post-transplant

Thin Basement Membrane Nephropathy (TBMN)

- Estimated to exist in 20–25% of those with asymptomatic haematuria
- 30–50% of those affected have family history of haematuria
- Diagnosed on renal biopsy showing extremely thin GBM

- Usually no association with CKD or hypertension and excellent long-term prognosis

Tuberous Sclerosis (TSC)
- Characterized by multiple benign hamartomas of the brain, eyes, heart, lung, liver, skin, and kidney along with renal cysts
- Caused by mutation in either the TSC1 gene (on chromosome 9) or the TSC2 gene (on chromosome 16), whose products are hamartin and tuberin, respectively
- Characteristic skin lesions, central nervous system benign tumours and epilepsy seen in 90% of patients, whilst 80% have renal angiomyolipomas and 44–65% have cognitive defects
- Surgery offered to those with renal and brain tumours, whilst mTOR inhibitors offered to those who are poor surgical candidates

Fabry Disease
- Fabry disease is the commonest lysosomal storage disorder
- X-linked inborn error of the glycosphingolipid metabolic pathway characterized by deficiency of the lysosomal hydrolase alpha-galactosidase A (alpha-Gal A)
- Males are affected more often and more severely
- Neurological, dermatological, and renal and/or cardiac manifestations appear by the second, third and fifth decades, respectively
- Treatment consists of replacing the deficient enzyme alpha-Gal A
- Kidney transplantation has excellent long-term renal prognosis

This chapter will discuss some of the more common hereditary and congenital renal diseases. There are broadly categorized into diseases associated with renal cysts and those presenting with haematuria.

Genetic cystic renal diseases:

- Autosomal-dominant polycystic kidney disease (ADPKD)
- Autosomal-recessive polycystic kidney disease (ARPKD)
- Tuberous sclerosis (TSC)
- von Hippel–Lindau disease (discussed in Chapter 5)

Genetic diseases presenting with haematuria:

- Alport's syndrome (AS)
- Thin basement membrane nephropathy (TBMN)

Autosomal-Dominant Polycystic Kidney Disease

ADPKD is a common disorder, occurring in approximately 1 in every 400–1000 live births, with more than half of the patients remaining undiagnosed during their lifetime [1]. It is a multisystem disorder characterized by enlarged kidneys with multiple and bilateral renal cysts, with cysts commonly seen in other organs such as liver and pancreas.

ADPKD is the fourth commonest cause of chronic kidney disease (CKD) after diabetes, hypertension, and glomerulonephritis. According to the US Renal Data System, ADPKD accounts for 2.2% of new cases of kidney failure each year in the USA [2].

Aetiology and Pathogenesis

The PKD1 (on chromosome 16) and PKD2 (on chromosome 4) genes encode proteins called polycystin-1 and polycystin-2 respectively. In 85% of patients and families with ADPKD there is an abnormality on chromosome 16 (PKD1 locus), whilst the rest have an abnormality on chromosome 4 (PKD2 locus) [3]. Mutations in PKD1 are associated with earlier clinical presentation and higher morbidity as well as mortality.

Polycystin-1 and -2 interact with each other to help primary cilia on the tubular epithelial cells sense the luminal environment, which in turn facilitates calcium (Ca^+) influx into the cells through polycystin-2 channels (Figure 12.1). Therefore, mutation in either of these proteins leads to defective ciliary function and reduced influx of Ca^+ into the tubular cells. Low intracellular Ca^+ leads to high cyclic adenosine monophosphate (cAMP) levels [4] in the ADPKD cells, which in turn leads to increased activity of the cystic fibrosis transmembrane conductance regulator (CFTR). The CFTR channel is localized on the apical membranes of ADPKD cells; that is, facing the cysts. Increased CFTR activity in these cells leads to

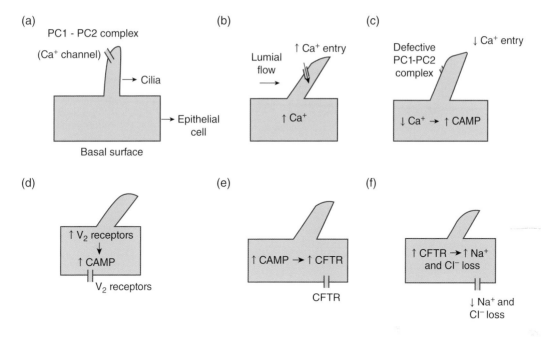

Figure 12.1 Pathogenesis of autosomal-dominant polycystic kidney disease. (a and b) PC1–PC2 complex aids the cilia on the tubular epithelial cell to sense the lumen environment and leads to Ca$^+$ influx into the cell. (c) Defect in PC1–PC2 complex leads to reduced Ca$^+$ entry into tubular cell, which leads to increased cellular cAMP levels. (d) Upregulation of V2 receptor on the tubular epithelial cells also leads to increased cellular cAMP levels. (e) Increased cAMP leads to increased activity of the CFTR channel. (f) Increased CFTR activity leads to increased secretion of NaCl and the resultant passive movement of water contributes to cyst growth. Ca$^+$, calcium; cAMP, cyclic adenosine monophosphate; CFTR, cystic fibrosis transmembrane conductance regulator; NaCL, sodium chloride; PC1, polycystin-1; PC2, polycystin-2; V2 receptor, vasopressin 2 receptor.

increased chloride secretion into the cysts. Since the negatively charged chloride is secreted along with positively charged sodium and water always follows sodium passively, chloride transport leads to increased water secretion into the cysts, with resultant enlargement of the cysts [5]. As one would expect, patients with both cystic fibrosis and ADPKD have less severe renal and liver cysts in comparison to those who have ADPKD without cystic fibrosis [6].

Upregulation of vasopressin V2 receptor and the resultant enhancement of action of vasopressin also contribute to high cAMP levels. Experiments on animal models have shown that administration of a vasopressin V2 receptor antagonist prevents renal enlargement and inhibits cyst formation by decreasing renal cAMP levels [7].

There appears to be a direct interaction between polycystin-1 and tuberin (whose mutation can lead to TSC, as discussed later) in kidney epithelial cells. Use of mammalian target of rapamycin (mTOR)-inhibitor rapamycin (sirolimus) preserved renal function and inhibited epithelial cell proliferation and fibrosis in a mouse model of ADPKD in which the PKD1 gene was conditionally deleted [8].

Clinical Presentation

Apart from the renal manifestations (Table 12.1), there are multiple extra-renal manifestations of ADPKD (Table 12.2) which can lead to significant morbidity and mortality. Patients usually present in their fourth to sixth decades. Patients with PKD1 mutation present earlier and usually have worse prognosis then those with PKD2 mutation.

Renal Manifestations

Pain

Acute flank and abdominal pain may be due to urinary tract and cyst infection, nephrolithiasis or cyst haemorrhage. Chronic pain is usually due to massively enlarged kidneys, leading to either stretching of the renal capsule or traction on the renal pedicle. Sometimes hepatic cysts may also cause pain.

Table 12.1 Renal manifestations of autosomal-dominant polycystic kidney disease

Abdominal and loin pain	Acute pain: urinary tract and cyst infection, nephrolithiasis, or cyst haemorrhage
	Chronic pain: mass effect of enlarged kidneys
Haematuria	Cyst haemorrhage, infection or nephrolithiasis
Hypertension	In up to 70% before decline in glomerular filtration rate
Urinary-concentrating defect	Polyuria, polydipsia, nocturia, and increased urinary frequency
End-stage renal disease	Kidneys by this stage are usually massively enlarged and full of cysts

Table 12.2 Extra-renal manifestations of autosomal-dominant polycystic kidney disease

Hepatic cysts seen in >90% of patients after the age of 35; usually do not cause liver problems
Other organ cysts: seminal vesicle (often bilateral and multiple) cysts in up to 40%, pancreatic cysts in 7–10%, rarely arachnoid membrane and prostate cysts
Cerebral aneurysm in up to 8% (maybe seen in up to 16% of those with family history)
Cardiac valvular abnormalities in 25–30% (most commonly mitral valve prolapse and aortic regurgitation)
Diverticula and hernia: colonic and duodenal diverticula and abdominal hernias more common than in the general population

Haematuria

Gross haematuria may be the initial presenting symptom and is seen in up to 40% of patients at some time in the course of the disease [9]. Most of the time haematuria is due to cyst haemorrhage and communication of the cyst with the collecting system. The haematuria generally settles down over two to seven days with conservative management and avoidance of heavy work. Often, though, the haemorrhaging cyst does not communicate with the collecting system and the patient presents with pain in the absence of haematuria. Other causes of haematuria include infection and stone.

Urinary Tract Infection and Cyst Infection

Cystitis, pyelonephritis, cyst infection, and perinephric abscesses are more common in patients with ADPKD compared to the general population. The route of infection in both pyelonephritis and cyst infection is usually retrograde from the bladder and therefore cystitis should be promptly treated in these patients.

When patients present with fever and flank pain and blood and urine cultures are negative, cyst aspiration under ultrasound or computed tomography (CT) guidance should be considered, to culture the organism and assist in the selection of antibiotic therapy.

Nephrolithiasis

Renal stones are seen in up to 20% of patients with ADPKD. In contrast to the predominance of calcium oxalate in patients without ADPKD, more than 50% of stones in ADPKD are composed of uric acid [10].

Hypertension

Hypertension is seen in up to 70% of patients with ADPKD before any significant reduction in glomerular filtration rate (GFR) occurs and is a major contributor to progression to CKD. Children and young adults diagnosed with ADPKD consistently have a higher ambulatory blood pressure and left ventricular mass index compared to age-matched controls [11]. Cyst expansion leads to focal areas of renal ischaemia, leading in turn to renin production and activation of the renin–angiotensin system. Poorly controlled hypertension in these patients can also increase the risk of aneurysmal bleed.

Urinary-Concentrating Defect

Most patients with ADPKD have a mild concentrating defect. They suffer from polydypsia, polyuria, nocturia, and urinary frequency. The symptoms worsen with age and patients may not mention them unless specifically asked.

End-Stage Renal Disease

Despite ongoing increase in kidney size due to relentless growth of the cysts, renal function is often maintained till the fourth or fifth decade of life. By the time renal function begins to decline, the kidneys are often massively enlarged and distorted with multiple cysts.

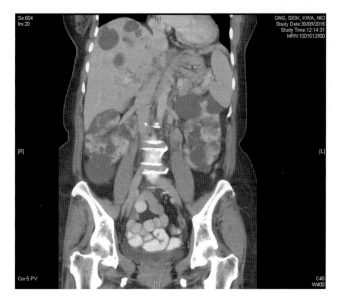

Figure 12.2 Abdominal computed tomography scan of patient with autosomal-dominant polycystic kidney disease showing multiple cysts in both kidneys and liver.

The following are risk factors for earlier progress to end-stage renal disease (ESRD):

- Male sex
- African race
- Diagnosis of ADPKD before the age of 30 years
- First episode of haematuria before the age of 30 years
- Onset of hypertension before the age of 35 years
- Hyperlipidaemia
- Sickle cell trait

Data from the Consortium for Radiologic Imaging of Polycystic Kidney Disease (CRISP) study, which followed up 241 patients over a period of 9.3 years, suggest that the decline in GFR correlates strongly with increasing kidney size and cyst volume.

Extra-renal Manifestations

Cerebral Aneurysm

This is the most dreaded complication and may be seen in up to 8% of patients with ADPKD. However, the prevalence may be as high as 16% in those with a family history of cerebral aneurysm. Screening is not indicated in every patient with ADPKD, as most cerebral aneurysms found on pre-symptomatic screening are small and have a low risk of rupture, with the risks associated with surgery clearly outweighing the risk of rupture. Indications for screening with magnetic resonance imaging (MRI) are:

- Family history of cerebral aneurysm or subarachnoid haemorrhage
- Previous aneurysmal rupture

- Preparation for surgery with potential for haemodynamic instability
- High-risk occupations, e.g. airline pilots
- Patients who require chronic anticoagulation, e.g. those with deep vein thrombosis or atrial fibrillation

If the initial scan is negative in this group of patients, then most clinicians rescreen them every five years.

Hepatic Cysts

As with renal cysts, the prevalence of hepatic cysts increases with age (Figure 12.2). Although hepatic cysts are seen in more than 90% of patients above the age of 35 years [12], they usually do not lead to liver failure or cirrhosis. Patients can have symptoms related to the mass effect of huge hepatomegaly, such as early satiety, dyspnoea or low back ache. Rarely, hepatic cyst haemorrhage or infection may be seen.

Other Organ Cysts

Seminal vesicle cysts, usually bilateral and multiple, can be seen in up to 40% of patients, whilst pancreatic cysts may be seen in 7–10% of patients with ADPKD. Arachnoid membrane and prostate cysts may also be seen.

Cardiac Abnormalities

Valvular abnormalities may be seen in 25–30% of patients with ADPKD. The most common valvular abnormalities are mitral valve prolapse and aortic regurgitation. Patients with ADPKD are also at an

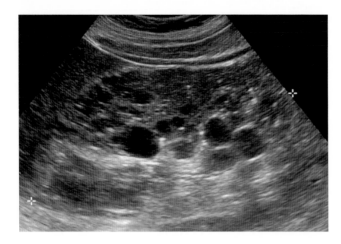

Figure 12.3 Abdominal computed tomography scan of patient with autosomal-dominant polycystic kidney disease showing multiple cysts in kidney.

increased risk for coronary artery aneurysm and dissection.

Diverticula and Hernia

Colonic and duodenal diverticula occur with more frequency in patients with ADPKD in comparison to the general population. Abdominal wall hernias are also more common in patients with ADPKD and CKD than in patients with CKD in the absence of ADPKD.

Diagnosis

The diagnosis of ADPKD rests on imaging revealing big kidneys with multiple cysts. Because of cost and safety, ultrasound is the imaging modality of choice (Figure 12.3). Rarely, patients with a strong family history but indeterminate imaging might need genetic testing.

Screening of asymptomatic children (below 18 years of age) by means of radiological or genetic testing is not advised. Adverse effects such as emotional, career or insurance issues probably outweigh the benefits of earlier diagnosis at an asymptomatic stage, given that we still do not have exact therapy to halt tumour growth.

Imaging diagnostic criterion for ADPKD are in Table 12.3 and include:

Patients with a positive family history:

- Between 15 and 39 years of age, at least three unilateral or bilateral kidney cysts.
- Between 40 and 59 years of age, at least two cysts in each kidney.
- For those 60 years or older, at least four cysts in each kidney.

Table 12.3 Ultrasound criteria for diagnosis of autosomal-dominant polycystic kidney disease in those with family history

Between 15 and 39 years of age	Between 40 and 59 years of age	60 years of age
At least 3 unilateral or bilateral kidney cysts	At least 2 cysts in each kidney	At least 4 cysts in each kidney

Patients with a negative family history:

- The diagnosis of ADPKD should be suspected in those with no known family history if there are 10 or more cysts in each kidney.
- These patients also mostly have bulky kidneys, with hepatic cysts often present.
- In up to 25% of cases, ADPKD is diagnosed in patients with no known family history.

However, one must remember that simple benign cysts are relatively common in the normal population. In a study in which renal ultrasonography was performed in 729 individuals with normal renal function who were referred for the investigation of symptoms unrelated to the urinary tract, 22% of those more than 70 years old had at least one cyst, whilst 9% in the same group had bilateral renal cysts [13]. It must also be remembered that CKD (particularly in patients on maintenance dialysis) is frequently associated with the development of multiple and bilateral renal cysts, which, though usually small, can at times reach sizes up to 2–3 cm. However, in patients with acquired cystic disease the kidneys are small to normal in size, as opposed to the extremely large kidneys found in all ADPKD individuals with renal insufficiency.

Management

Treatment of ADPKD includes non-specific measures, such as strict blood pressure control, low-salt diet and statins, which may prevent the progression of disease and reduce cardiovascular mortality. No therapy has yet proven to definitely stop the progression of cysts, although there are promising therapies on the horizon, including vasopressin receptor antagonists, somatostatin analogues, and mTOR inhibitors.

Whilst treating cyst infections it is important to remember that many antibiotics are not lipophilic and hence do not penetrate the cyst wall effectively. Trimethoprim-sulfamethoxazole and fluoroquinolones achieve good intracystic concentration and are usually the antibiotics of choice.

Cyst haemorrhage usually responds to conservative management with bed rest, analgesics, and adequate hydration. Rarely, bleeding may be severe or persistent, needing arterial embolization or surgery.

If there are no contraindications, then angiotensin-converting–enzyme (ACE) inhibitors or angiotensin II–receptor blockers (ARBs) are the preferred first-line antihypertensive agents. As shown by the HALT-PKD trial, there is no advantage in combining an ACE inhibitor with an ARB. The HALT A-PKD trial also showed that a blood pressure target of <110/75 mmHg led to a lower total kidney volume, lower albuminuria, and lower left ventricular mass index, when compared with a blood pressure target of 120–130/80 mmHg in relatively young, healthy individuals with preserved kidney function [14].

Vasopressin Receptor Antagonists

As discussed under the pathogenesis of ADPKD, vasopressin leads to high cAMP levels, which in turn lead to cyst growth. Multiple animal and human studies have shown that tolvaptan, as compared with placebo, slows the increase in total kidney volume and the decline in kidney function [7, 15].

Increased fluid intake to suppress endogenous vasopressin secretion is considered as a possible treatment to inhibit cyst growth.

Somatostatin Analogues

Multiple studies have shown that somatostatin analogues such as octreotide lead to decreased cyst growth in patients with ADPKD [16, 17]. However,

larger multicentre studies are required to determine the long-term benefit of somatostatin.

mTOR Inhibitors

Although there is some interest in the use of this group of drugs, trials have indicated conflicting results. One also has to be aware of the potential side effect of these drugs [18, 19].

Occasional patients with ADPKD may require nephrectomy of one or both kidneys for recurrent urinary tract infection, chronic pain, chronic haematuria requiring ongoing transfusions or to accommodate the transplant kidney.

Autosomal Recessive Polycystic Kidney Disease

ARPKD is characterized by cystic dilations of the renal collecting ducts (unlike cystic dilatation of any part of nephron in the more common ADPKD) and varying degrees of congenital hepatic fibrosis. It is caused by mutations in the PKHD1 (polycystic kidney and hepatic disease) gene located on chromosome 6. The majority of cases are identified either in utero or at birth, with ultrasonographic evidence of markedly enlarged kidneys. More severely affected neonates generally present with respiratory distress due to pulmonary insufficiency, whilst others present in early childhood with progressive renal failure and signs of portal hypertension.

Diagnosis is usually made on the basis of ultrasound evidence of large echogenic kidneys with poor corticomedullary differentiation and coexisting liver disease. Genetic testing may be offered in cases of uncertainty or for prenatal diagnosis. However, one must be aware that because of the large size of the PKHD1 gene and the large number of possible mutations, is possible that genetic testing could miss the diagnosis.

Renal transplantation should be offered to children with ESRD, because there is no disease recurrence and the prognosis is excellent.

Alport's Syndrome

AS is the commonest form of hereditary nephritis and is commonly associated with sensorineural deafness and ocular abnormalities. It is caused by mutations that affect type IV collagen and has a prevalence of approximately 1 in 50 000 live births [20, 21].

Before discussing the pathophysiology of AS, it is helpful to revise the following relevant terminology:

- Basement membrane is a thin, extracellular layer of tissue that separates the epithelium (lining skin, respiratory tract, gastrointestinal and genitourinary tract), mesothelium (lining pleural, peritoneal and pericardial cavity), and endothelium (lining blood vessels) from underlying connective tissue. It is rich in collagen type IV.
- Collagen is the most abundant protein in the human body. It consists of three polypeptides called alpha-chains which wrap around each other in a triple helix, forming a rope-like structure. The alpha-chains have roughly 1400 amino acids and are repeating sequences of Gly-X-Y, where Gly (glycine) is the smallest amino acid and X is frequently proline, whilst Y is hydroxyproline or hydroxylysine. Collagen molecule has a C terminal non-collagenous domain (NC1) of about 230 amino acids and a smaller N terminal non-collagenous domain of about 20 amino acids. The four major types of collagen are:
  - Type I: found in skin, bone, tendon, and cornea
  - Type II: found in cartilage, intervertebral disc, and vitreous body
  - Type III: found in blood vessels and foetal skin
  - Type IV: found in basement membrane.
- Six distinct type IV collagen chains are encoded by six different genes:

  - COL4A1 and COL4A2 at chromosome 13 (encode for alpha1 and alpha2 chains, respectively)
  - COL4A3 and COL4A4 at chromosome 2 (encode for alpha3 and alpha4 chains, respectively)
  - COL4A5 and COL4A6 on chromosome X (encode for alpha5 and alpha6 chains, respectively).
- Tissue distribution of three different forms of type IV collagen is:

  - Alpha1-alpha1-alpha2: ubiquitous and found in all basement membranes
  - Alpha3-alpha4-alpha5: exclusively in glomerular basement membrane (GBM), tubular basement membrane, eye (Descemet membrane, Bruch membrane and anterior lens capsule), lungs, cochlea
  - Alpha5-alpha5-alpha6: epidermal basement membranes, distal tubular basement membrane (*but not GBM*).

Pathogenesis

AS, which is genetically heterogeneous, is caused by defects in the genes encoding alpha3, alpha4 or alpha5 chains of type IV collagen of the basement membranes. The three forms of AS identified are:

- *X-linked AS (*XLAS*)*: caused by mutations in the COL4A5 (alpha5 chain) is the predominant form accounting for up to 80% of patients [22]. Females are generally less severely affected.
- *Autosomal-recessive AS (ARAS)*: caused by mutations affecting both the alleles of COL4A3 (alpha3 chain) or COL4A4 (alpha4 chain), ARAS is seen in up to 15% of patients [23]. Both males and females tend to be severely affected.
- *Autosomal-dominant AS (ADAS)*: heterozygous mutation in either COL4A3 or COL4A4 causes a less severe disease [24].

Clinical Manifestations

The classic presentation as described here is for males with XLAS (the disease is generally milder in females with XLAS).

Renal Manifestations

Haematuria is the cardinal finding in AS. Males often have persistent microscopic haematuria, with episodes of gross haematuria precipitated by upper respiratory infections in the first two decades of life. Eventually patients developed proteinuria, hypertension, and progressive renal insufficiency. ESRD develops in 90% of XLAS males by the age of 40 (compared with 12% in females with XLAS) [25].

Hearing Loss

Bilateral sensorineural hearing loss may be detected by audiometry in 85% of males and 18% of females with XLAS by 15 years of age. Hearing loss begins in the high-frequency range and progresses over time to frequencies in the range of normal conversation.

Ocular Defects

Ocular defects are seen in 30–40% of XLAS males and 15% of XLAS females [25]. Anterior lenticonus, which is anterior conical protrusion of the lens, is pathognomic of AS and seen in up to half of patients with ocular manifestations. Other ocular presentations include maculopathy and corneal defects.

Leiomyomatosis

XLAS is rarely associated with diffuse leiomyomatosis, a benign hypertrophy of the visceral smooth muscle in gastrointestinal, respiratory, and female reproductive tracts [26].

Women with X-Linked Alport's Syndrome

Women with XLAS are generally heterozygous carriers of the disease. Female carriers with asymptomatic microscopic haematuria have a very small risk of progression to ESRD. Risk factors for CKD in female carriers include age over 60 years, development of deafness, and onset or progression of proteinuria [25].

Pathology

Light microscopy does not show any characteristic features to define AS. Electron microscopy reveals typical findings of variable thickening, thinning, basket-weaving pattern, and lamellation of the GBM. Immunostaining for type IV collagen demonstrates absence of or an abnormal distribution of the alpha3, alpha4, and/or alpha5(IV) chains in the GBM, thus confirming the diagnosis.

Diagnosis

AS should always be considered in the differential diagnosis of a young patient presenting with ongoing haematuria once structural abnormalities have been ruled out. A carefully taken family history, ophthalmic evaluation, and audiometry are often helpful. Renal biopsy and/or molecular genetic testing are diagnostic. Skin biopsy may be helpful in the male child with a known family history of XLAS by showing a complete absence of alpha5(IV) chain on immunostaining (alpha5-alpha5-alpha6 make up the type IV collagen found on basement membrane in skin).

Treatment

There is no specific treatment for AS. As in other causes of chronic renal disease, ACE inhibitors or ARBs are useful to slow down the progress of proteinuria. Renal transplantation is the only available therapy. The disease does not recur as the donor kidney has normal GBM.

Patients with AS who receive renal transplant generally do well. However, a post-transplant anti-GBM like disease affects up to 5% of these patients [27]. As defects in the COL4A5 gene are responsible for most cases of AS, and the alpha5(IV) chains in the GBM of the trasplanted kidney becomes a target for the anti-GBM alloantibodies in the recipient. As a reminder, native anti-GBM disease is characterized by anti-GBM alloantibodies against the NC1 domain of alpha3(IV) chains in the GBM.

Thin Basement Membrane Nephropathy

TBMN is a histological diagnosis defined by excessively thin GBMs. It is estimated that 20–25% of patients who have renal biopsy for asymptomatic haematuria have TBMN. It is often familial, with a family history of haematuria being noted in 30–50% of cases. Some but not all patients with TBMN have mutations of the type IV collagen genes COL4A3 and COL4A4 [28]. Urinary protein excretion and blood pressure are typically normal in these patients and long-term renal prognosis is excellent.

Tuberous Sclerosis

TSC is a disease characterized by multiple benign hamartomas of the brain, eyes, heart, lung, liver, skin, and kidney along with renal cysts. Hamartomas are focal but disorganized collection of normal tissue that grow at the same rate as normal tissue; they often cause problems by virtue of their location and size.

TSC is an autosomal-dominant genetic disorder with an incidence of approximately 1 in 12 000–14 000 in children under the age of 10 years in the UK [29, 30]. According to TSC Australia, there are more than 2000 affected individuals in Australia, giving an incidence of 1 in 12 000 adults.

TSC can be caused by a mutation in either the TSC1 gene or the TSC2 gene. De novo mutations account for approximately 80% of TSC cases. TSC2 mutations are four times more common in de novo cases, whilst the prevalence of TSC1 and TSC2 mutations is approximately equal amongst familial TSC cases.

Pathogenesis

The disease is believed to be due to uninhibited activity of mTOR leading to excessive cell proliferation and the resultant hamartomas.

The TSC1 gene on chromosome 9 encodes a protein called hamartin, whilst the TSC2 gene on chromosome 16 encodes tuberin. Normally RHEB (Ras homologue enriched in brain) activates mammalian mTOR, which in turn drives cell cycle progression and increases cell proliferation. Under physiological conditions the hamartin–tuberin complex by its intrinsic GTPase activity deactivates RHEB by causing guanosine triphosphate (GTP) to be cleaved from it and thereby inhibits mTOR. Mutation in either hamartin or tuberin interferes with the normal inhibition of RHEB, leading to excessive activation of mTOR.

The PKD gene product polycystin-1 by interaction with tuberin also plays a role in inhibiting mTOR.

Clinical Presentation

Table 12.4 lists the major and minor clinical features of TSC. From 81 to 95% of patients with TSC have characteristic skin lesions [30], which include:

Table 12.4 Diagnostic criteria for tuberous sclerosis (TSC)

Major features

1. Facial angiofibromas or forehead plaque
2. Non-traumatic ungual or periungual fibroma
3. Hypomelanotic macules (more than three)
4. Shagreen patch (connective tissue nevus)
5. Multiple retinal nodular hamartomas
6. Cortical tuber
7. Subependymal nodule
8. Subependymal giant cell astrocytoma
9. Cardiac rhabdomyoma, single or multiple
10. Lymphangiomyomatosis
11. Renal angiomyolipoma

Minor features

1. Multiple randomly distributed pits in dental enamel
2. Hamartomatous rectal polyps
3. Bone cysts
4. Cerebral white matter migration lines
5. Gingival fibromas
6. Non-renal hamartomas
7. Retinal achromic patch
8. 'Confetti' skin lesions
9. Multiple renal cysts

Definite TSC: Either 2 major features or 1 major feature with 2 minor features.
Probable TSC: One major feature and one minor feature.
Possible TSC: Either 1 major feature or 2 or more minor features.
Note: When both lymphangiomyomatosis and renal angiomyolipomas are present, other features of TSC should be present before a definitive diagnosis is assigned.

- *Hypopigmented macules*: also called ash-leaf spots, usually elliptic-shaped white spots on the skin. For a diagnosis of TSC the patient should have three or more of them.
- *Angiofibromas* (sometimes called fibroadenomas): small, raised lesions usually scattered on the face, especially on the nose and cheeks, and sometimes on the forehead, eyelids, and chin. They typically involve the malar regions.
- *Shagreen patch*: an area of thickened, elevated pebbly skin seen most commonly over the lower trunk.
- *Distinctive brown fibrous plaque on the forehead*: this may be the first and most readily recognized feature of TSC to be appreciated on physical examination in children.

Cortical glioneuronal hamartomas and subependymal nodules are present on brain MRI in approximately 90% of children with TSC [31]. Subependymal giant cell astrocytoma, by their position in the region of the foramen of Monro, can lead to presentation with obstructive hydrocephalous.

Epilepsy affects up to 90% of these patients, whilst cognitive defects may be seen in 44–65% of patients [30].

From 10 to 40% of patients develop lymphangioleiomyomatosis, which is a multicystic lung disease that can cause significant limitation in pulmonary function and lead to pneumothorax.

Renal involvement is seen in more than half of cases of TSC, with the principal manifestations being angiomyolipomas (85%), renal cysts (45%), and malignant neoplasms, which are mostly malignant epithelioid angiomyolipomas (4%).

Diagnosis

Major and minor criteria, as described in Table 12.4, help in the diagnosis of TSC. Genetic testing is helpful in confirming diagnosis in individuals with possible TSC who do not meet the criteria for definite TSC by clinical evaluation. Genetic tests are also helpful in prenatal diagnosis and in identifying whether other at-risk relatives (e.g. parents or siblings) carry the mutation [29, 31].

Treatment

Treatment consists of both periodic evaluation and management of the various manifestations of TSC, which include seizures, neuropsychiatric disorders, brain tumours, skin lesions, renal disease, pulmonary disease, and cardiac involvement. This includes regular electroencephalogram (EEG), brain MRI, psychiatric evaluation, dermatological evaluation, renal ultrasound or CT scan, high-resolution CT (HRCT) scan of the lung, echocardiogram, ophthalmological examination, and annual serum creatinine. Surgery is offered to those with brain and renal tumours. Medical therapy with mTOR inhibitors is offered to those patients who are poor surgical candidates.

Fabry Disease

Fabry disease is the commonest lysosomal storage disorder. It is an X-linked inborn error of the glycosphingolipid metabolic pathway, characterized by deficiency of the lysosomal hydrolase alpha-galactosidase A (alpha-Gal A), which catalyses the hydrolytic cleavage of the terminal galactose from globotriaosylceramide (Gb3). The condition has an estimated incidence of 1 in 117000 live births for males [32]. Approximately 80% of males have neurological, dermatological, and renal and/or cardiac manifestations by the second, third, and fifth decades, respectively. Females may be asymptomatic or less severely affected. Proteinuria is present in >90% of males by the age of 50 years and a significant proportion of these patients develop ESRD. Many patients develop proximal renal tubular acidosis and Fanconi syndrome.

Light microscopy shows characteristic vacuolization of the podocytes and distal tubular epithelial cells, whilst electron microscopy shows lamellated membranous structures called myeloid or zebra bodies (enlarged lysosomes full of Gb3).

Treatment consists of enzyme replacement therapy (ERT); that is, replacing the deficient enzyme, alpha-Gal A.

Although survival is lower in Fabry disease patients with renal failure than in non-Fabry controls, overall survival of patients undergoing maintenance dialysis is relatively good. Whilst histological examination of renal allograft tissue may show deposition of Gb3 in tubular epithelial and endothelial cells, these deposits appear to be insufficient to compromise allograft function [33]. Overall, kidney transplantation has an excellent long-term outcome in these patients [34].

References

1. Davies, F., Coles, G.A., Harper, P.S. et al. (1991). Polycystic kidney disease re-evaluated: a population-based study. *Q. J. Med.* 79 (290): 477–485.
2. United States Renal Data System (2013). *2012 Annual Data Report: Atlas of Chronic Kidney Disease and End-Stage Renal Disease in the United States*, vol. 2. Bethesda, MD: National Institute of Diabetes and Digestive and Kidney Diseases.
3. Grantham, J.J. (2008, 2008). Autosomal dominant polycystic kidney disease. *N. Engl. J. Med.* 359: 1477–1485 October 2. https://doi.org/10.1056/NEJMcp0804458.
4. Cooper, D.M.F., Mons, N., and Karpen, J.W. (30 March 1994). Adenylyl cyclases and the interaction between calcium and cAMP signalling. *Nature* 374: 421–424. https://doi.org/10.1038/374421a0.
5. Davidow, C.J., Maser, R.L., Rome, L.A. et al. (1996). The cystic fibrosis transmembrane conductance regulator mediates transepithelial fluid secretion by human autosomal dominant polycystic kidney disease epithelium in vitro. *Kidney Int.* 50 (1): 208.
6. O'Sullivan, D.A., Torres, V.E., Gabow, P.A. et al. (1998). Cystic fibrosis and the phenotypic expression of autosomal dominant polycystic kidney disease. *Am. J. Kidney Dis.* 32 (6): 976.
7. Torres, V.E., Wang, X., Qian, Q. et al. (2004). Effective treatment of an orthologous model of autosomal dominant polycystic kidney disease. *Nat. Med.* 10 (4): 363.
8. Shillingford, J.M., Piontek, K.B., Germino, G.G., and Weimbs, T. (2010). Rapamycin ameliorates PKD resulting from conditional inactivation of Pkd1. *J. Am. Soc. Nephrol.* 21 (3): 489.
9. Ajay Srivastava, M.D. and Neel Patel, M.D. (2014 Sep 1). Autosomal dominant polycystic kidney disease. *Am. Fam. Physician.* 90 (5): 303–307.
10. Torres, V.E., Wilson, D.M., Hattery, R.R., and Segura, J.W. (1993). Renal stone disease in autosomal dominant polycystic kidney disease. *Am. J. Kidney Dis.* 22 (4): 513.
11. Almeida, E.A., Oliveira, E.I., Lopes, J.A. et al. (2006). Tissue Doppler imaging in the evaluation of left ventricular function in young adults with autosomal dominant polycystic kidney disease. *Am. J. Kidney Dis.* 47 (4): 587.
12. Bae, K.T., Zhu, F., Chapman, A.B. et al. (2006). Magnetic resonance imaging evaluation of hepatic cysts in early autosomal-dominant polycystic kidney disease: the consortium for radiologic imaging studies of polycystic kidney disease cohort. *Clin. J. Am. Soc. Nephrol.* 1 (1): 64.
13. Ravine, D., Gibson, R.N., Donlan, J., and Sheffield, L.J. (1993). An ultrasound renal cyst prevalence survey: specificity data for inherited renal cystic diseases. *Am. J. Kidney Dis.* 22 (6): 803.

14. Schrier, R.W., Abebe, K.Z., Perrone, R.D. et al. (2255). Blood pressure in early autosomal dominant polycystic kidney disease. *N. Engl. J. Med.* 371 (24): 2014.

15. Torres, V.E., Chapman, A.B., Devuyst, O. et al. (2012). Tolvaptan in patients with autosomal dominant polycystic kidney disease. *N. Engl. J. Med.* 367: 2407–2418. https://doi.org/10.1056/NEJMoa1205511.

16. Caroli, A., Antiga, L., Cafaro, M. et al. (2010). Reducing polycystic liver volume in ADPKD: effects of somatostatin analogue octreotide. *Clin. J. Am. Soc. Nephrol.* 5 (5): 783.

17. Caroli, A., Perico, N., Perna, A. et al. (2013). Effect of longacting somatostatin analogue on kidney and cyst growth in autosomal dominant polycystic kidney disease (ALADIN): a randomised, placebo-controlled, multicentre trial. *Lancet* 382 (9903): 1485.

18. Qian, Q., Du, H., King, B.F. et al. (2008). Sirolimus reduces polycystic liver volume in ADPKD patients. *J. Am. Soc. Nephrol.* 19 (3): 631.

19. Serra, A.L., Poster, D., Kistler, A.D. et al. (2010). Sirolimus and kidney growth in autosomal dominant polycystic kidney disease. *N. Engl. J. Med.* 363 (9): 820.

20. Hudson, B.G., Tryggvason, K., Sundaramoorthy, M., and Neilson, E.G. (2003). Alport's syndrome, Goodpasture's syndrome, and type IV collagen. *N. Engl. J. Med.* 348: 2543–2556. https://doi.org/10.1056/NEJMra022296.

21. Levy, M. and Feingold, J. (2000). Estimating prevalence in single-gene kidney diseases progressing to renal failure. *Kidney Int.* 58 (3): 925.

22. Martin, P., Heiskari, N., Zhou, J. et al. (1998). High mutation detection rate in the COL4A5 collagen gene in suspected Alport syndrome using PCR and direct DNA sequencing. *J. Am. Soc. Nephrol.* 9: 2291–2301.

23. Mochizuki, T., Lemmink, H.H., Mariyama, M. et al. (1994). Identification of mutations in the alpha 3(IV) and alpha 4(IV) collagen genes in autosomal recessive Alport syndrome. *Nat. Genet.* 8: 77–81.

24. Longo, I., Porcedda, P., Mari, F. et al. (2002). COL4A3/COL4A4 mutations: from familial hematuria to autosomal-dominant or recessive Alport syndrome. *Kidney Int.* 61: 1947–1956.

25. Jais, J.P., Knebelmann, B., Giatras, I. et al. (2000). X-linked Alport syndrome: natural history in 195 families and genotype-phenotype correlations in males. *J. Am. Soc. Nephrol.* 11: 649–657.

26. Uliana, V., Marcocci, E., Mucciolo, M. et al. (2011). Alport syndrome and leiomyomatosis: the first deletion extending beyond COL4A6 intron 2. *Pediatr. Nephrol.* 26 (5): 717.

27. Browne, G., Brown, P.A.J., Tomson, C.R.V. et al. (2004). Retransplantation in Alport post-transplant anti-GBM disease. *Kidney Int.* 65: 675–681.

28. Rana, K., Wang, Y.Y., Powell, H. et al. (2005). Persistent familial hematuria in children and the locus for thin basement membrane nephropathy. *Pediatr. Nephrol.* 20 (12): 1729.

29. Curatolo, P., Bombardieri, R., and Jozwiak, S. (2008). Tuberous sclerosis. *Lancet* 372 (9639): 657.

30. Webb, D.W., Clarke, A., Fryer, A., and Osborne, J.P. (1996). The cutaneous features of tuberous sclerosis: a population study. *Br. J. Dermatol.* 135 (1): 1.

31. Yates, J.R., Maclean, C., Higgins, J.N. et al. (2011 Nov). The tuberous sclerosis 2000 study: presentation, initial assessments and implications for diagnosis and management. *Arch. Dis. Child.* 96 (11): 1020–1025. Epub 2011 Aug 3.

32. El Dib, R., Gomaa, H., Ortiz, A. et al. (2017). Enzyme replacement therapy for Anderson-Fabry disease: a complementary overview of a Cochrane publication through a linear regression and a pooled analysis of proportions from cohort studies. *PLoS One* 12 (3): e0173358. Published online. doi: https://doi.org/10.1371/journal.pone.0173358.

33. Gantenbein, H., Bruder, E., Burger, H.R. et al. (1995). Recurrence of Fabry's disease in a renal allograft 14 years after transplantation. *Nephrol. Dial. Transplant.* 10 (2): 287.

34. Ersözlü, S., Desnick, R.J. et al. (November 2018). Long-term outcomes of kidney transplantation in Fabry disease. *Transplantation* 102 (11): 1924–1933. https://doi.org/10.1097/TP.0000000000002252.

Questions and Answers

Questions

1. The incidence of ADPKD in the general population is:
a. 1 in 50 000
b. 1 in a million
c. 1 in 500–1000
d. 1 in 100 000
e. 1 in 50

2. The pathogenesis of ADPKD is linked to:
a. Decreased intracellular cyclic AMP
b. Increased intracellular cyclic AMP
c. Low intracellular calcium
d. High intracellular calcium
e. b and c

3. Antibiotic of choice while pending culture reports in a suspected case of pyelonephritis with suspected cyst infection in patient with ADPKD is:
a. Tazocin
b. Ceftriaxone
c. High-dose penicillin
d. Ciprofloxacin
e. Aminoglycoside

4. Indication for screening for intracranial aneurysm in patients with ADPKD does not include:
a. Patients with history of previous rupture
b. A positive family history of an intracerebral bleed
c. High-risk professional such as aviation pilot
d. Children diagnosed to have ADPKD at an age below 18 years
e. Those who need warfarin for ischaemic heart disease

5. All of the following have been suggested to predict progression to ESRD in patients with ADPKD except:
a. Increased fluid intake
b. Male sex
c. Onset of hypertension before the age of 35 years
d. African race
e. First episode of haematuria before the age of 30 years

6. The commonest diagnosis seen on renal biopsy of patients with asymptomatic haematuria is:
a. Thin basement membrane nephropathy
b. Alport's syndrome
c. Postinfectious glomerulonephritis
d. IgA nephropathy
e. Lupus nephritis

7. Tuberous sclerosis is characterized by hamartomas in multiple organs. Hamartomas are best defined as:
a. Highly metastatic tumours
b. Benign tumours starting in the epithelial tissue of a gland or gland-like structure
c. Low-grade malignant tumours
d. Tumours of fibrous or connective tissue that can grow in any organ
e. Focal but disorganized collection of normal tissue that grow at the same rate as normal tissue

Answers

1. c. ADPKD is a common disorder, occurring in approximately 1 in every 400–1000 live births with more than half the patients remaining undiagnosed during their lifetime.

2. e. Mutation in Polycystin 1 and 2 results in low intracellular Ca, which in turn leads to cAMP activation. The raised intracellular cAMP leads to activation of CFTR which are characteristically found on the apical membranes of ADPKD cells. Active chloride transport across CFTR leads to increased water secretion into the cysts with resultant enlargement of the cysts.

3. d. Trimethoprim-sulfamethoxazole and fluoroquinolones by virtue of their lipophilic nature are able to cross the lipid-rich cyst wall and achieve good intracystic concentration.

4. d. Routine screening for cerebral aneurysm is not indicated in every patient with ADPKD as most cerebral aneurysms found on presymptomatic screening are small and have a low risk to rupture with the risks associated with surgery clearly outweighing risk of rupture. Indications for screening with MRI include:

   - Family history of cerebral aneurysm or sub arachnoid haemorrhage
   - Previous aneurysmal rupture
   - Preparation for surgery with potential for hemodynamic instability
   - High-risk occupations, e.g. airline pilots
   - Patients who require chronic anticoagulation, e.g. those with DVT or AF

5. a. Upregulation of vasopressin V2 receptor and high circulating levels of vasopressin seen in patients with ADPKD leads to high intracellular cAMP, which in turn is postulated to lead to cyst growth. Increased fluid intake leads to lower vasopressin levels and is suggested as a part of treatment to slow down cyst growth. As per the findings of the CRISP study, increasing cyst and renal size have a direct co-relation with decline in GFR. Other risk factors for progression to ESRD in patients with ADPKD include:

   - Male sex
   - African race
   - Diagnosis of ADPKD before the age of 30 years
   - First episode of haematuria before the age of 30 years
   - Onset of hypertension before the age of 35 years
   - Hyperlipidaemia
   - Sickle cell trait

6. a. It is estimated that 20–25% of patients who have renal biopsy for asymptomatic haematuria have thin basement membrane nephropathy. IgA nephropathy is the commonest cause of glomerulonephritis worldwide but the question was for patients with asymptomatic haematuria and not glomerulonephritis. Patients with postinfectious glomerulonephritis and lupus nephritis are unlikely to present with just asymptomatic haematuria. Though Alport's syndrome is the commonest cause of hereditary nephritis and can present with asymptomatic haematuria, it is much less common than thin basement membrane nephropathy overall.

7. e. Hamartomas are focal but disorganized collection of normal tissue that grows at the same rate as normal tissue; they often cause problems by virtue of their location. Choice b describes adenoma while d is fibroma.

13

Hepatorenal Syndrome

Surjit Tarafdar

Summary

- Hepatorenal syndrome (HRS) is a reversible and functional renal failure with extremely poor prognosis that occurs in patients with acute or chronic liver disease and portal hypertension
- Inefficient clearance of endotoxins or bacterial DNA from the gut leads to their translocation into the blood stream, which stimulates nitric oxide (NO) production
- NO leads to splanchnic vasodilatation and low systemic mean arterial pressure
- Unopposed renal production of vasoconstrictors triggers HRS
- The kidneys in HRS are histologically normal
- HRS is a diagnosis of exclusion
- Pharmacotherapy with systemic vasoconstrictors is based on the understanding that splanchnic vasodilatation is responsible for renal failure in HRS
- Liver transplantation is the only curative treatment for HRS

Hepatorenal syndrome (HRS) is a reversible and functional renal failure that occurs in patients with acute or chronic liver disease and portal hypertension. It is essentially the outcome of a sequence of reductions in renal perfusion induced by increasingly severe hepatic injury.

Widespread splanchnic and systemic vasodilatation, together with intense renal vasoconstriction, is the pathophysiological hallmark of HRS. Although HRS is associated with an extremely poor prognosis, the histological appearance of the kidneys is normal, and the kidney function often improves following liver transplantation [1]. The reported incidence of HRS in cirrhotic patients with normal renal function is 18% and 39%, at one and five years respectively, making it a common condition [2]. It must be remembered, though, that HRS is only one of the many causes of renal failure in patients with acute or chronic liver disease. It is also important to bear in

mind that HRS is a diagnosis of exclusion, and there is no single gold standard diagnostic test.

Pathogenesis

Onset of portal hypertension and the subsequent development of ascites predate the development of HRS.

Splanchnic vasodilatation associated with portal hypertension plays the central role in the pathogenesis of HRS (Figure 13.1). In patients with portal hypertension, bacterial products such as endotoxins or bacterial DNA are not cleared efficiently and enter the systemic circulation due to portal-systemic shunting. The presence of these agents stimulates increased production of nitric oxide (NO) by both the endothelium and peritoneal macrophages. NO in turn leads to

Lecture Notes Nephrology: A Comprehensive Guide to Renal Medicine, First Edition. Edited by Surjit Tarafdar.
© 2020 John Wiley & Sons Ltd. Published 2020 by John Wiley & Sons Ltd.

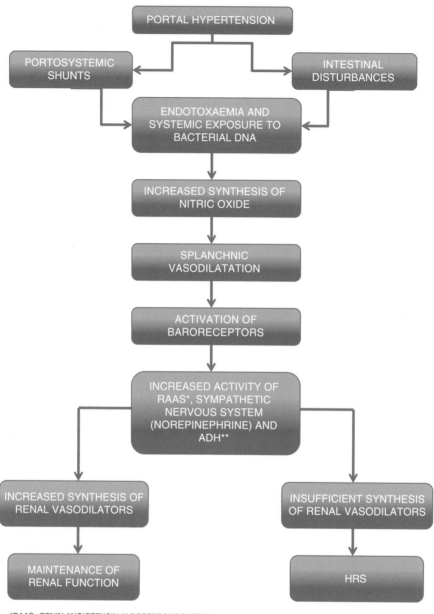

Figure 13.1 Pathogenesis of hepatorenal syndrome (HRS). ADH, antidiuretic syndrome; RAAS, renin–angiotensin–aldosterone system.

significant splanchnic vasodilatation, with a profound reduction in the systemic vascular resistance and mean arterial pressure (MAP) [3]. The ongoing vasodilatation stimulates the carotid and renal volume receptors, which leads to compensatory activation of vasoconstrictor systems, namely the renin–angiotensin–aldosterone system (RAAS), sympathetic nervous system (norepinephrine), and antidiuretic hormone (ADH). These local vasoconstrictors could potentially lead to a reduction in glomerular filtration rate (GFR), but the kidney counters this effect by increased production of local vasodilators such as prostaglandin E2, prostacyclin, and kallikrein. However, with ongoing or worsening hepatic injury, the kidneys are unable to sustain the generation of enough local vasodilators. Reduction of renal vasodilators with unopposed action of renal vasoconstrictors is the final event that leads to the development of HRS.

Clinical Presentation

HRS is characterized by the following features in a patient who has established acute or chronic liver disease with portal hypertension:

- A progressive rise in serum creatinine
- Absence of significant haematuria and proteinuria of less than 500 mg/day
- A very low rate of sodium excretion (urine sodium concentration <10 mEq/l)
- Oliguria

HRS is classified into two groups, depending on the severity of presentation:

Type 1 HRS:
- Associated with doubling of serum creatinine to greater than 2.5 mg/dl (220 µmol/l) or a 50% reduction in GFR to less than 20 ml/min in less than two weeks
- Median survival without treatment is two weeks

Type 2 HRS:
- Associated with a much less rapid decline in renal function and often presents with refractory ascites
- Median survival without treatment is four to six months [4]

Type 1 HRS is characterized by a rapid decline in kidney function and is most often observed in patients suffering from acute liver failure, acute alcoholic hepatitis or acute decompensation on a background of cirrhosis. These patients often have multiorgan failure with low blood pressure and hyponatraemia. At times, a clear precipitating event such as spontaneous bacterial peritonitis, sepsis, gastrointestinal bleeding, vigorous diuretic therapy, abdominal paracentesis or administration of nonsteroidal anti-inflammatory drugs (NSAIDs) might be identified. Whilst patients may not be oliguric at presentation, the urine output tends to drop with disease progression.

Type 2 HRS presents with a more insidious onset. Patients usually have refractory ascites and low to normal blood pressure. Usually no precipitating cause is identified and the condition reflects the natural course of the disease.

Urea is the major disposal form of amino acids, which in turn are derived from protein breakdown. The urea cycle occurs in the liver and therefore patients with advanced liver disease have a low urea generation. These patients are also likely to have reduced meat intake and decreased muscle mass, often leading to a lower than expected serum creatinine level. Hence, patients with HRS often have a renal dysfunction that is significantly more severe than is suggested by the serum urea and creatinine levels.

Diagnosis

HRS should always be suspected in any patient with acute or chronic liver disease and portal hypertension who develops progressive renal impairment. Table 13.1 lists the diagnostic criteria for HRS.

It is important to appreciate that HRS is a diagnosis of exclusion. Patients with cirrhosis may develop acute kidney injury (AKI) due to prerenal disease (such as variceal bleeding), vigorous diuresis, administration of a radiocontrast agent, sepsis or acute tubular necrosis (ATN) after aminoglycoside or NSAID therapy [5]. Prerenal disease or ATN is usually suspected from the history and a rapid rise in serum creatinine, which is in contrast to the somewhat more gradual rise in HRS. Prerenal disease is also usually reversible when diuretics or nephrotoxins are withheld, or when the acute precipitating event is addressed.

Table 13.1 Diagnostic criteria for hepatorenal syndrome

- Cirrhosis with ascites
- Serum creatinine >133 µmol/l (1.5 mg/dl)
- Absence of renal tract obstruction on ultrasound
- Absence of shock
- Not on current and recent nephrotoxic drugs
- Absence of intrinsic renal pathology, evidenced by urine red cell excretion of fewer than 50 cells per high power field and proteinuria less than 500 mg/day
- No improvement in renal function after volume expansion with intravenous albumin (1 g/kg of body weight per day up to 100 g/day) for at least two days and withdrawal of diuretics

Table 13.2 Medical treatment of hepatorenal syndrome albumin is an essential part of the treatment options

Therapy	Mechanism of action
Terlipressin with albumin	Terlipressin is a vasopressin analogue which reverses splanchnic vasodilatation
Midodrine, octreotide and albumin	Midodrine is an alpha-1 adrenergic agonist, which leads to systemic vasoconstriction. Octreotide inhibits multiple endogenous vasodilators
Norepinephrine with albumin	Norepinephrine causes vasoconstriction by its effect on alpha-1 receptors

Treatment

The initial treatment for HRS should include improvement of liver function through management of the underlying condition, such as abstinence in alcoholic hepatitis or treatment of decompensated hepatitis B with effective antiviral therapy. However, improvement in liver function is often not possible in the short term, and medical therapy needs to be instituted in an attempt to reverse the AKI associated with HRS. Once the diagnosis of HRS is made, suitable candidates, especially those suffering from HRS type 1, should be placed on the urgent waiting list for cadaveric or living donor liver transplantation.

Pharmacotherapy with systemic vasoconstrictors is based on the understanding that systemic vasodilatation, especially in the splanchnic circulation, is responsible for the renal failure in HRS. Vasoconstriction increases the effective arterial blood volume and leads to better renal perfusion and some reversal of the condition [2].

The three pharmacotherapy options for the management of HRS are (shown in Table 13.2).

Terlipressin with Albumin

Terlipressin is a vasopressin analogue which reverses splanchnic vasodilatation. The administration of terlipressin and albumin is associated with a significant improvement in GFR, increase in MAP, and reduction of serum creatinine in 42–77% of cases [6–9]. Although the optimum duration of therapy is not clear, it is usually continued for 15 days or until serum creatinine decreases to less than 133 μmol/l (1.5 mg/dl) [10].

Midodrine, Octreotide, and Albumin

In many countries including the USA, terlipressin is not available and the combination of midodrine, octreotide, and albumin is a reasonable alternative. Midodrine, by its alpha-1 adrenergic agonist activity, is a systemic vasoconstrictor, whilst octreotide is an inhibitor of endogenous vasodilators [11, 12].

Norepinephrine with Albumin

In patients with HRS who are admitted to the Intensive Care Unit with hypotension, a norepinephrine infusion (with the aim of raising the MAP by at least 10 mmHg) along with intravenous albumin for at least two days is another option [13].

Treatment options for patients who do not respond to one of the medical therapies listed here include a transjugular intrahepatic portosystemic shunt (TIPS) and dialysis. However, many patients with HRS are too ill to undergo TIPS or dialysis. It is important to realize that the definitive treatment for HRS is liver transplantation [6]. Without treatment, the median survival rates for type 1 and type 2 HRS are two weeks and four to six months, respectively.

References

1. Boyer, T.D., Sanyal, A.J., Garcia-Tsao, G. et al. (2011). Impact of liver transplantation on the survival of patients treated for hepatorenal syndrome type 1. *Liver Transpl.* 17 (11): 1328–1332. https://doi.org/10.1002/lt.22395.

2. Gines, A., Escorsell, A., Gines, P. et al. (1993). Incidence, preventive factors and prognosis of the

hepatorenal syndrome in cirrhosis with ascites. *Gastroenterology* 105 (1): 229.

3. Abelmann, W.H. (1994). Hyperdynamic circulation in cirrhosis: a historical perspective. *Hepatology* 20 (5): 1356.

4. Martín-Llahí, M., Guevara, M., Torre, A. et al. (2011). Prognostic importance of the cause of renal failure in patients with cirrhosis. *Gastroenterology* 140 (2): 488.

5. Ginès, P. and Schrier, R.W. (2009). Renal failure in cirrhosis. *N. Engl. J. Med.* 361 (13): 1279.

6. Ortega, R., Gines, P., Uriz, J. et al. (2002). Terlipressin therapy with and without albumin for patients with hepatorenal syndrome: results of a prospective, nonrandomized study. *Hepatology* 36: 941–948.

7. Uriz, J., Gines, P., Cardenas, A. et al. (2000). Terlipressin plus albumin infusion: an effective and safe therapy of hepatorenal syndrome. *J. Hepatol.* 33: 43–48.

8. Alessandria, C., Venon, W.D., Marzano, A. et al. (2002). Renal failure in cirrhotic patients: role of terlipressin in clinical approach to hepatorenal syndrome type 2. *Eur. J. Gastroenterol. Hepatol.* 14: 1363–1368.

9. Solanki, P., Chawla, A., Garg, R. et al. (2003). Beneficial effects of terlipressin in hepatorenal syndrome: a prospective, randomized placebo-controlled clinical trial. *J. Gastroenterol. Hepatol.* 18: 152–156.

10. Moreau, R., Durand, F., Poynard, T. et al. (2002). Terlipressin in patients with cirrhosis and type 1 hepatorenal syndrome: a retrospective multicenter study. *Gastroenterology* 122: 923–930.

11. Wadei, H.M., Mai, M.L., Ahsan, N., and Gonwa, T.A. (2006). Hepatorenal syndrome: pathophysiology and management. *Clin. J. Am. Soc. Nephrol.* 1 (5): 1066–1079. https://doi.org/10.2215/CJN.01340406.

12. Kalambokis, G., Economou, M., Fotopoulos, A. et al. (2005). The effects of chronic treatment with octreotide versus octreotide plus midodrine on systemic hemodynamics and renal hemodynamics and function in nonazotemic cirrhotic patients with ascites. *Am. J. Gastroenterol.* 100 (4): 879.

13. Duvoux, C., Zanditenas, D., Hézode, C. et al. (2002). Effects of noradrenalin and albumin in patients with type I hepatorenal syndrome: a pilot study. *Hepatology* 36 (2): 374–380.

Questions and Answers

Questions

1. Which is true about the pathogenesis of ascites in cirrhosis?
   a. Caused by splanchnic vasoconstriction due to norepinephrine
   b. Caused by splanchnic vasodilatation due to epinephrine
   c. Caused by splanchnic vasodilatation due to vasopressin
   d. Caused by splanchnic vasodilatation due to nitric oxide (NO)
   e. Caused by splanchnic vasoconstriction due to prostacyclin

2. Which is true about HRS?
   a. Caused by imbalance between splanchnic vasodilatation and vasoconstriction
   b. Caused by imbalance between renal vasodilatation and vasoconstriction
   c. Caused by imbalance between renal vasodilatation and splanchnic vasoconstriction
   d. Caused by ongoing splanchnic vasodilatation and renal vasoconstriction
   e. Caused by renal inability to generate renin due to damage to macula densa

3. The incidence of HRS in cirrhotic patients with portal hypertension at five years is:
   a. About 15%
   b. About 25%
   c. About 10%
   d. About 5%
   e. About 40%

4. The following are needed to diagnose HRS except:
   a. Lack of improvement in renal function after 48 hours of intravenous albumin and withholding diuretics and nephrotoxins
   b. Urine red cell excretion of less than 50 cells per high power field
   c. Protein excretion less than 500 mg/day
   d. History of exposure to radiocontrast material
   e. No evidence of hydronephrosis

5. Terlipressin is proposed to help in the treatment of HRS by:
   a. Causing renal vasoconstriction
   b. Increasing renin release
   c. Reversing splanchnic vasodilatation
   d. Increasing sympathetic activity
   e. Increasing splanchnic vasodilatation

6. Which of the following is true about the diagnosis of HRS?
   a. It can be definitively diagnosed only with renal biopsy
   b. Urinary eosinophils with worsening renal function is virtually diagnostic
   c. A liver biopsy can be helpful in establishing the diagnosis
   d. White cell casts in urine are diagnostic
   e. It is a diagnosis of exclusion

Answers

1. d. In patients with portal hypertension, bacterial products such as endotoxins or bacterial DNA enter the systemic circulation due to portal-systemic shunting and lead to increased production of the vasodilatory NO. Ascites is predominantly due to splanchnic vasodilatation and the resultant reduction in SVR induced by NO. The opening of portasystemic collaterals leads to further reduction in SVR and probably contributes to the pathogenesis of ascites.

2. d. Splanchnic vasodilatation characteristically seen in HRS leads to activation of the vasoconstrictor systems, namely the renin-angiotensin-aldosterone system (RAAS), sympathetic nervous system (norepinephrine), and antidiuretic hormone (ADH). These local vasoconstrictors could potentially lead to reduction in GFR, but the kidney counters this effect by increased production of local vasodilators such as prostaglandin E2, prostacyclin, and kallikrein. HRS develops when the kidney is not able to generate enough local vasodilators to combat the vasoconstrictors.

3. e. The reported incidence of HRS in cirrhotic patients with normal renal function is 18 and 39%, at one and five years, respectively.

4. d. Lack of improvement in renal function after fluid replacement helps to rule out a prerenal cause of renal failure, while the absence of significant haematuria and proteinuria helps to rule out a renal cause.

5. c. Terlipressin is a vasopressin analogue and reverses splanchnic vasodilatation by a direct vasoconstrictor effect without any inotropic or chronotropic effects.

6. e. There is no histological abnormality in the HRS kidney and the disease is due to unopposed renal vasoconstriction. Any significant findings on renal biopsy or urine examination should make one look for a cause other than HRS causing the renal failure.

14

Infections of the Kidney

Surjit Tarafdar and Alexander Gilbert

Summary

Urinary tract infections (UTIs)

- Urinary tract infections include cystitis (infection of urinary bladder/lower urinary tract) and pyelonephritis (infection of the kidney/upper urinary tract)
- Colonization of the urethral meatus and urethra by bacteria from the faecal flora followed by ascent into the urinary bladder causes cystitis, whilst further ascent via the ureter to the kidney causes pyelonephritis
- The presence of high fever, symptoms of systemic illness (including chills or rigors), flank pain or costovertebral angle tenderness (suggesting pyelonephritis), pelvic or perineal pain in men (which can suggest accompanying prostatitis) in the presence of UTI are all grouped together as acute complicated cystitis
- *Escherichia coli* is the most frequent microbial cause of both complicated and uncomplicated cystitis
- Risk factors for both uncomplicated and complicated UTI with multidrug-resistant (MDR) organisms include recent broad-spectrum antimicrobial use, healthcare exposures, and travel to parts of the world where MDR organisms are prevalent, e.g. India, Israel, Spain, and Mexico
- Complications of pyelonephritis include renal abscess, perinephric abscess, emphysematous pyelonephritis, and papillary necrosis

Urogenital Tuberculosis (TB)

- Urogenital TB is the second most common form of extra-pulmonary TB after tuberculous lymph node involvement
- The classical presentation primarily involves the urinary collecting system (including renal pelvis, calyces, ureters, and bladder), with the much less common renal parenchymal involvement presenting as interstitial nephritis or glomerulonephritis
- Patients who develop amyloid A amyloidosis due to TB may present with nephrotic syndrome and cardiomyopathy

Human Immunodeficiency Virus (HIV) and the Kidneys

- The prevalence of chronic kidney disease (CKD) in patients with HIV has decreased substantially since the introduction of combination antiretroviral therapy (ART), with most recent studies showing estimates between 3.5 and 10%
- Risk factors for development of renal disease in HIV include older age, hypertension, diabetes mellitus, lower CD4 count, high viral load, and African descent (perhaps due to APOL1 gene variants)
- The classic kidney disease of HIV infection, HIV-associated nephropathy (HIVAN), usually presents with heavy proteinuria, a rapid decline in glomerular filtration rate (GFR), and increased echogenicity of kidneys on ultrasound, typically without hypertension or oedema
- Histologically, HIVAN is characterized by collapsing focal segmental glomerulosclerosis
- HIV immune complex disease of the kidney (HIVCK) comprises a number of disease subtypes including membranous nephropathy, membranoproliferative and mesangial proliferative glomerulonephritis, 'lupus-like' proliferative

Lecture Notes Nephrology: A Comprehensive Guide to Renal Medicine, First Edition. Edited by Surjit Tarafdar.
© 2020 John Wiley & Sons Ltd. Published 2020 by John Wiley & Sons Ltd.

glomerulonephritis, and, rarely, immunoglobulin A nephropathy
- HIVCK generally manifests with sub-nephrotic-range proteinuria, active urinary sediment (haematuria and red cell casts), hypocomplementaemia, and a progressive reduction in GFR
- Identification of CKD in the setting of HIV should prompt commencement of ART

Leptospirosis
- Leptospirosis is a common disease worldwide and is spread to humans by animal urine (most commonly rodent urine)

- People at risk are those who have close contact with animals or who are exposed to water, mud, soil or vegetation that has been contaminated with animal urine
- The condition can occasionally lead to acute kidney injury
- Treatment consists of oral doxycycline or azithromycin for mild cases and intravenous penicillin or third-generation cephalosporins for severe cases

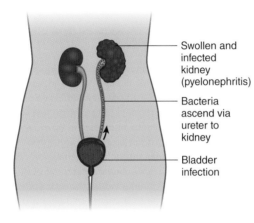

Swollen and infected kidney (pyelonephritis)

Bacteria ascend via ureter to kidney

Bladder infection

Figure 14.1 Ascension of bacteria via urethra to urinary bladder causes cystitis; further ascent of bacteria from urinary bladder to kidney via ureter causes pyelonephritis.

Urinary tract infections (UTIs) include cystitis (infection of the urinary bladder/lower urinary tract) and pyelonephritis (infection of the kidney/upper urinary tract). UTIs initially start with colonization of the urethral meatus and urethra by bacteria from the faecal flora. This is followed by ascension of the bacteria via the urethra into the urinary bladder, causing cystitis; pyelonephritis develops if the bacteria ascend via the ureters to the kidney (Figure 14.1). Pyelonephritis can also develop if there is bacterial seeding of the kidneys in bacteraemia.

Cystitis

Cystitis is classified as follows:

- *Uncomplicated cystitis*: acute infection involving and limited to urinary bladder.

- *Complicated cystitis*: cystitis which has spread beyond the urinary bladder and is suggested by the following features:
  - High fever
  - Other signs or symptoms of systemic illness (including chills or rigors)
  - Flank pain
  - Costovertebral angle tenderness
  - Pelvic or perineal pain in men suggesting prostatitis.

By the above criteria, pyelonephritis is a complicated UTI, regardless of patient characteristics. This differentiation is important, because treatment strategies are more aggressive with complicated cystitis, usually warranting parenteral antibiotic therapy. Also, some of the antibiotics used in uncomplicated cystitis are not of much use in complicated cystitis as they do not achieve adequate levels in tissue.

Unlike in the past, the presence of diabetes mellitus, underlying urological abnormalities (such as nephrolithiasis, strictures, stents or urinary diversions), and immunocompromised conditions (such as neutropenia or advanced HIV infection) are not enough to classify cystitis into the complicated category.

Acute Uncomplicated Cystitis in Adults

This condition is more common in women because of the shorter distance from the anus to the urethral opening and the bladder [1]. Amongst healthy women (Table 14.1), risk factors for cystitis include recent sexual intercourse, history of UTIs, use of spermicide-coated condoms, diaphragms, spermicides, structural or functional urinary tract abnormalities, indwelling urinary catheter, oestrogen deficiency in postmenopausal women, and obesity.

Table 14.1 Risk factors for urinary tract infections (UTIs) in women

Recent sexual intercourse
History of UTIs
Use of spermicide-coated condoms, diaphragms, and spermicides
Structural or functional urinary tract abnormalities
Indwelling urinary catheter
Oestrogen deficiency in postmenopausal women
Obesity

Table 14.2 Risk factors for developing urinary tract infections (UTIs) with multidrug-resistant organisms

Recent use of a broad-spectrum antibiotic (e.g. fluoroquinolone, trimethoprim-sulfamethoxazole, third or later generation cephalosporin)
Inpatient stay at a healthcare facility (e.g. hospital, nursing home, long-term acute care facility)
Travel to parts of the world where multidrug-resistant organisms are prevalent, e.g. India, Israel, Spain, and Mexico
History of multidrug-resistant urinary isolate

In men, recurrent cystitis or the presence of co-existent pelvic or perineal pain should always lead to suspicion of prostatitis.

Microbiology

Escherichia coli is the most frequent microbial cause of cystitis (75–85% of cases), with another 5% caused by *Staphylococcus saprophyticus* [2, 3]. Occasional infections are caused by other species of *Enterobacteriaceae* such as *Klebsiella pneumoniae* and *Proteus mirabilis*, whilst other gram-negative bacilli (e.g. *Pseudomonas*), *enterococci* and fungi may be identified in those with recent antimicrobial or other healthcare exposures. An increase in cystitis due to extended-spectrum beta-lactamase (ESBL)-producing strains of *E. coli* is being seen worldwide.

Risk factors for both uncomplicated and complicated UTI with multidrug-resistant (MDR) organisms include recent broad-spectrum antimicrobial use, healthcare exposures, and travel to parts of the world where MDR organisms are prevalent, such as India, Israel, Spain, and Mexico (Table 14.2).

Presentation

The usual presentation in uncomplicated cystitis is with dysuria, urinary frequency, urinary urgency, suprapubic pain, and often haematuria. Presentation can be quite subtle, especially in the elderly.

Investigation

Blood or urine investigations are usually not necessary in women who present with the classic symptoms of uncomplicated cystitis. However, when the presentation is atypical, urine examination with both dipstick and microscopy aids in diagnosis. All men with suspected cystitis should have urine examination.

Urine dipstick can detect the presence of leukocyte esterase (an enzyme released by leukocytes, reflecting pyuria) and nitrite (reflecting the presence of *Enterobacteriaceae*, which convert urinary nitrate to nitrite); it has a sensitivity of 75% and a specificity of 82%. Microscopy reveals ≥10 leukocytes/µl in unspun voided midstream urine.

Treatment

The antibiotic of choice for treatment for those patients who do not have risk factors for MDR is nitrofurantoin, trimethoprim/sulfamethoxazole, fosfomycin or pivmecillinam (Table 14.3). If the patient has risk factors for MDR infection, urine should be sent for culture and susceptibility testing before starting therapy. Empirical therapy whilst waiting for the urine culture report consists of nitrofurantoin, fosfomycin or pivmecillinam.

A fluoroquinolone (e.g. ciprofloxacin) is indicated if prostatitis is suspected in men with cystitis.

Acute Complicated Cystitis, Including Pyelonephritis, in Adults

The presence of high fever, symptoms of systemic illness (including chills or rigors), flank pain, costovertebral angle tenderness, pelvic or perineal pain in men (which can suggest accompanying prostatitis) in

Table 14.3 First-line antimicrobial choices and doses for uncomplicated cystitis

Nitrofurantoin	100 mg orally twice daily for five days
Trimethoprim/sulfamethoxazole	One double-strength tablet (160/800 mg) orally twice daily for three days
Fosfomycin	3 g of powder mixed in water as a single oral dose
Pivmecillinam	400 mg orally twice daily for five to seven days

the presence of a UTI are all grouped together as acute complicated cystitis. The differentiation is important to ensure the appropriateness of antimicrobial therapy.

Microbiology

Amongst young healthy women, specific virulent clones of *E. coli* account for more than 90% of pyelonephritis [4]. In contrast, amongst men, elderly women and institutionalized patients, less-virulent *E. coli* strains, non-*E. coli* gram-negative bacilli, gram-positive organisms and candida are more prevalent, although infections with *E. coli* still predominate [5, 6].

Presentation

The spectrum for complicated UTI includes both complicated cystitis and pyelonephritis:

- Apart from the signs and symptoms of uncomplicated cystitis already discussed, patients also have fever or other features of systemic illness (including chills or rigors), which suggest that infection has extended beyond the bladder.
- Patients with pyelonephritis present with fever, chills, flank pain, costovertebral angle tenderness, and nausea/vomiting. Symptoms of cystitis are often but not always present. Up to 20% of patients do not have bladder symptoms, and some patients do not have fever [7].

Investigations

Patients with suspected acute complicated UTI, including pyelonephritis, should have urinalysis (either by microscopy or by dipstick) and urine culture with susceptibility testing. Urine culture typically yields 10 000 or more colony-forming units of uropathogen per millilitre of urine, although lower counts may be seen if the patient has received previous antimicrobial therapy, has extremely acidic urine or has urinary tract obstruction [8].

Patients should have routine blood testing including electrolytes, full blood count, and C-reactive protein, along with blood cultures if febrile.

Most patients with acute complicated UTI do not warrant imaging studies for diagnosis or management. Imaging is generally reserved for those who are severely ill, have persistent clinical symptoms despite 48–72 hours of appropriate antimicrobial therapy, have known or suspected urolithiasis or have suspected urinary tract obstruction (e.g. if the renal function has declined below baseline or if there is a precipitous decline in the urinary output). Computed tomography (CT) scanning of the abdomen and pelvis (with and without contrast) is generally the study of choice to detect anatomical or physiological factors associated with acute complicated UTI [9]. Whilst renal ultrasound is used where exposure to contrast or radiation needs to be avoided, its sensitivity is lower than that of CT.

Complications

Patients with acute complicated UTI can present with bacteraemia, sepsis/shock, multiple organ system dysfunction, and acute kidney injury (AKI). This is more likely in patients with urinary tract obstruction or other urinary tract abnormalities, recent urinary tract instrumentation, the elderly or those who have diabetes mellitus. Other complications of acute pyelonephritis include renal abscess, perinephric abscess, emphysematous pyelonephritis, and papillary necrosis.

Chronic pyelonephritis, which is not very common and is usually seen in the setting of chronically obstructing kidney stone [10] or vesicoureteral reflux (especially in children), can lead to chronic tubulointerstitial disease and chronic kidney disease (CKD).

Treatment

Empirical antibiotic therapy should be initiated straightaway, taking into consideration any recent positive urine cultures with known drug sensitivity.

The following group of patients need to be admitted in hospital:

- Persistently high fever
- Severe pain
- Marked debility
- Inability to maintain oral hydration or take oral medications
- Suspicion of urinary tract obstruction

Hospitalized patients who are not critically unwell can be treated with ceftriaxone or piperacillin-tazobactam. Oral or parenteral fluoroquinolones (ciprofloxacin or levofloxacin) are also reasonable alternatives if there is no history of resistance to fluoroquinolones in the prior three months and the community prevalence of E. coli fluoroquinolone resistance is not known to be higher than 10%.

Patients who are critically unwell or have risk factors for MDR infection are usually started on treatment with carbapenems. If drug-resistant gram-positive organisms are suspected because of previous urinary isolates or other risk factors, vancomycin (for methicillin-resistant *Staphylococcus aureus*, MRSA), linezolid or daptomycin (for vancomycin-resistant *Enterococcus*, VRE) should be added. In case of a suspicion of *Pseudomonas aeruginosa* (e.g. with previous history or febrile neutropenia), piperacillin-tazobactam or a fluoroquinolone should be chosen. Other useful anti-pseudomonal agents include the cephalosporins, cefepime, and ceftazidime.

Complications of Pyelonephritis

Renal and Perinephric Abscess

Both renal abscesses (which include cortical and corticomedullary abscesses) and perinephric abscesses present with a similar clinical picture of fever, chills, back or abdominal pain, and costovertebral tenderness.

Cortical abscess is often caused by haematogenous spread of *Staphylococcus aureus* [11]. There may be no urinary symptoms if the cortical abscess does not communicate with the urinary collecting system. A corticomedullary abscess, on the other hand, is mostly caused by ascending UTI in association with an underlying urinary tract abnormality, such as obstructive uropathy or vesicoureteral reflux; usual causative organisms are E. coli and other coliforms.

Perinephric abscess can result from either local or haematogenous spread. Thus, perinephric abscesses may result from outward diffusion of a renal infection (generally due to gram-negative organisms) to the perirenal fat, a renal abscess that ruptures through the capsule [12] or haematogenous spread (mostly staphylococcal).

Whilst ultrasound can help make the diagnosis, CT with contrast medium enhancement is the best imaging procedure for evaluation of renal or perinephric abscesses and for evaluating the extension of perinephric abscess to adjacent structures, such as liver or diaphragm.

The choice of empirical antibiotic therapy depends on the suspected pathogenesis of the abscess; that is, target *Enterobacteriaceae* in a case of associated pyelonephritis and anti-staphylococcal in a case of *Staphylococcus* bacteraemia.

Whilst percutaneous therapeutic drainage (CT or ultrasound guided) is usually indicated in renal abscesses bigger than 5 cm, the smaller ones are only drained if not responding appropriately after several days of antimicrobial therapy. Perinephric abscesses often need percutaneous drainage for diagnostic purposes. Therapeutic drainage is generally needed for larger perinephric abscesses or when medical therapy alone is not sufficient.

Urgent urological intervention with surgical drainage and/or rescue nephrectomy may be required in the following scenarios:

- Urological obstruction that needs relief
- Abscess occurring in the context of an anatomical abnormality (such as large, obstructing renal stones or vesicoureteral reflux)
- Abscess too large for percutaneous drainage

Nephrectomy may be indicated in the setting of a renal abscess in a small, scarred, chronically pyelonephritic, and poorly functioning kidney destroyed by previous episodes of infection.

Acute lobar nephronia is used to describe a non-suppurative, focal form of acute bacterial infection, generally affecting one or more renal lobules. Ultrasound or CT scan demonstrates a wedge-shaped or round, poorly defined area, unlike the well-defined cavities seen with renal abscess. Treatment consists of antibiotic therapy (usually two to three weeks).

Emphysematous Pyelonephritis

Emphysematous pyelonephritis is a rare, gas-forming, severe infection of renal parenchyma and its surrounding areas [13]. The condition is diagnosed by radiological evidence of air in the renal parenchyma or bladder. Up to 90% of patients have diabetes mellitus, and dehydration and ketoacidosis are common. Most of the cases are caused by *E. coli*, followed by *K. pneumoniae* and, rarely, *P. aeruginosa* or *P. mirabilis*.

Treatment consists of systemic antibiotics together with percutaneous catheter drainage, whilst some patients may need nephrectomy [14]. Failure to treat these patients adequately is associated with a high mortality rate.

Renal Papillary Necrosis

This condition, which is characterized by necrosis of the renal papilla, is usually diagnosed on imaging such as CT scan with contrast or retrograde pyelography [15]. More than half of these patients have diabetes, but the condition is also associated with analgesic abuse, sickle cell disease, and obstruction. Renal papillae are particularly vulnerable to ischaemia because of the sluggish blood flow in the vasa recta. Passage of sloughed papillae into the ureter may cause renal colic, obstruction, and even renal failure. Papillary necrosis in the setting of pyelonephritis is associated with pyuria and positive urine culture. Spiral CT scan shows irregular papillary tip, dilated calyceal fornix, extension of contrast material into the parenchyma and a separated crescent-shaped papilla surrounded by contrast material (called the ring sign). Broad-spectrum antibiotics are indicated and papillae obstructing the ureter may require cystoscopic removal.

Asymptomatic Bacteriuria

Asymptomatic bacteriuria is defined as the isolation of a single organism of $\geq 10^5$ cfu/ml in two consecutive clean-catch voided urine specimens in asymptomatic women; a single specimen in asymptomatic men is sufficient to label it as asymptomatic bacteriuria [16]. In both asymptomatic catheterized men and women, a single urine specimen is sufficient to diagnose asymptomatic bacteriuria if the single organism count is $\geq 10^5$ cfu/ml [17].

Whilst asymptomatic bacteriuria is rare in healthy young males, it may be seen in 2–7% of sexually active women (similar rates are observed in both pregnant and non-pregnant women). Populations with structural or functional abnormalities of the genitourinary tract have a high prevalence of asymptomatic bacteriuria [18]. Asymptomatic bacteriuria is seldom associated with adverse outcome and treatment is generally not advised. Screening for asymptomatic bacteriuria and treatment are generally recommended only in pregnant women or patients undergoing urological surgery. Although screening is routinely performed in transplant patients, there is not much evidence of its usefulness.

Urogenital Tuberculosis

Urogenital tuberculosis (TB) is the second most common form of extra-pulmonary tuberculosis after tuberculous lymph node involvement [19]. Mycobacterial seeding of the urogenital tract via haematogenous spread can occur at the time of pulmonary infection or in the setting of reactivation of TB or miliary disease. Urogenital TB may be seen in 2–20% of those affected with pulmonary TB and can present as:

- The commoner classic presentation, primarily involving the urinary collecting system (including renal pelvis, calyces, ureters, and bladder).
- The much less common renal parenchymal involvement, which can present as interstitial nephritis or glomerulonephritis [20].
- In men, genital TB can affect the entire male genital tract, including the prostate, seminal vesicles, vas deferens, epididymis, testicles, and penis. In women it can affect the fallopian tubes, endometrium, and ovaries, but generally spares the myometrium. Whilst most cases of genital TB occur because of seeding from haematogenous spread, TB of the female genital tract can develop after sexual intercourse with a man with TB of the penis or epididymis.

Initial symptoms of urogenital TB may be non-specific, and pyuria and/or microscopic haematuria may be observed as incidental findings. Once the disease has progressed to involve the bladder, symptoms of frequency, dysuria, urgency, and nocturia are often seen. An elevated plasma creatinine concentration may be observed in the setting of bilateral renal involvement and/or in the setting of interstitial nephritis or glomerulonephritis.

Patients who develop amyloid A amyloidosis due to TB may present with nephrotic syndrome and cardiomyopathy [21].

HIV-Associated Renal Disease

Human immunodeficiency virus (HIV) infection is associated with an increased risk of both acute and chronic kidney injury through a variety of mechanisms [22]. The epidemiology of HIV-related kidney disease has changed dramatically following the introduction of highly effective combination anti-retroviral therapy (cART) in the mid-1990s. The reported prevalence of CKD, defined by an estimated glomerular filtration rate (eGFR) <60 ml/min, in most recent studies is between 3.5 and 10% of HIV patients [23–25]. Risk factors associated with the development of renal disease in HIV include older age, hypertension, diabetes mellitus, lower CD4 count, high viral load, and African descent (perhaps due to APOL1 gene variants) [25–27].

The most common renal diseases attributed to HIV are HIV-associated nephropathy (HIVAN) and HIV immune complex disease of the kidney (HIVCK). Both are mediated by exposure of renal cells to viral antigens.

HIVAN usually presents with heavy proteinuria, a rapid decline in GFR and increased echogenicity of kidneys on ultrasound, typically without hypertension or oedema. It is strongly associated with those of African descent, and is most common in untreated or advanced HIV disease [28]. Histologically, HIVAN is characterized by collapsing focal segmental glomerulosclerosis. Additionally, microcystic tubular dilatation, interstitial inflammation, and endothelial tubuloreticular inclusion bodies are observed [29]. Whilst previously HIVAN was the predominant cause of CKD in HIV patients, the incidence has decreased in the post-cART era [30]. HIVAN is not seen in patients on cART who have a normal CD4 cell count and an undetectable HIV viral load.

HIVCK comprises a number of disease subtypes including membranous nephropathy, membranoproliferative glomerulonephritis (MPGN), mesangial proliferative glomerulonephritis, 'lupus-like' proliferative glomerulonephritis, and rarely immunoglobulin A nephropathy. HIVCK generally manifests with sub-nephrotic-range proteinuria, active urinary sediment (haematuria and red cell casts), hypocomplementaemia, and a progressive reduction in GFR [31].

Other HIV-associated renal diseases include thrombotic microangiopathy and membranous nephropathy or MPGN associated with hepatitis B or C co-infection. Though improving patient survival, many of the antiretroviral drugs used to treat HIV carry a risk of nephrotoxicity. Protease inhibitors, such as indinavir and atazanavir can cause crystalluria and AKI. Tenofovir, a nucleoside reverse transcriptase inhibitor, can lead to AKI and/or proximal tubular dysfunction (with Fanconi syndrome in severe cases) [32].

Screening

The 2014 Infectious Diseases Society of America guidelines suggest monitoring serum creatinine, eGFR, urinalysis, and quantitative urinary protein estimation at HIV diagnosis and prior to initiation of cART. Subsequently, HIV-positive individuals should have their GFR estimated at least twice yearly and a quantitative assessment of urinary protein excretion at least once yearly, in order to monitor for the development of kidney disease [28]. A 2014 Australian consensus statement advocated for testing of renal function at three-monthly intervals for the first year in patients on tenofovir therapy, with yearly screening following this.

Treatment

Identification of CKD in the setting of HIV, regardless of CD4 count, should prompt commencement of cART, with evidence demonstrating improvement in GFR associated with suppression of plasma viraemia [33]. Medication doses should be adjusted for the level of GFR, with particular attention to nucleoside and nucleotide reverse transcriptase inhibitors. In addition, optimization of other renal risk factors, including hypertension and diabetes, is critical.

Renin-angiotensin system inhibition with angiotensin-converting enzyme inhibitors has been demonstrated to improve proteinuria and long-term renal survival in biopsy-proven HIVAN or those with significant proteinuria [34–36]. There is also limited evidence for the efficacy of glucocorticoids in the reduction of proteinuria and limiting the progression of decline in renal function in biopsy-proven HIVAN [37].

Dialysis and renal transplantation are both viable renal replacement options for HIV patients with end-stage renal failure (ESRF). There appears to be no significant difference in survival rates between patients on haemodialysis and peritoneal dialysis [38].

Although large-cohort studies have demonstrated the safety and efficacy of renal transplantation in ESRF patients with HIV, the rate of rejection is higher than in the non-HIV population [39].

Leptospirosis

Leptospirosis is a bacterial disease of humans and animals caused by *Leptospira* bacteria found in infected animal urine and animal tissues. It is a widespread disease, with prevalence in the tropics being approximately 10 times higher than in temperate regions [40]. Rodents are the most important reservoirs for maintaining transmission, with organisms shed in their urine remaining viable for days to months in soil and water.

Portals of entry into humans include cuts or abraded skin, mucous membranes or conjunctivae, and rarely contaminated food. People at risk are those who have close contact with animals or who are exposed to water, mud, soil or vegetation that has been contaminated with animal urine.

Most cases are mild and self-limited, but the disease can be severe and potentially fatal. Following an incubation period of 2–26 days, the disease usually presents with fever, rigours, myalgia, non-productive cough, nausea, vomiting, and diarrhoea. Leptospirosis may be complicated by jaundice and renal failure (Weil's disease), acute respiratory distress syndrome, uveitis, optic neuritis, peripheral neuropathy, myocarditis, and rhabdomyolysis.

Renal failure is often non-oliguric and associated with hypokalaemia. Though renal replacement therapy may be needed in severe cases, the renal prognosis is generally very good.

Serological tests are used for the diagnosis of leptospirosis, though they may not be very useful in the acute setting due to the endemicity of the bacteria. Paired samples are needed to establish diagnosis. Molecular techniques such as real-time polymerase chain reaction (PCR) and loop-mediated isothermal amplification (LAMP) are being used more and more and have the advantage of being useful for rapid and accurate diagnosis of acute leptospirosis.

Both oral doxycycline and azithromycin can be used in mild to moderate cases, whilst intravenous penicillin or third-generation cephalosporins are useful in severe cases [41].

References

1. Foxman, B. (2014). Urinary tract infection syndromes: occurrence, recurrence, bacteriology, risk factors, and disease burden. *Infect. Dis. Clin. N. Am.* 28 (1): 1.

2. Czaja, C.A., Scholes, D., Hooton, T.M., and Stamm, W.E. (2007). Population-based epidemiologic analysis of acute pyelonephritis. *Clin. Infect. Dis.* 45 (3): 281–283.

3. Echols, R.M., Tosiello, R.L., Haverstock, D.C., and Tice, A.D. (1999). Demographic, clinical, and treatment parameters influencing the outcome of acute cystitis. *Clin. Infect. Dis.* 29 (1): 113.

4. Stamm, W.E., Hooton, T.M., Johnson, J.R. et al. (1989). Urinary tract infections: from pathogenesis to treatment. *J. Infect. Dis.* 159: 400–406.

5. Johnson, J.R. and Russo, T.A. (2018). Acute pyelonephritis in adults. *N. Engl. J. Med.* 378: 48–59. https://doi.org/10.1056/NEJMcp1702758.

6. Talan, D.A., Takhar, S.S., Krishnadasan, A. et al. (2016). Fluoroquinolone-resistant and extended-spectrum β-lactamase-producing *Escherichia coli* infections in patients with pyelonephritis, United States. *Emerg. Infect. Dis.* 22: 1594–1603.

7. Piccoli, G.B., Consiglio, V., Colla, L. et al. (2006). Antibiotic treatment for acute 'uncomplicated' or 'primary' pyelonephritis: a systematic, 'semantic revision'. *Int. J. Antimicrob. Agents* 28 (Suppl 1): S49–S63.

8. Platt, R. (1983). Quantitative definition of bacteriuria. *Am. J. Med.* 75 (1B): 44–52.

9. van Nieuwkoop, C., Hoppe, B.P., Bonten, T.N. et al. (2010). Predicting the need for radiologic imaging in adults with febrile urinary tract infection. *Clin. Infect. Dis.* 51: 1266–1272.

10. Oosterhof, G.O. and Delaere, K.P. (1986). Xanthogranulomatous pyelonephritis. A review with 2 case reports. *Urol. Int.* 41 (3): 180.

11. Dembry, L.M. and Andriole, V.T. (1997). Renal and perirenal abscesses. *Infect. Dis. Clin. N. Am.* 11 (3): 663.

12. Hill, G.S. (1989). Renal infection. In: *Uropathology*, 1e (ed. G.S. Hill), 33. New York: Churchill Livingstone.

13. Huang, J.J. and Tseng, C.C. (2000). Emphysematous pyelonephritis: clinicoradiological classification, management, prognosis, and pathogenesis. *Arch. Intern. Med.* 160 (6): 79.

14. Chen, M.T., Huang, C.N., Chou, Y.H. et al. (1997). Percutaneous drainage in the treatment of emphysematous pyelonephritis: 10-year experience. *J. Urol.* 157 (5): 1569.

15. Kim, S.H. (2011). *Radiology Illustrated: Uroradiology*, 472. Springer Science & Business Media.

16. Nicolle, L.E., Bradley, S., Colgan, R. et al. (2005). Infectious Diseases Society of America guidelines for the diagnosis and treatment of asymptomatic bacteriuria in adults. *Clin. Infect. Dis.* 40 (5): 643.

17. Hooton, T.M., Bradley, S.F., Cardenas, D.D. et al. (2010). Diagnosis, prevention, and treatment of catheter-associated urinary tract infection in adults: 2009 international clinical practice guidelines from the Infectious Diseases Society of America. *Clin. Infect. Dis.* 50 (5): 625.

18. Nicolle, L.E. (2003). Asymptomatic bacteriuria: when to screen and when to treat. *Infect. Dis. Clin. N. Am.* 17 (2): 367.

19. Figueiredo, A.A., Lucon, A.M., and Srougi, M. (2017). Urogenital Tuberculosis. *Microbiol Spectr.* 5 (1).

20. Chapagain, A., Dobbie, H., Sheaff, M., and Yaqoob, M.M. (2011). Presentation, diagnosis, and treatment outcome of tuberculous-mediated tubulointerstitial nephritis. *Kidney Int.* 79 (6): 671.

21. Dubrey, S.W., Hawkins, P.N., and Falk, R.H. (2011). Amyloid diseases of the heart: assessment, diagnosis, and referral. *Heart* 97 (1): 75.

22. Wyatt, C.M., Arons, R.R., Kltoman, P.E., and Klotman, M.E. (2006). Acute renal failure in hospitalised patients with HIV: risk factors and impact on in-hospital mortality. *AIDS* 20 (4): 561–565. https://doi.org/10.1097/01.aids.0000210610.52836.07.

23. Gracey, D., Chan, D., Bailey, M. et al. (2012). Screening and management of renal disease in human immunodeficiency virus-infected patients in Australia. *Intern. Med. J.* 43 (4): 410–216. https://doi.org/10.1111/j.1445-5994.2012.02933.x.

24. Juega-Marino, J., Bonjoch, A., Perez-Alvarez, N. et al. (2017). Prevalence, evolution, and related risk factors of kidney disease among Spanish HIV-infected individuals. *Medicine (Baltimore)* 96 (37): e7421. https://doi.org/10.1097/MD.0000000000007421.

25. Mocroft, A., Kirk, O., Gatell, J. et al. (2007). Chronic renal failure among HIV-1 infected patients. *AIDS* 21 (9): 1119–1127. https://doi.org/10.1097/QAD.0b013e3280f774ee.

26. Gupta, S.K., Smurzynski, M., Franceschini, N. et al. (2009). The effects of HIV-1 viral suppression and non-viral factors on quantitative proteinuria in the HAART era. *Antivir. Ther.* 14 (4): 543–549.

27. Choi, A.I., Rodriguez, R.A., Bacchetti, P. et al. (2007). Racial differences in end-stage renal disease rates in HIV infection versus diabetes. *J. Am. Soc. Nephrol.* 18 (11): 2968–2974. https://doi.org/10.1681/ASN.2007040402.

28. Lucas, G.M., Ross, M.J., Stock, P.G. et al. (2014). Clinical practice guideline for the management of chronic kidney disease in patients infected with HIV: 2014 update by the HIV Medicine Association of the Infectious Diseases Society of America. *Clin. Infect. Dis.* 59 (9): e96–e138. https://doi.org/10.1093/cid/ciu617.

29. Wyatt, C.M., Klotman, P.E., and D'Agati, V.D. (2008). HIV-associated nephropathy: clinical presentation, pathology, and epidemiology in the era of antiretroviral therapy. *Semin. Nephrol.* 28 (6): 513–522. https://doi.org/10.1016/j.semnephrol.2008.08.005.

30. Berliner, A.R., Fine, D.M., Lucas, G.M. et al. (2008). Observations on a cohort of HIV-infected patients undergoing native renal biopsy. *Am. J. Nephrol.* 28 (3): 478–486. https://doi.org/10.1159/000112851.

31. Cohen, S.D., Kopp, J.B., and Kimmel, P.L. (2017). Kidney diseases associated with human immunodeficiency virus infection. *N. Engl. J. Med.* 377 (24): 2363–2374. https://doi.org/10.1056/NEJMra1508467.

32. Hall, A.M., Hendry, B.M., Nitsch, D., and Connolly, J.O. (2011). Tenofovir-associated kidney toxicity in HIV-infected patients: a review of the evidence. *Am. J. Kidney Dis.* 57 (5): 773–780. https://doi.org/10.1053/j.ajkd.2011.01.022.

33. Kalayjian, R.C., Franceschini, N., Gupta, S.K. et al. (2008). Suppression of HIV-1 replication by antiretroviral therapy improves renal function in persons with low CD4 cell counts and chronic kidney disease. *AIDS* 22 (4): 481–487. https://doi.org/10.1097/QAD.0b013e3282f4706d.

34. Wei, A., Burns, G.C., Williams, B.A. et al. (2003). Long-term renal survival in HIV-associated nephropathy with angiotensin-converting enzyme inhibition. *Kidney Int.* 64 (4): 1462–1471.

35. Kimmel, P.L., Mishkin, G.J., and Umana, W.O. (1996). Captopril and renal survival in patients with human immunodeficiency virus nephropathy. *Am. J. Kidney Dis.* 28 (2): 202–208.

36. Burns, G.C., Paul, S.K., Toth, I.R., and Sivak, S.L. (1997). Effect of angiotensin-converting enzyme inhibition in HIV-associated nephropathy. *J. Am. Soc. Nephrol.* 8 (7): 1140–1146.

37. Eustace, J.A., Nuermberger, E., Choi, M. et al. (2000). Cohort study of the treatment of severe HIV-associated nephropathy with corticosteroids. *Kidney Int.* 58 (3): 1253–1260. https://doi.org/10.1046/j.1523-1755.2000.00280.x.

38. Ahuja, T.S., Collinge, N., Grady, J., and Khan, S. (2003). Is dialysis modality a factor in survival of patients with ESRD and HIV-associated nephropathy? *Am. J. Kidney Dis.* 41 (5): 1060–1064. https://doi.org/10.1016/S0272-6386(03)00204-X.

39. Stock, P.G., Barin, B., Murphy, B. et al. (2010). Outcomes of kidney transplantation in HIV-infected recipients. *N. Engl. J. Med.* 363 (21): 2004–2014. https://doi.org/10.1056/NEJMoa 1001197.

40. Hartskeerl, R.A., Collares-Pereira, M., and Ellis, W.A. (2011). Emergence, control and re-emerging leptospirosis: dynamics of infection in the changing world. *Clin. Microbiol. Infect.* 17 (4): 494–501.

41. Forbes, A.E., Zochowski, W.J., Dubrey, S.W., and Sivaprakasam, V. (2012). Leptospirosis and Weil's disease in the UK. *QJM* 105 (12): 1151–1162. https://doi.org/10.1093/qjmed/hcs145.

Questions and Answers

Questions

1. Co-existence of which of the following conditions automatically classifies patients with UTI to have complicated cystitis?
   a. Diabetes mellitus
   b. HIV infection
   c. Nephrolithiasis
   d. Urinary diversions
   e. None of the above

2. Patients of UTI who are susceptible to papillary necrosis include those with:
   a. Renal cancer
   b. Hypertension
   c. History of analgesic abuse
   d. Obesity
   e. Renal artery stenosis

3. Which of the following is not a risk factor for developing multidrug resistant (MDR) cystitis?
   a. HIV
   b. Recent use of a broad-spectrum antibiotic
   c. Nursing home resident
   d. Recent visit to Spain
   e. Recent hospital admission for community acquired pneumonia

4. Commonest causative organism leading to emphysematous pyelonephritis is:
   a. *Klebsiella pneumoniae*
   b. *Staphylococcus aureus*
   c. *Pseudomonas aeruginosa*
   d. *E. coli*
   e. MRSA

5. Screening for asymptomatic bacteriuria is suggested in the following conditions:
   a. Patients with history of more than two UTIs in a year
   b. Diabetes
   c. Sexually active women
   d. Pregnancy
   e. End-stage renal disease

6. HIV-associated nephropathy (HIVAN) typically presents with nephrotic range proteinuria and histologically resembles:
   a. IgA nephropathy
   b. Membranoproliferative glomerulonephritis
   c. Membranous nephropathy
   d. Minimal change disease
   e. Focal segmental glomerulosclerosis

Answers

1. e. Patients with underlying urologic abnormalities (such as nephrolithiasis, strictures, stents, or urinary diversions), immunocompromising conditions (such as neutropenia or advanced HIV infection), or poorly controlled diabetes mellitus are not automatically considered to have complicated cystitis. Among healthy women, risk factors for cystitis include recent sexual intercourse, history of UTI, use of spermicide-coated condoms, diaphragms, spermicides, structural or functional urinary tract abnormalities, indwelling urinary catheter, estrogen deficiency in post-menopausal women, and obesity.

2. c. More than half of the patients with papillary necrosis have diabetes, but the condition is also associated with analgesic abuse, sickle cell disease, and obstruction.

3. a. Risk factors for both uncomplicated and complicated UTI with multidrug resistant (MDR) organisms include recent broad-spectrum antimicrobial use, health care exposures, and travel to parts of the world where multidrug-resistant organisms are prevalent, e.g. India, Israel, Spain, and Mexico.

4. d. Most of the cases of emphysematous pyelonephritis are caused by *E. coli*, followed by *K. pneumoniae*. Rarer causes include *P. aeruginosa* and *Proteus mirabilis*. The condition is diagnosed by radiological evidence of air in the renal parenchyma or bladder and up to 90% of the patients have diabetes mellitus.

5. d. Screening for asymptomatic bacteriuria and treatment is generally recommended only in pregnant women or patients undergoing urologic surgery. Some centres screen for the condition in their transplant patients. While asymptomatic bacteriuria is rare in healthy young males, it may be seen in 2–7% of sexually active women (similar rates are observed in both pregnant and non-pregnant women).

6. e. Histologically, HIVAN is characterized by 'collapsing' variant of focal segmental glomerulosclerosis. HIVAN usually presents with heavy proteinuria, a rapid decline in GFR, and increased echogenicity of kidneys on ultrasound; typically without hypertension or edema. It is strongly associated with black race, and is most common in untreated or advanced HIV disease. Patients with HIV may develop HIV immune complex disease of the kidney (HIVCK) which comprises a number of disease-subtypes including membranous nephropathy, membranoproliferative (MPGN) and mesangial proliferative glomerulonephritis, 'lupus-like' proliferative glomerulonephritis, and rarely IgA nephropathy.

15

Diabetic Nephropathy

Mark McLean and Rajini Jayaballa

Summary

- Diabetic nephropathy (DN) is the commonest cause of end-stage renal disease (ESRD) requiring dialysis or transplantation in industrialized nations
- DN is characterized by persistent proteinuria and progressive decline in renal function leading to ESRD
- DN occurs with similar frequency in both type 1 and type 2 diabetes, suggesting that hyperglycaemia is the major factor in its causation
- The three major histological changes in the glomeruli in DN are mesangial expansion, glomerular basement membrane thickening, and glomerulosclerosis
- Glomerular hypertension and resultant hyperfiltration are key early elements in the development of DN
- Good blood pressure control helps to prevent or delay progression of DN

Diabetic nephropathy (DN) is a chronic glomerulopathy characterized by persistent proteinuria and a progressive decline in renal function, potentially leading to end-stage renal disease (ESRD). DN is associated with both type 1 and type 2 diabetes and is almost always accompanied by other microvascular complications of diabetes; that is, retinopathy and peripheral neuropathy.

DN is now the single most common cause of ESRD requiring dialysis or transplantation in industrialized nations. The natural history of the condition follows a gradual and often predictable course over many years: starting with microalbuminuria (also termed moderately increased albuminuria), evolving to nephrotic-range proteinuria and/or chronic kidney disease (CKD), and eventually ESRD. This process typically begins between 5 and 10 years after the onset of diabetes, and its rate of progression is influenced by both glycaemic and blood pressure control [1].

Epidemiology

The fact that DN occurs with similar frequency in both type 1 and type 2 diabetes suggests that hyperglycaemia is the major factor in its causation. Males and females are equally affected, and the incidence is higher in non-Caucasians, including African Americans, Asians, and Australian Aborigines. Approximately one-third of people with diabetes develop significant nephropathy, with the incidence peaking about 10 years after the onset of diabetes. Nephropathy is strongly associated with systemic vasculopathy in diabetes, including coronary artery disease and stroke. In fact, the excess of cardiovascular morbidity and mortality seen in type 1 and type 2 diabetes is almost entirely confined to those with evidence of diabetic kidney disease.

Lecture Notes Nephrology: A Comprehensive Guide to Renal Medicine, First Edition. Edited by Surjit Tarafdar.
© 2020 John Wiley & Sons Ltd. Published 2020 by John Wiley & Sons Ltd.

Pathology of Diabetic Nephropathy

The three major histological changes in the glomeruli in DN are mesangial expansion, glomerular basement membrane (GBM) thickening, and glomerulosclerosis [2]. The glomerulosclerosis may be diffuse, affecting the basement membranes of glomerular capillaries as well as the tubules and arterioles, or it may take a periodic acid–Schiff (PAS)-positive nodular appearance (Kimmelstiel–Wilson lesion), typically seen in the mesangium. The classic Kimmelstiel–Wilson lesion is pathognomonic of DN but is only seen in approximately half of cases (Figures 15.1 and 15.2).

In 2010, the Renal Pathologic Society proposed the following histological classification of DN [2]:

- *Class I*: isolated GBM thickening with no evidence of mesangial expansion or glomerulosclerosis.
- *Class II*: mild (class IIa) or severe (class IIb) mesangial expansion. A lesion is considered severe if areas of expansion larger than the mean area of a capillary lumen are present in >25% of the total mesangium.
- *Class III*: at least one Kimmelstiel–Wilson lesion is observed and there is <50% global glomerulosclerosis.
- *Class IV*: >50% global glomerulosclerosis.

The Renal Pathology Society also classifies the interstitial and vascular lesions in DN as follows:

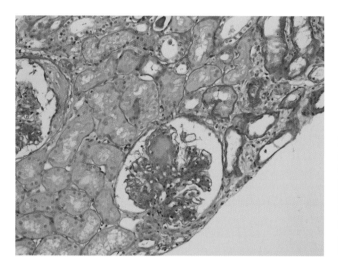

Figure 15.1 Light microscopy image with periodic acid–Schiff (PAS) staining showing nodular appearance of the glomeruli in diabetic nephropathy (Kimmelstiel–Wilson lesion). Nodules seen in light chain deposition disease, amyloidosis, and mesangiocapillary glomerulonephritis stain very weakly with PAS and trichrome stain.

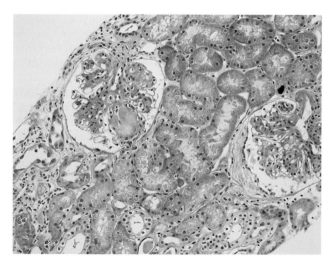

Figure 15.2 Light microscopy image of diabetic nephropathy with trichrome staining showing Kimmelstiel–Wilson nodular lesions in the glomeruli.

- A score of 0 was assigned if the interstitium had no areas of interstitial fibrosis and tubular atrophy (IFTA); a score of 1, 2, or 3 was assigned if areas of IFTA were <25, 25–50 or >50%, respectively
- A score of 0, 1, or 2 was assigned if no arteriolar hyalinosis, one arteriole or more than one arteriole with hyalinosis was present. In addition, the most severely affected arteriole was assigned a score of 0, 1, or 2 if there was no intimal thickening, intimal thickening < thickness of media or intimal thickening > thickness of media, respectively.

Pathogenesis

Although blood glucose control is a strong predictor of the risk of DN, there is significant intra-individual variation. Some patients may not develop nephropathy even after decades of poor diabetes control, whilst others will have advanced microangiopathy despite seemingly good blood glucose control. Therefore, other factors clearly contribute to causation (Table 15.1). Genetic predisposition seems to influence the susceptibility to hyperglycaemic injury, as evidenced by familial clustering of DN in both type 1 and type 2 diabetes. Arterial hypertension and atherosclerosis are also crucial contributors. An important predisposing factor is a low nephron number at birth, which may be associated with low birthweight babies born to mothers who had been hyperglycaemic during pregnancy. This seems to be associated with increased single-nephron glomerular filtration rate (GFR) from early life, with a consequent increased susceptibility to hyperfiltration injury to the glomerulus [3].

Thickening of the GBM is often the first change in DN that can be quantitated. This may be accompanied or followed by mesangial expansion, which may be diffuse or nodular (Kimmelstiel–Wilson nodule).

Table 15.1 Key elements in the pathogenesis of diabetic nephropathy
- Glomerular hypertension and resultant hyperfiltration
- Mesangial expansion and injury – glomerulosclerosis
- Role of growth factors, cytokines, and advanced glycation end products
- Progressive proteinuria
- Tubulointerstitial fibrosis and tubular atrophy

Glomerular Hyperfiltration and Mesangial Expansion

A 25–50% elevation in the GFR is seen early in the course of disease in up to one-half of patients with both type 1 and type 2 diabetes [3, 4]. The rise in GFR is accompanied by glomerular hypertrophy and increased renal size. This early phase of DN is characterized by relative dilatation of the afferent and constriction of the efferent glomerular arterioles, reflecting increased angiotensin II activity. The consequent rise in glomerular capillary pressure induces glomerular hyperfiltration, and at the same time increases mechanical stress on the mesangial matrix, leading to increased mesangial matrix production and an element of mesangial cellular expansion (Figure 15.3). The following factors are implicated in the development of glomerular hyperfiltration and mesangial expansion:

- *Insulin-like growth factor 1* (IGF1): although the exact pathogenetic role of IGF1 is unproven, infusion of this hormone in normal subjects can replicate the glomerular hypertension and hyperfiltration seen in DN. IGF1 is also postulated to lead to decreased mesangial degradation because of its inhibitory effect on the metalloproteinase-2 [5].
- *Sorbitol*: under normal conditions only a small amount of glucose that enters cells is metabolized to sorbitol by the enzyme aldose reductase. However, glucose conversion to sorbitol is more pronounced with chronic hyperglycaemia. Sorbitol is postulated to increase intracellular osmolarity and decrease Na^+-K^+-ATPase activity. An aldose reductase inhibitor, sorbinil, has been shown to minimize albuminuria and GBM thickening in diabetic rats [6].
- *Advanced glycation end products* (AGEs): in chronic hyperglycaemia, some of the excess circulating glucose combines with free amino acids on circulating or tissue proteins. This non-enzymatic glycation leads to the production of AGEs, which may be formed in situ in the kidney or may arrive as circulating glycated proteins filtered at the glomerulus. By cross-linking with collagen, they may promote expansion of extracellular mesangial matrix and, by recruiting factors such as transforming growth factor-beta (TGF-β), mediate further mesangial cell proliferation and matrix deposition. AGEs may also impair endothelial function, reducing nitric oxide-mediated vasodilation and thereby altering glomerular haemodynamics.

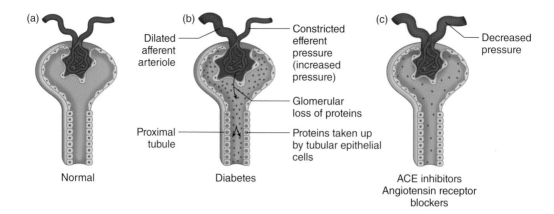

Figure 15.3 Comparison of (a) a normal nephron, (b) a nephron in diabetic nephropathy (DN), and (c) a nephron in DN after administration of angiotensin-converting enzyme inhibitor or angiotensin receptor blocker.

- *Cytokine activation*: increased expression of vascular endothelial growth factor (VEGF) and TGF-β leads to mesangial cellular hypertrophy and matrix expansion [7]. DN is also associated with a reduction in the expression of factors that counter the actions of these proliferative cytokines. The net result is cellular hyperplasia, enhanced collagen synthesis and expansion of the connective tissue matrix, which are defining characteristics of DN.

The mesangial expansion is, for the most part, due to an increase in the mesangial matrix, with a lesser contribution from increased mesangial cellularity. Mesangial expansion out of proportion to glomerular expansion is strongly correlated with a decreased peripheral GBM filtration surface area and hence decreased GFR.

Proteinuria

In the normal glomerulus, a highly electronegative filtration barrier, which consists of the endothelium, GBM, and podocytes, prevents negatively charged proteins in blood (e.g. albumin) from leaking into urine. DN is characterized by loss of negatively charged heparin sulphate from the GBM, and reduced transcription of nephrin, one of the chief negatively charged proteins on the slit diaphragm of the podocytes [8], by the following mechanisms:

- The characteristic widening of GBM in DN is associated with accumulation of type IV collagen at the cost of reduced heparin sulphate.
- Transcription of nephrin is reduced by the elevated levels of angiotensin II and restored by inhibitors of the renin–angiotensin system (RAS).

- In addition, in DN, podocyte apoptosis is triggered by various factors like angiotensin II and TGF-β. Both absolute podocyte number and podocyte density are reduced, which contributes to the proteinuria.

Tubulointerstitial Fibrosis and Tubular Atrophy

Tubulointerstitial pathology begins early during DN and correlates with prognosis. The mechanisms underlying tubulointerstitial fibrosis and tubular atrophy are similar to those in non-diabetic progressive kidney damage. Reabsorption of the filtered protein by renal tubular cells damages these cells, causing them to express proinflammatory and profibrotic factors such as TGF-β and epidermal growth factor. These factors cause the tubulointerstitial cells to change their phenotypes and become fibroblasts. Additionally, renal hypoxia due to anaemia, which is seen in CKD, causes induction of fibroblastic factors such as VEGF, leading to further aggravation of interstitial fibrosis. Treatment of anaemia early in the course of renal failure with erythropoietin slows down the progress of DN.

Clinical Features and Natural History

The first phase of nephropathy, characterized by glomerular hyperfiltration, may begin soon after the diagnosis of type 1 or type 2 diabetes. At this stage, which has no symptomatic or clinical manifestations, albuminuria is not present, but a supra-normal GFR and a raised intraglomerular pressure can be demonstrated.

The second phase of the disease is characterized by the appearance of 'moderately increased albuminuria', formerly called 'microalbuminuria' (defined as urinary albumin excretion between 30 and 300 mg/day or between 30 and 300 mg/g creatinine on a random urine sample). At this stage, glomerular hyperfiltration may persist, or GFR may decline to the normal range. Structural changes in the glomerulus are already evident by this time, but may be reversible. Progression to renal failure can be prevented by achievement of good glycaemic control and by pharmacological therapy to reduce intra-glomerular pressure, using drugs that block the action of the renin–angiotensin axis. Therefore, angiotensin-converting enzyme (ACE) inhibitors or angiotensin receptor blockers (ARBs) are the mainstay of management for this stage of the condition.

The onset of 'severely increased albuminuria', formerly called 'macroalbuminuria' (defined as urinary albumin excretion above 300 mg/day or above 300 mg/g creatinine on a random urine sample), in the absence of effective therapy is often followed by a progressive decline in GFR and, given enough time, ESRD.

The onset of proteinuria is accompanied by a steady progression of glomerular pathology (already described) and declining GFR. Hypertension, which is frequently coexistent, contributes to a further decline in GFR. Clinically, patients with DN demonstrate parallel development of diabetic retinopathy and peripheral neuropathy, and progressive glomerulosclerosis is characteristic on renal biopsy. The incidence is substantially higher in certain ethnic groups, including Australian Aborigines [9].

Diabetic Nephropathy and Cardiovascular Disease

The presence of DN is an important marker of systemic cardiovascular disease (CVD) in a patient with diabetes. In patients with diabetes, those with albuminuria are consistently observed to have substantially elevated mortality rates, primarily due to myocardial infarction or stroke. Albuminuria and decreasing GFR are independently and additively associated with increased risks of CVD events and all-cause mortality [10]. In both type 1 and type 2 diabetes

cohorts, the excess risks of mortality and CVD compared to the non-diabetic population are almost entirely limited to patients who have evidence of DN. Diabetic patients with normal levels of albuminuria and GFR have risks similar to the general non-diabetic population [11, 12]. These observations suggest that the recognition of early DN in a patient with diabetes should lead to a therapeutic focus on mitigating the high CVD risk for such patients. This involves the combined targeting of blood glucose, blood pressure, serum lipids, smoking cessation, and other factors known to have impacts on CVD outcomes.

Screening for Diabetic Nephropathy

All patients with diabetes should be screened on a regular basis for evidence of early DN, so that interventions may be undertaken to prevent or delay its progression. Since DN is an asymptomatic condition, it is essential to establish a regular screening protocol. Increased urinary protein excretion, initially consisting almost entirely of albumin, is the earliest clinical manifestation of DN. Urine dipstick testing is an insensitive marker for the early stage of DN and does not become positive until protein excretion reaches >300 mg/day, by which time glomerular pathology is fairly advanced. Use of a specific assay for albumin is therefore necessary to ensure sufficient sensitivity of detection of early nephropathy.

The normal rate of albumin excretion is less than 30 mg/day. Persistent albumin excretion of 30–300 mg/day is termed moderately increased albuminuria (formerly termed microalbuminuria). Detection of DN at the microalbuminuria stage allows interventions which have been shown to slow the progression of the condition. The most accurate quantitation of albumin excretion is obtained from a timed urine sample, collected over 24 hours. However, this involves considerable inconvenience for the patient. A 'spot' urine sample can be used for nephropathy screening if the albumin concentration is expressed as a ratio to the urinary creatinine concentration (the urinary albumin to creatinine ratio). This corrects for variation in the albumin concentration caused by fluctuations in urine volume and dilution by free water excretion. The upper limit of the normal range for this ratio is 2.5 mg of albumin per mmol of creatinine. An albumin to creatinine ratio between 3.5 and 35 mg/mmol correlates with albumin excretion in the moderately increased albuminuria range when compared with timed collections. A urinary albumin to creatinine ratio of greater than 35 mg/mmol likely indicates severely increased albuminuria.

The within-patient variability of urine albumin excretion is very low, making it an ideal test for screening. The accuracy of the test is minimally affected by the time of day, but albumin excretion can be increased (producing a false positive test) after vigorous exercise, or in the presence of a urinary tract infection. A normal test result has a high negative predictive value, thereby excluding DN. A positive test should be confirmed by repeat measurement, or by undertaking a timed urinary albumin excretion test, before embarking on pharmacological intervention.

In patients with type 1 diabetes, screening for DN with urine albumin estimation is recommended to commence five years after the diagnosis of diabetes. In patients with type 2 diabetes, it is possible that the patient has had undiagnosed hyperglycaemia for a prolonged period prior to the diagnosis. Up to one-third of patients with type 2 diabetes will have moderately increased albuminuria already present at the time of diagnosis. Therefore, screening should be undertaken as soon as diabetes is recognized in patients with type 2 diabetes. Persons with type 1 or type 2 diabetes and moderately severe proteinuria should continue to be tested for albuminuria annually to monitor disease progression and response to therapy [13].

Diagnosis

The diagnosis of DN is often entertained in a patient with known diabetes who has proteinuria, or in patients with diabetes who have an elevated serum creatinine concentration. However, it must be remembered that a patient with diabetes may develop renal disease from other causes, and diabetes actually increases the likelihood of coexisting hypertension, renal artery atherosclerosis, CVD leading to renal hypoperfusion and urinary tract infection. An analysis of the National Health and Nutrition Examination Survey (NHANES) suggests that approximately 30% of patients with diabetes and impaired renal function have a non-diabetic primary cause for their kidney dysfunction [14, 15]. The challenge is, therefore, to recognize the positive features of DN, and also to exclude other causes of renal impairment (Table 15.2).

DN has characteristic clinical features, which assist in its recognition. It is invariably associated with

---

Table 15.2 Approach to diagnosis of deteriorating renal function in a patient with diabetes

- What is the temporal trend in glomerular filtration rate and serum creatinine? A sudden deterioration suggests a non-diabetic cause
- Are other microvascular diabetes complications present? Their absence makes diabetic nephropathy (DN) unlikely
- Consider prerenal factors and nephrotoxins
- Urine culture – treat urinary tract infection and reassess
- Urine microscopy – an active sediment (white blood cell, red blood cell [RBC] cast or dysmorphic RBC) suggests a non-diabetic cause
- Renal ultrasound – exclude obstruction; renal size is usually not reduced in DN

---

proteinuria, which progresses with a falling GFR. By this time DN is almost always accompanied by evidence of other microvascular complications of diabetes, including retinopathy and peripheral neuropathy. Therefore, if a patient with diabetes has deteriorating renal function in the absence of these characteristic features, DN is unlikely and an alternative diagnosis should be sought. Microscopy should be performed on the urinary sediment from a freshly collected and centrifuged urine sample. In DN the sediment is typically bland, with no evidence of inflammatory disease (dysmorphic red blood cells or casts, white blood cells), although microscopic haematuria can be present in some patients. The presence of an 'active' urinary sediment is suggestive of a non DN renal pathology.

Renal tract ultrasound should be performed to exclude obstructive uropathy and assess renal size. In CKD due to DN, the kidneys are usually of normal size, compared with the reduced renal volume typically seen in chronic glomerulonephritis. In patients with diabetes and deteriorating renal function, a presumptive diagnosis of DN can be made if the clinical and laboratory features are all consistent with that diagnosis and no alternative diagnosis is evident. However, where atypical features exist, a renal biopsy may be indicated.

The onset of DN is gradual and its progression is slow and insidious. If a patient with diabetes experiences a sudden deterioration in renal function, it is unlikely to be due to DN alone. Other contributing factors, which might be reversible, should then be looked for. These include prerenal insults (hypovolaemia, hypotension, poor cardiac output), nephrotoxins such as non-steroidal anti-inflammatory drugs (NSAIDs), ACE inhibitors or ARB drugs, antibiotics, contrast media and renal tract obstruction.

Monitoring Renal Function in Patients with Diabetes

Whilst the estimation of urinary albumin is useful in the diagnosis of DN and albumin excretion may decrease in response to treatment (see later), once nephropathy is established, the level of proteinuria is not a very reliable predictor of the progression of the disease. Serum creatinine levels are similarly unreliable, since they remain normal until at least 50% of renal function has been lost [16]. In diabetic patients with albuminuria or overt nephropathy, measurement of GFR, either directly or by indirect inference, provides the best assessment of the progress of the condition. Once the condition has progressed to the macroproteinuric stage, the rate of decline in GFR for an individual patient tends to remain quite constant over time. This makes it possible to predict the likely time that will elapse before renal replacement therapy will be required.

Once nephropathy has become established, there is limited value in continuing to monitor an individual patient's urinary albumin or protein excretion, and it is a poor predictor of prognosis. As end-stage renal failure approaches, the rate of albumin excretion declines, reflecting severely restricted glomerular filtration.

Incidence and Progression

The United Kingdom Prospective Diabetes Study (UKPDS) has reported data from 5097 patients followed from the time of diagnosis of type 2 diabetes. Amongst those without any degree of albuminuria at baseline, progression to microalbuminuria occurred at 2.0% per year, from microalbuminuria to macroalbuminuria at 2.8% per year, and from macroalbuminuria to elevated plasma creatinine or ESRD at 2.3% per year. Ten years following diagnosis of diabetes, the prevalence of microalbuminuria was 24.9%, macroalbuminuria was 5.3%, and elevated plasma

creatinine or renal replacement therapy was observed in 0.8% [17]. These data demonstrate that though the development of microalbuminuria is common, many patients do not progress to more serious degrees of renal impairment.

The incidence of nephropathy in type 1 diabetes is similar to that in type 2 diabetes. A systematic review of nine published longitudinal studies with 7938 patients reported the overall incidence of microalbuminuria as 28% at 15 years after diagnosis [18]. There is no substantial difference in the risk of nephropathy between males and females. The cardinal risk factors for the development of microalbuminuria and impaired kidney function are poor glycaemic control, presence of hypertension, cigarette smoking, and hyperlipidaemia.

Regression of microalbuminuria to normoalbuminuria is not infrequent, even in the absence of specific treatment. In various longitudinal studies, reversion to normal urine albumin excretion has been reported in between 15 and 60% of patients and is similar for type 1 and type 2 diabetes. There is a consistent finding that regression of urine albumin excretion is likely to be associated with improved blood glucose control, lower blood pressure, and in individuals with lower baseline albumin excretion rates. However, once nephropathy has progressed to the stage of overt proteinuria, subsequent regression of the disease is very uncommon.

Effect of Glycaemic Control on Nephropathy

Poor blood glucose control, as often evidenced by an increased glycosylated haemoglobin level, is the primary risk factor for the development of microalbuminuria and progression to DN. Two landmark prospective clinical studies have clearly demonstrated the association of glycosylated haemoglobin levels with the risk of development and progression of DN. The Diabetes Control and Complications Trial (DCCT) of type 1 diabetes [19] and the UKPDS of newly diagnosed type 2 diabetes [17] compared groups of patients randomly allocated to either tight blood glucose control ('intensive treatment') or more lenient blood glucose targets ('conventional treatment'). Both studies demonstrated the benefit of tight blood glucose control on the risk of developing new-onset microalbuminuria, or advanced nephropathy. In UKPDS, intensive treatment (median haemoglobin

A1c [HbA1c] 7.0%), compared with conventional control (median HbA1c 7.9%), resulted in a 33% reduction in the relative risk of developing microalbuminuria or proteinuria at 12 years from diagnosis, and a significant reduction in the proportion of patients who experienced doubling of their plasma creatinine (0.9 versus 3.5%). In DCCT, intensive treatment (median HbA1c of 7.2%, versus 9.1% in the conventional treatment group) was associated with a 34% reduction in the relative risk of new-onset microalbuminuria, and a 54% reduction in the risk of heavy proteinuria (>300 mg/day). Thus, achievement of good blood glucose targets reduces the onset and progress of DN. Importantly, blood glucose control similarly improves the risk of other microvascular diabetic complications, whilst having a more modest benefit for prevention of macrovascular disease.

In type 2 diabetes, the benefit of improved blood glucose control occurs independently of whether insulin or oral hypoglycaemic agents are used. It is also similar in males and females, and regardless of age at diagnosis of diabetes.

Effect of Control of Blood Pressure

Hypertension is present in 40% of type 1 and 70% of type 2 diabetic patients with normoalbuminuria. Strict arterial blood pressure control has proven to be one of the most important factors in preventing or delaying the progression of DN and other cardiovascular complications. The effect of treatment of hypertension in diabetic patients has been assessed in three major randomized trials: UKPDS, the Hypertension Optimal Treatment (HOT) trial, and the ADVANCE trial [17, 20, 21]. Each of these studies, together with meta-analysis of combined trials, supports the conclusion that a target blood pressure for diabetic patients of less than 140/90 mmHg is associated with a significant reduction in total cardiovascular risk. The benefit is most marked for prevention of stroke and total cardiovascular mortality, with likely benefits for renal failure and myocardial infarction.

These studies lend support to the recommendation that all patients with diabetes should be treated for hypertension with a target blood pressure of less than 140/90 mmHg. In patients with coexisting microalbuminuria, a more intensive blood pressure target of 130/80 mmHg is supported by some additional studies. Most diabetic patients with hypertension will require more than one antihypertensive drug to achieve this goal.

Effect of Renin-Angiotensin Blockade, Calcium Channel Blockade, and Sodium-Glucose Co-transporter 2 Inhibitors

In addition to the general benefit of the reduction of arterial blood pressure, there seem to be specific renal protective effects from the use of drugs that block the renin–angiotensin axis; that is, ACE inhibitors and ARBs. It is likely that the specific benefits of these drugs relate to their ability to alter intraglomerular pressure, owing to the influence of angiotensin on glomerular efferent arteriolar tone. The stage of microalbuminuria appears to be the time at which treatment with an ACE inhibitor or ARB can most favourably influence the progression of DN. Many randomized controlled trials, and meta-analysis of combined trials, have demonstrated that monotherapy with an ACE inhibitor or ARB produces a greater reduction in protein excretion and better preservation of GFR compared with a placebo treatment, and even with other hypertensive agents that produce a similar reduction in blood pressure [22]. For example, the addition of an ACE inhibitor or ARB will usually lower urinary protein excretion in patients already being treated with a beta-blocker or thiazide diuretic.

Amongst the other antihypertensive drugs, the non-dihydropyridine calcium channel blockers (diltiazem and verapamil) appear to be approximately equally effective to ACE inhibitors or ARB drugs in lowering protein excretion in diabetic patients [23–25]. The beneficial effects of verapamil and ACE inhibitors also appeared to be additive in at least one study. The dihydropyridine calcium channel blockers (amlodipine and nifedipine) and beta-blockers seem inferior to ACE inhibitors or ARBs in their influence on the natural history of DN, despite a similar reduction in blood pressure [26, 27].

Sodium-glucose co-transporter 2 (SGLT2) inhibitors act by reducing the proximal tubular reabsorption of filtered glucose. Although they are not considered first-line oral hypoglycaemic agents, multiple trials including the CANVAS programme and the EMPA-REG OUTCOME trial have shown their beneficial effect in reducing cardiovascular morbidity and mortality in patients with type 2 diabetes, as well as a decreased need for renal replacement therapy or death from renal causes in these patients.

Other Treatments

Dietary Protein Restriction

In experimental animal models and in limited human clinical studies, the restriction of dietary protein intake (e.g. to 0.6 g/kg body weight/day, compared with normal daily intake of 0.8 g/kg) has been associated with a reduction in proteinuria and a diminished rate of deterioration in GFR. However, the clinical benefit of protein restriction is relatively modest, is not proven to be sustained, and places a significant burden on the patient, who is already trying to comply with dietary recommendations for control of blood glucose, lipids, and body weight [28].

Avoidance of Other Renal Insults

Consideration should be given to minimization of additional insults to the kidney in patients with established DN. Nephrotoxic drugs (including NSAIDs, contrast agents, proton pump inhibitors, aminoglycoside antibiotics) and cigarette smoking should be eliminated whenever possible.

Treatment of Diabetes in the Presence of Renal Failure

Development of advanced renal failure introduces significant challenges for the preservation of good blood glucose control. The renal handling of drugs used in the treatment of diabetes also adds complexity to therapy choices. Additionally, uraemia often causes deterioration in appetite, and a further propensity for hypoglycaemia. Hypoglycaemia is to be avoided because it can result in falls and injury, seizure, myocardial infarction, stroke, or death. The risk is greatest in patients who are older and frail, or who have inconsistent eating habits. Patients with advanced DN frequently also have diabetic autonomic neuropathy, which may result in a lack of sympathetic-mediated warning symptoms of hypoglycaemia. Recurrent hypoglycaemic episodes constitute an independent risk factor for CVD, especially myocardial infarction, in this group of patients who have a very high incidence of coexisting coronary artery disease. This combination of factors makes maintenance of blood glucose control difficult in diabetic patients entering ESRD.

Metformin is associated with a small risk of lactic acidosis. Whilst this risk is negligible in the presence of normal renal and hepatic function, it rises significantly in the presence of CKD. Most clinical practice guidelines stipulate that that metformin should be stopped once serum creatinine exceeds 150 µmol/l (1.7 mg/dl) or eGFR falls below 30 ml/min per 1.73 m^2 [29, 30]. The safety of newer antidiabetic agents, such as SGLT2 inhibitors or glucagon-like peptide-1 (GLP-1) agonists, in advanced renal failure is less clear. Hence, most oral diabetes drugs need to be stopped in patients with advanced renal failure, and insulin becomes the mainstay of treatment for maintaining blood glucose control. Linagliptin is the only dipeptidyl peptidase-4 (DPP4) inhibitor which by virtue of non-renal elimination can be safely used in CKD.

After renal failure ensues, the benefit of intense blood glucose control is unproven and the risks of hypoglycaemia are significantly higher. Therefore, easing of strict blood glucose targets may be appropriate in patients with advanced DN. There are insufficient research data on the ideal glycaemic target in CKD stage 3 or more, and individualizing goals for each patient is important to optimize the risk to benefit ratio [31].

Monitoring glycaemic control in CKD can be difficult. HbA1c may be a less valid index of blood glucose flux due to factors such as anaemia, haemolysis, iron deficiency or blood transfusions. HbA1c can be falsely high from carbamylation of haemoglobin or in the presence of acidosis. Fructosamine, a measure of multiple glycated serum proteins, is an alternative measure of glycaemic control, but has not proven to be superior to HbA1c in patients with CKD. Therefore, HbA1c remains widely used in these patients [32]. Regular self-monitored finger-prick blood glucose readings are the most useful data for insulin dose titration.

Alterations in Insulin Action in Renal Failure

The kidney normally plays a pivotal role in the clearance and degradation of circulating insulin. Insulin secreted by the pancreas enters the portal vein and approximately half is cleared during the first pass through the liver. Of the remaining insulin that subsequently enters the systemic circulation, most is cleared on passage through the kidney, with a short half-life of only four to six minutes [33]. In patients with diabetes who inject exogenous insulin, the absorption is entirely into the systemic (not portal) venous system, so that the relative contribution of the kidney to insulin metabolism is even greater. Insulin is a 51-amino acid peptide hormone with a molecular weight of approximately 6000 Da (about one-tenth the size of albumin) and it is freely filtered at the glomerulus. Insulin in the tubular lumen is taken up into proximal tubular cells by carrier-mediated endocytosis and then undergoes proteolytic breakdown to oligopeptides and amino acids. Consequently, less than 1% of filtered insulin appears in the urine. However, there is a process of active transport of insulin from peritubular capillaries into tubular cells, with consequent tubular secretion. The net effect of the tubular secretion of insulin is that the total rate of renal clearance of insulin at 200 ml/min exceeds GFR (120 ml/min) by approximately 50%.

In CKD, impairment of the renal clearance of insulin substantially prolongs the half-life of circulating insulin; particularly that of exogenously administered insulin. This explains the clinical observation of a substantial decrease in the insulin requirement and increased incidence of hypoglycaemia in diabetic patients with worsening CKD.

Dialysis in Patients with Diabetes

Diabetes is now the leading cause of ESRD requiring dialysis in Australia, accounting for one in three new cases in 2011 [34]. The choice of dialysis modality for patients with diabetes is therefore an important question. Considerations include the impact of dialysis method on blood glucose control, and the effect of diabetes and its cardiovascular complications on dialysis efficacy. The survival for those with diabetes on dialysis is poor, at 78.3% and 37.9% at one and five years, respectively [35]. Survival of those with diabetes on dialysis is lower than those without diabetes on dialysis, with CVD being the main cause of morbidity and mortality [36]. The pathophysiology of CVD in advanced DN is a complex interaction of atherosclerotic arterial disease, left ventricular hypertrophy, chronic volume overload, anaemia, inflammation, oxidant stress, elevated homocysteine, and other aspects of the uraemic milieu [37].

Whilst the choice between haemodialysis (HD) and peritoneal dialysis (PD) often depends on non-medical factors (cost, location, independence and motivation of the patient, manual dexterity, and visual acuity), a patient with diabetes is more likely to have additional medical factors which influence choice of dialysis method, compared to patients with non-diabetic renal disease (Table 15.3). The presence of advanced CVD or severe diabetic neuropathy also affects the choice regarding the modality of dialysis. Additionally, the effect of absorption of glucose from PD fluids can have a significant impact on blood glucose control.

Autonomic neuropathy, a complication of diabetes, can result in increased risk of hypotension due to an inability of the autonomic nervous system to compensate for the changes in circulating volume which are associated with dialysis. Since fluid shifts are more gradual with PD, it may be better tolerated than HD. The presence of severe peripheral arterial disease in patients with diabetes may limit the ability to form a functional arterio-venous anastomosis or may decrease effective flow rates and compromise HD efficiency. Patients with advanced DN usually have coexisting retinopathy, which may severely limit vision and the patient's capacity for the self-management of dialysis.

PD is less expensive and does not require vascular access. Though PD may seem to provide a survival advantage over HD in the first two to four years of treatment, many studies, mainly retrospective and observational, have found conflicting or no differences in the mortality of PD versus HD. Few patients choose home HD, which is generally associated with the highest survival rates.

Table 15.3 Potential benefits of peritoneal dialysis (PD) versus haemodialysis (HD) in patients with end-stage renal failure due to diabetic nephropathy

Potential benefits of PD	Potential benefits of HD
<ul><li>Home-based therapy</li><li>Greater autonomy and independence than HD</li><li>No need for vascular access or pain from needle puncture</li><li>Gradual fluid shifts and less risk of hypotension</li></ul>	<ul><li>Faster fluid removal</li><li>Faster correction of potassium</li><li>Less risk of non-compliance</li><li>Less impact on glycaemic management than PD</li></ul>

In PD, a high glucose concentration in the dialysate fluid creates an osmotic effect to draw interstitial fluid and solutes into the peritoneal cavity. However, the peritoneum provides a large surface area for the absorption of intra-peritoneal glucose. Depending on dialysate glucose concentration and dwell-time, the amount of glucose absorbed may constitute 12–34% of total caloric intake, which is enough to have a significant impact on blood glucose control and nutritional status [38]. Variation in glucose absorption from PD fluid, due to alterations in fluid prescription or altered peritoneal absorption, can contribute to blood glucose instability in PD patients. The addition of insulin directly to PD fluid to correct hyperglycaemia has been common practice in the past. It is no longer recommended because of high insulin requirements due to losses in dialysate and binding to PD bags and tubes, complicated insulin regimens, risk of bacterial contamination of dialysate, an associated risk of peritoneal fibroblastic proliferation and, possibly, risk of hepatic steatosis [39, 40]. The subcutaneous route remains the preferred method of insulin administration in all patients.

Kidney Transplantation in Patients with Diabetes

Renal transplant is the preferred form of renal replacement therapy in ESRD. Of those with ESRD who receive renal transplantation, quality of life, and overall survival are significantly higher (85% at five years versus 36–42% with HD/PD) [35]. However, comorbidities or complications of diabetes can pose a problem when a patient is being considered for a renal transplant. The incidence of CVD, and hence of adverse cardiac events in the early and late post-transplant period is higher in diabetic transplant recipients [41]. Clinically silent coronary artery or cerebrovascular disease is highly prevalent, and all patients should undergo non-invasive or angiographic evaluation as part of a pre-transplant workup. Coronary or carotid revascularization should be considered prior to transplant, when indicated.

After transplantation, the risk of fungal and bacterial infections is elevated in those with diabetes and is additive to the risks of pharmacological immune suppression. Steroid-based regimens also have a negative impact on blood glucose control. Requirement for a glucocorticoid dose greater than

prednisone 5 mg daily or equivalent is associated with insulin resistance and hyperglycaemia. This has important implications for the risk of recurrence of diabetic lesions in the transplanted kidney [41, 42], as well as the progression of other diabetes complications. The commonly used post-transplant medications, calcineurin inhibitors (cyclosporine and tacrolimus), are diabetogenic and can cause worsening of blood sugar control in the diabetic patient.

A simultaneous pancreas–kidney transplant (SPKT) is theoretically an ideal solution to deal with patients with type 1 diabetes and ESRD, but not for the more numerous cases of type 2 diabetes (where insulin resistance, not pancreatic failure, is implicated in the pathogenesis). Some studies have suggested increased survival in SPKT for appropriate patient cohorts [43]. However, the disadvantages of SPKT include the scarcity of donor organs (no live donors for pancreas transplantation, and only one organ per cadaveric donor) and the increased complexity of surgery. Other options such as pancreas-after-kidney transplant and islet cell transplantation have also been utilized in type 1 diabetes. However, access to such programmes remains severely limited, and relapse of diabetes due to chronic pancreatic rejection remains a significant problem.

Pregnancy in Diabetic Nephropathy

Women with ESRD are usually anovulatory and infertile. However, women with early DN characterized by albuminuria or mild renal impairment can generally conceive spontaneously or with assisted fertility measures.

DN complicates 5–10% of pregnancies in women with type 1 or type 2 diabetes. It may adversely affect the outcome of pregnancy by three mechanisms: development of severe hypertension with deterioration of maternal renal function, preterm delivery due to hypertension and preeclampsia, and foetal intrauterine growth restriction and foetal distress caused by placental dysfunction [44]. A slightly higher prevalence of severe congenital malformations has been described in women with DN compared with women with diabetes and normal kidney function [45].

Renal function can decline during the course of pregnancy. Pregnancy is associated with increased renal blood flow and increased GFR, which can

Table 15.4 Pre-pregnancy planning for women with diabetic nephropathy

- Counselling for couples
- Start high-dose folic acid 5 mg daily to reduce neurocongenital defects
- Attain a pre-conception haemoglobin A1c <7%
- Stop antidiabetic medications and use insulin and/or metformin
- Screen and treat for retinopathy and coronary artery disease prior to conception
- Stop statins
- Stop angiotensin-converting enzyme inhibitors and angiotensin receptor blockers and replace with pregnancy-safe antihypertensives

accelerate renal decline in women who have nephropathy, likely due to glomerular hyperfiltration and increased renal vasodilation. Generally, women with microalbuminuria and normal GFR have a low risk of worsening of renal function in pregnancy, but may have a transient increase in albuminuria [46]. On the other hand, those with poorly controlled hypertension, reduced GFR or high-range proteinuria at the start of pregnancy have higher perinatal risks of decline in maternal kidney function leading to ESRD, preeclampsia, preterm delivery, and perinatal mortality [47]. Therefore, assessment for the extent of DN is an important part of a pre-conception workup for women with diabetes (Table 15.4). It is necessary to provide careful counselling for the woman and her partner of the pregnancy risks before they consider pregnancy. In women presenting with unplanned pregnancy, assessment of proteinuria, blood pressure control, and GFR allows stratification of risk.

It is vital to achieve strict control of blood glucose levels and blood pressure during pregnancy to reduce maternal and foetal complications. The choice of antihypertensive therapy in pregnancy is limited due to the potential for teratogenicity. ACE inhibitors and ARBs are contraindicated in pregnancy and should be stopped in women planning pregnancy, or immediately after diagnosis of an unplanned pregnancy. Antihypertensive drugs with an established safety record for pregnancy include labetalol, oxprenolol, hydralazine, and methyldopa. Use of aspirin before pregnancy and/or after foetal organogenesis may prevent preeclampsia [48]. Insulin is the mainstay of diabetes management in pregnancy, and insulin requirements increase substantially in the second and third trimesters due to the insulin-resistance effect of placental hormones. Most oral antidiabetic medications are contraindicated for use in pregnancy, although recent evidence suggests that metformin may be safely used in women with gestational diabetes or type 2 diabetes, where it has an insulin-sparing effect and also minimizes excess maternal weight gain.

References

1. Afkarian, M., Sachs, M., Kestenbaum, B. et al. (2013). Kidney disease and increased mortality risk in type 2 diabetes. *J. Am. Soc. Nephrol.* 24 (2): 302–308.
2. Tervaert, T., Mooyaart, A., Amann, K. et al. (2010). Pathologic classification of diabetic nephropathy. *J. Am. Soc. Nephrol.* 21 (4): 556–563.
3. Luychx, V.A. and Brenner, B.M. (2005). Low birth weight, nephron number and kidney disease. *Kidney Int.* 68: S68–S77.
4. Tuttle, K.R., Bruton, J.L., Perusek, M.C. et al. (1991). Effect of strict glycemic control on renal haemodynamic response to aminoacids and renal enlargement in insulin-dependent diabetes mellitus. *N. Engl. J. Med.* 324 (23): 1626.
5. Lupia, E., Elliot, S.J., Lenz, O. et al. (1999). IGF-1 decreases collagen degradation in diabetic NOD mesangial cells: implications for diabetic nephropathy. *Diabetes* 48 (8): 1638–1644.
6. Kassab, J.P., Guillot, R., Andre, J. et al. (1994). Renal and microvascular effects of an aldose reductase inhibitor in experimental diabetes. Biochemical, functional and ultrastructural studies. *Biochem. Pharmacol.* 48 (5): 1003–1008.
7. Wolf, G. and Ziyadeh, F. (1999). Molecular mechanisms of diabetic renal hypertrophy. *Kidney Int.* 56 (2): 393–405.
8. Benigni, A., Gagliardini, E., Tomasoni, S. et al. (2004). Selective impairment of gene expression and assembly of nephrin in human diabetic nephropathy. *Kidney Int.* 65 (6): 2193–2200.
9. Evans, T. and Capell, P. (2000). Diabetic nephropathy. *Clin. Diabetes.* 18 (1): 7.
10. Fox, C.S., Matsushita, K., Woodward, M. et al. (2012). Chronic Kidney Disease Prognosis Consortium. Associations of kidney disease measures with mortality and end-stage renal disease in individuals with and without diabetes: a meta-analysis. *Lancet* 380: 1662–1673.
11. Groop, P.-H., Thomas, M.C., Moran, J.L. et al. (2009). FinnDiane Study Group. The presence and severity of chronic kidney disease predicts all-cause mortality in type 1 diabetes. *Diabetes* 58: 1651–1658.

12. Afkarian, M., Sachs, M.C., Kestenbaum, B. et al. (2013). Kidney disease and increased mortality risk in type 2 diabetes. *J. Am. Soc. Nephrol.* 24: 302–308.

13. American Diabetes Association (2010). Executive summary: standards of medical care in diabetes – 2011. *Diabetes Care* 34 (Supplement_1): S4–S10.

14. Brunner, F.P. and Selwood, N.H. (1992). Profile of patients on RRT in Europe and death rates due to major causes of death groups. The EDTA Registration Committee. *Kidney Int. Supplement* 38: S4.

15. Kramer, H.J., Nguyen, Q.D., Curhan, G., and Hsu, C.Y. (2003). Renal insufficiency in the absence of albuminuria and retinopathy among adults with type 2 diabetes mellitus. *JAMA* 289: 3273.

16. Levey, A. (2003). National Kidney Foundation practice guidelines for chronic kidney disease: evaluation, classification, and stratification. *Ann. Intern. Med.* 139 (2): 137.

17. UK Prospective Diabetes Study (UKPDS) Group (1998). Intensive blood-glucose control with sulphonylureas or insulin compared with conventional treatment and risk of complications in patients with type 2 diabetes (UKPDS 33). *Lancet* 352: 837.

18. Microalbuminuria Collaborative Study Group (1992). Microalbuminuria in type I diabetic patients. Prevalence and clinical characteristics. *Diabetes Care* 15: 495.

19. Diabetes Control and Complications Trial Research Group (DCCT) (1993). The effect of intensive treatment of diabetes on the development and progression of long-term complications in insulin-dependent diabetes mellitus. *N. Engl. J. Med.* 329: 977.

20. Cruickshank, J.M. (1998). Hypertension Optimal Treatment (HOT) trial. *Lancet* 352: 573–574.

21. ADVANCE Collaborative Group, Patel, A., MacMahon, S. et al. (2560). Intensive blood glucose control and vascular outcomes in patients with type 2 diabetes. *N. Engl. J. Med.* 2008: 358.

22. Kunz, R., Friedrich, C., Wolbers, M., and Mann, J.F. (2008). Meta-analysis: effect of monotherapy and combination therapy with inhibitors of the renin angiotensin system on proteinuria in renal disease. *Ann. Intern. Med.* 148: 30.

23. Bakris, G.L. (1990). Effects of diltiazem or lisinopril on massive proteinuria associated with diabetes mellitus. *Ann. Intern. Med.* 112: 707.

24. Böhlen, L., de Courten, M., and Weidmann, P. (1994). Comparative study of the effect of ACE-inhibitors and other antihypertensive agents on proteinuria in diabetic patients. *Am. J. Hypertens.* 7: 84S.

25. Bakris, G.L., Copley, J.B., Vicknair, N. et al. (1996). Calcium channel blockers versus other antihypertensive therapies on progression of NIDDM associated nephropathy. *Kidney Int.* 50: 1641.

26. Bakris, G.L., Weir, M.R., Secic, M. et al. (2004). Differential effects of calcium antagonist subclasses on markers of nephropathy progression. *Kidney Int.* 65: 1991.

27. Agodoa, L.Y., Appel, L., Bakris, G.L. et al. (2001). Effect of ramipril vs amlodipine on renal outcomes in hypertensive nephrosclerosis: a randomized controlled trial. *JAMA* 285: 2719.

28. Menon, V., Kopple, J.D., Wang, X. et al. (2009). Effect of a very low-protein diet on outcomes: long-term follow-up of the Modification of Diet in Renal Disease (MDRD) study. *Am. J. Kidney Dis.* 53: 208.

29. Lipska, K.J., Bailey, C.J., and Inzucchi, S.E. (2011). Use of metformin in the setting of mild-to-moderate renal insufficiency. *Diabetes Care* 34 (6): 1431–1437.

30. Sambol, N.C., Chiang, J., Lin, E.T. et al. (1995). Kidney function and age are both predictors of pharmacokinetics of metformin. *J. Clin. Pharmacol.* 35: 1094–1102.

31. KDOQI (Kidney Disease Outcomes Quality Initiative) (2012). Clinical practice guideline for diabetes and CKD: 2012 update. *Am. J. Kidney Dis.* 60: 850–886.

32. Freedman, B.I., Shenoy, R.N., Planer, J.A. et al. (2010). Comparison of glycated albumin and hemoglobin A1c concentrations in diabetic subjects on peritoneal and hemodialysis. *Perit. Dial. Int.* 30: 72–79.

33. Duckworth, W.C., Bennett, R.G., and Hamel, F.G. (1998). Insulin degradation: progress and potential. *Endocr. Rev.* 19 (5): 608–624.

34. ANZ DATA (2013). Australia and New Zealand Dialysis and Transplant Registry. www.anzdata. org.au/anzdata/AnzdataReport/36thReport/ 2013c02_newpatients_v1.7.pdf (accessed 23 October 2016).

35. Cardiovascular Disease in Patients with ESRD. (2015). United States Renal Data System. https:// www.usrds.org/2015/download/vol2_09_ CVD_15.pdf (accessed 23 October 2016).

36. Dikow, R. and Ritz, E. (2003). Cardiovascular complications in the diabetic patient with renal disease: an update in 2003. *Nephrol. Dial. Transpl.* 18: 1993.

37. Meeus, F.K.O., Guerin, A.P., Gaudry, C. et al. (2000). Pathophysiology of cardiovascular disease in hemodialysis patients. *Kidney Int.* 76: S140–S147.

38. Grodstein, G.P., Blumenkrantz, M.J., Kopple, J.D. et al. (1981). Glucose absorption during continuous ambulatory peritoneal dialysis. *Kidney Int.* 19 (4): 564–567.

39. Diaz-Buxo, J.A. (1993). Blood glucose control in diabetics: I. *Semin. Dialy* 6: 392.

40. Quellhorst, E. (2002). Insulin therapy during peritoneal dialysis: pros and cons of various forms of administration. *J. Am. Soc. Nephrol.* 13 (Suppl 1): S92.

41. Lentine, K.L., Rocca Rey, L.A., Kolli, S. et al. (2008). Variations in the risk for cerebrovascular events after kidney transplant compared with experience on the waiting list and after graft failure. *Clin. J. Am. Soc. Nephro.* 3: 1090–1101.

42. Gill, J.S., Tonelli, M., Johnson, N., and Pereira, B.J. (2004). Why do preemptive kidney transplant recipients have an allograft survival advantage? *Transplantation* 78: 873–879.

43. Ojo, A.O., Meier-Kriesche, H.U., Hanson, J.A. et al. (2001). The impact of simultaneous pancreas-kidney transplantation on long-term patient survival. *Transplantation* 71 (1): 82–90.

44. Nevis, I.F., Reitsma, A., Dominic, A. et al. (2011). Pregnancy outcomes in women with chronic kidney disease: a systematic review. *Clin. J. Am. Soc. Nephrol.* 6 (11): 2587–2598.

45. Bell, R., Glinianaia, S., Tennant, P. et al. (2012). Peri-conception hyperglycaemia and nephropathy are associated with risk of congenital anomaly in women with pre-existing diabetes: a population-based cohort study. *Diabetologia* 55 (4): 936–947.

46. Vérier-Mine, O., Chaturvedi, N., Webb, D., and Fuller, J.H. (2005). Is pregnancy a risk factor for microvascular complications? The EURODIAB prospective complications study. *Diabetic Med.* 22: 1503.

47. Biesenbach, G., Stöger, H., and Zazgornik, J. (1992). Influence of pregnancy on progression of diabetic nephropathy and subsequent requirement of renal replacement therapy in female type I diabetic patients with impaired renal function. *Nephrol. Dial. Transpl.* 7: 105.

48. Duley, L., Henderson-Smart, D.J., Meher, S., and King, J.F. (2007). Antiplatelet agents for preventing pre-eclampsia and its complications. *Cochrane Database Syst. Rev* 2: CD004659. https://doi.org/10.1002/14651858.CD004659. pub2.

Questions and Answers

Questions

1. A 52-year-old man has T2DM for nearly 10 years. He has been on metformin therapy for five years. His general practitioner noticed that his renal function has been slowly declining over the years and suspects diabetic nephropathy. Below what eGFR should he consider ceasing metformin?
   a. $15\,ml/min/1.73\,m^2$
   b. $30\,ml/min/1.73\,m^2$
   c. $45\,ml/min/1.73\,m^2$
   d. $60\,ml/min/1.73\,m^2$
   e. No need to stop at any eGFR

2. A 65-year-old lady presents to her general practitioner for an annual review. She has a four-year history of T2DM. Her blood pressure was $150/90\,mmHg$. Spot urine test revealed microalbuminuria of $50\,mg/mmol$ Cr. Which antihypertensive is most appropriate for this patient?
   a. Perindopril
   b. Metoprolol
   c. Amlodipine
   d. Nifedipine
   e. No need for antihypertensive

3. Which one or more of following statements regarding DN are true:
   a. Glomerulosclerosis is a histological feature.
   b. It occurs only in those with type 1 DM.
   c. It usually presents as a sudden deterioration in renal function.

   d. Only those with poor blood pressure control should be screened for DN.
   e. It can lead to ESRD.

4. Which of the following medications is most suitable in a patient with very poorly controlled T2DM with an HbA1c of 12% and has an eGFR of $10\,ml/min/1.73\,m^2$?
   a. Metformin
   b. Dapagliflozin
   c. Acarbose
   d. Exenatide
   e. Insulin

5. Which one of the following is a risk factor for developing DN?
   a. Poorly controlled diabetes
   b. Hypertension
   c. Genetic predisposition
   d. Elevated lipid levels
   e. All of the above

6. A 39-year-old female with DN is now planning pregnancy. Which of the following is an inappropriate action?
   a. Provide counselling to her and her partner on the pregnancy risks
   b. High-dose folic acid 5 mg daily
   c. Achieve pre-conception glycaemic control of HbA1c <7%
   d. Blood pressure control with ACE-I or ARB
   e. Screen and treat for retinopathy and coronary artery disease prior to conception

Answers

1. b. Metformin can be used in dose reductions down to an eGFR of <30 ml/min/1.73 m², after which it is advisable to be stopped, mainly to reduce the risk of lactic acidosis.

2. a. Strict arterial blood pressure control has proven to be one of the most important factors in preventing or delaying progression of diabetic nephropathy, and other cardiovascular complications. Studies support the recommendation that all patients with diabetes should be treated for hypertension with a target blood pressure of less than 140/90 mmHg. In patients with coexisting microalbuminuria, a more intensive blood pressure target of 130/80 is supported by some additional studies. In addition to the general benefit of the reduction of arterial blood pressure, there appears to be specific renal protective effects with the use of drugs that block the renin-angiotensin axis; angiotensin converting enzyme inhibitors (ACE-I) and angiotensin receptor blockers (ARB). It is likely that the specific benefits of these drugs relate to their ability to alter intraglomerular pressure, owing to the role of angiotensin in causing efferent arteriolar vasoconstriction.

3. a and e. The three major histologic changes in the glomeruli in DN are mesangial expansion, GBM thickening, and glomerulosclerosis. DN can occur in both types 1 and 2 diabetes with similar incidence. The onset of DN is gradual and its progression is slow and insidious. If a patient with diabetes experiences a sudden deterioration in renal function, it is unlikely to be due to diabetic nephropathy alone. All patients with diabetes should be screened on a regular basis for evidence of early diabetic nephropathy so that interventions may be undertaken to prevent or delay its progression.

DN can eventually result in ESRD. Diabetes is now the leading cause of ESRD in Australia, accounting for 1 in 3 new cases in 2011.

4. e. The choice of medications used in CKD requires knowledge in which ones can be used safely. It is important to note that many antidiabetic medications are renally cleared. Hence, a dose reduction or cessation may be necessary in renal failure. Metformin can be used in dose reductions down to an eGFR of <30 ml/min/1.73 m², after which it is advisable to be stopped, mainly to reduce the risk of lactic acidosis. The safety of the newer agents such as SGLT2 inhibitors or GLP-1 agonists in renal failure is less clear. Linagliptin is the only DPP4-inhibitor which by virtue of non-renal elimination can be safely used in CKD. Sulphonylureas can be used but run a higher risk of causing hypoglycaemia given the reduced renal clearance. Insulin is the mainstay of treatment.

5. e. Blood glucose control is a strong predictor of the risk of diabetic nephropathy, though there is significant intra-individual variation. Genetic predisposition seems to influence the susceptibility to hyperglycaemic injury as evidenced by familial clustering of DN in both types 1 and 2 diabetes. Arterial hypertension and atherosclerosis are also crucial contributors. Smoking habits, and the amount and origin of dietary protein also seem to play a role as risk factors.

6. d. It is vital to strictly control blood glucose levels and blood pressure during pregnancy to reduce maternal and foetal complications. Choice of antihypertensive medication use in pregnancy is limited due to potential for teratogenicity. ACE inhibitors and ARBs are contraindicated in pregnancy and should be stopped in women planning pregnancy, or immediately after diagnosis of an unplanned pregnancy.

16

Kidney Disease in Myeloma and Other Monoclonal Gammopathies

M.K. Phanish and Vinay Sakhuja

Summary

- Plasma cell dyscrasias are a heterogenous group of disorders characterized by the proliferation of monoclonal bone marrow plasma cells.
- Whilst the paraprotein produced can be free light chains, heavy chains or intact immunoglobulins, there is always an excess of free light chain production.
- Common renal disorders associated with monoclonal plasma cell disorders are myeloma cast nephropathy (myeloma kidney), amyloid light chain (AL) amyloidosis, light/heavy chain deposition disease, and cryoglobulinaemia.
- The recently coined term monoclonal gammopathy of renal significance refers to renal disease attributable to paraprotein (on histological evidence) in the absence of other criteria for the diagnosis of myeloma.
- Serum free light chain assay is a useful adjunct to protein electrophoresis and immunofixation for improved diagnostic sensitivity and monitoring response to therapy.
- Slightly elevated serum kappa/lambda ratio is common in chronic kidney disease due to reduced glomerular filtration rate.
- Common clinical presentations include acute kidney injury (myeloma cast nephropathy, sepsis, dehydration and hypercalcaemia) and nephrotic syndrome (AL amyloidosis, light chain deposition disease).
- Chemotherapy followed by autologous stem cell transplantation in appropriate patients is the treatment of choice for multiple myeloma and AL amyloidosis.

Lecture Notes Nephrology: A Comprehensive Guide to Renal Medicine, First Edition. Edited by Surjit Tarafdar.
© 2020 John Wiley & Sons Ltd. Published 2020 by John Wiley & Sons Ltd.

Plasma cell dyscrasias are a heterogenous group of disorders characterized by the proliferation of monoclonal bone marrow plasma cells. Clinical manifestations can range from relatively benign presentation with an incidental discovery of paraprotein to an aggressive malignant disease. These diseases are often associated with kidney disease, and advanced kidney disease can limit treatment options, making early diagnosis and treatment an essential aspect of care given to these patients.

Monoclonal disorders of plasma cells include:

- Monoclonal gammopathy of uncertain/undetermined significance (MGUS)
- Monoclonal gammopathy of renal significance (MGRS)
- Multiple myeloma (MM)
- Waldenström's macroglobulinaemia
- Solitary plasmacytoma
- Amyloid light chain (AL) amyloidosis

The commonest plasma cell disorder that a nephrologist deals with is MM, a malignant disorder of immunoglobulin producing plasma cells derived from a single clone (monoclonal) of B lymphocytes [1]. The plasma cells proliferate in the bone marrow and can cause extensive skeletal damage. Myeloma usually presents as one or more of the following clinical presentations:

- Bone pain with lytic lesions discovered on routine skeletal films.
- Unexplained anaemia.
- Hypercalcaemia, which is either symptomatic or discovered incidentally.
- Acute renal failure with a bland urinalysis (rarely with urinary dysmorphic red blood cells (RBCs)/ RBC casts in case of membranoproliferative glomerulonephritis (MPGN) or cryoglobulinaemic vasculitis), or less commonly nephrotic syndrome due to concurrent AL amyloidosis or light chain deposition disease.

The hyperglobulinaemia in MM is monoclonal, in contrast to the polyclonal hyperglobulinaemia seen in infective or inflammatory conditions due to excessive proliferation of normal plasma cells.

Myeloma accounts for around 13% of all haematological cancers and is characterized by dysregulated overproduction of immunoglobulins by a single clone of malignant plasma cells. Paraproteins produced are immunoglobulin (Ig) G in 52%, IgA in 21%, kappa or lambda light chain only (Bence-Jones protein) in 16%, IgD in 2%, biclonal in 2%, IgM in 0.5%, negative (non-secretory) in 6.5% of cases. The malignant cells always make an excess of light chains irrespective of whether the primary paraprotein being produced is a full Ig molecule or the light chain. Light chains, by virtue of their smaller size, are freely filtered across the glomeruli and hence cause nephrotoxicity, as discussed later. The disease is cytogenetically heterogeneous and is commonly preceded by an asymptomatic premalignant stage called MGUS (IgG MGUS in about 80% of cases and 20% from light chain MGUS [1, 2]). MM is predominantly a disorder of older individuals, but increasing numbers of younger patients diagnosed with myeloma are being seen in clinical practice, with 37% patients younger than 65 years at the time of diagnosis [3].

Renal involvement is an important feature of myeloma and primary amyloidosis and forms an important component of the CRAB features (hye**r**calcaemia, **r**enal failure, **a**naemia, **b**one lesions) required for the diagnosis of MM. In 2014, the International Myeloma Working Group updated the criteria for the diagnosis of MM [2]; these are summarized in Table 16.1.

Renal Involvement in Monoclonal Plasma Cell Disorders

Epidemiology

Whilst 20–40% of newly diagnosed myeloma patients will have acute kidney injury (AKI) or chronic kidney disease (CKD) on presentation, almost 50% will have AKI or CKD at some stage during their disease [4]. Up to 10% of patients present in severe renal failure needing dialysis and only 15–30% of these patients can discontinue dialysis. Prognosis in MM is inversely related to the severity of renal dysfunction. Whilst bortezomib-based therapy has improved survival in MM patients with renal involvement, the median survival of those needing dialysis is 28 months, versus 90 months for those not needing dialysis.

Types of Renal Disease in Monoclonal Plasma Cell Disorders

Tubular disorders are more often responsible for renal failure than glomerular pathologies in patients with MM. The various renal pathologies seen in this condition (Table 16.2) are:

- **Tubular:**

- Light chain cast nephropathy (myeloma kidney): 30–50%
- Interstitial nephritis/fibrosis: 20–30%

Table 16.1 Revised International Myeloma Working Group diagnostic criteria for multiple myeloma, smouldering multiple myeloma and monoclonal gammopathy of undetermined significance [2]

Definition of multiple myeloma
Clonal bone marrow plasma cells ≥10% or biopsy-proven bony or extramedullary plasmacytoma and any one or more of the following myeloma-defining events:
1. Evidence of end-organ damage that can be attributed to the underlying plasma cell proliferative disorder, specifically:
• Hypercalcaemia: serum calcium >0.25 mmol/l (>1 mg/dl) higher than the upper limit of normal or >2.75 mmol/l (>11 mg/dl)
• Renal insufficiency: creatinine clearance <40 ml per min or serum creatinine >177 μmol/l (>2 mg/dl)
• Anaemia: haemoglobin value of >20 g/l below the lower limit of normal, or a haemoglobin value <100 g/l
• Bone lesions: one or more osteolytic lesions on skeletal radiography, computed tomography (CT), or positron emission tomography-CT (PET-CT)
2. Any one or more of the following:
• Clonal bone marrow plasma cell ≥60%
• Involved: uninvolved serum free light chain ratio ≥100
• >1 focal lesions on magnetic resonance imaging studies
Definition of smouldering multiple myeloma
Both criteria must be met:
• Serum monoclonal protein ≥30 g/l or urinary monoclonal protein ≥500 mg/24 hours and/or clonal bone marrow plasma cells 10–60%
• Absence of myeloma defining events or amyloidosis
Definition of monoclonal gammopathy of undetermined significance
All three criteria must be met:
• Serum monoclonal protein <30 g/l
• Bone marrow plasma cells <10%
• Absence of myeloma-defining events or amyloidosis (or Waldenström's macroglobulinemia in the case of immunoglobulin M monoclonal gammopathy of uncertain/undetermined significance)

- Acute tubular necrosis: 10%
- Fanconi syndrome (rare)

- **Glomerular:**

- Amyloidosis: 10%
- Monoclonal immunoglobulin deposition disease (mostly light chain deposition disease): 5%
- Rarely, cryoglobulinaemia, MPGN, dense deposit disease, fibrillary glomerulopathy, and immunotactoid glomerulopathy

- **Others:**

- Hypercalcaemia, urate nephropathy, Fanconi syndrome

Pathogenesis of Acute Kidney Injury in Monoclonal Plasma Cell Disorders

Free light chains, which are always produced in excess in patents with myeloma, are extensively filtered across the glomeruli, unlike the non-filterable bigger immunoglobulin molecules. The filtered light chains are reabsorbed by the proximal convoluted tubular (PCT) cells. Once endocytosed, the free light chains are toxic to the PCT cells, and this leads to the picture of proximal renal tubular acidosis and Fanconi syndrome. Injury to the PCT cells allows overflow of free light

Table 16.2 Histological lesions present with distinct clinical entities in monoclonal plasma cell disorders

Histology	Renal function	Clinical presentation and urinalysis
Cast nephropathy (30–50%)	Reduced glomerular filtration rate (GFR)	Acute kidney injury (AKI) Tubular proteinuria (generally <1–2g/day), light chains in urine, no haematuria
Acute tubular necrosis (10%)	Reduced GFR	AKI Normal urinalysis
Monoclonal immunoglobulin deposition disease (5%)	Normal or reduced GFR	Nephrotic syndrome; AKI Nephrotic-range proteinuria (>3–3.5g/day), light chains in the urine, no haematuria
AL amyloidosis (10%)	Normal or reduced GFR	Nephrotic syndrome Nephrotic-range proteinuria (>3–3.5g/day), light chains in the urine, no haematuria Hypotension is commonly seen secondary to autonomic nervous system and/or cardiac involvement
Cryoglobulinaemic glomerulonephritis and membranoproliferative glomerulonephritis (<1%)	Reduced GFR	AKI, rapidly progressive glomerulonephritis Haematuria, proteinuria, casts

chains to the ascending limb of the loop of Henle, where they bind to the Tamm–Horsfall protein, leading to the formation of tubular casts. These tubular casts occlude the tubular lumen, leading to cast nephropathy (myeloma kidney) and the resultant renal failure. The greater the urinary excretion of free light chains, the greater is the risk for renal failure. The obstructing casts elicit a surrounding interstitial inflammatory reaction with or without multinucleated giant cells and at times lead to tubular rupture, allowing escape of the light chains into the interstitium and leading to an interstitial inflammatory process.

Factors that may promote intratubular cast formation are:

- Volume depletion, by slowing down the flow within the tubules, which can promote cast formation.
- Metabolic acidosis, which by lowering the urinary pH promotes the binding of free light chains to Tamm–Horsfall protein.
- Loop diuretics (which are sometimes used to treat the hypercalcaemia or to promote diuresis in AKI), promote the binding of free light chains to Tamm–Horsfall protein.
- Radiocontrast agents, which may interact with light chains and promote intratubular obstruction.

Hypercalcaemia, which may be seen in up to 15% of patients with myeloma, can precipitate AKI by causing renal vasoconstriction, promoting intratubular calcium deposition or causing volume depletion due to polyuria (resulting in prerenal AKI and/or promotion of tubular cast formation, as already discussed).

Myeloma Cast Nephropathy (Myeloma Kidney)

Cast nephropathy is the commonest cause of AKI in myeloma. The amount of filtered free light chains (light chain load) is a critical factor for the development of cast nephropathy. Excessive monoclonal light chains freely filtered by the glomerulus lead to intratubular cast formation and elicit an inflammatory reaction. The risk of renal failure is twice as high in patients with pure light chain myeloma. More than 70% of patients who secrete >10g/day of light chains develop renal failure [5]. Whilst both kappa and lambda light chains can cause renal injury, some

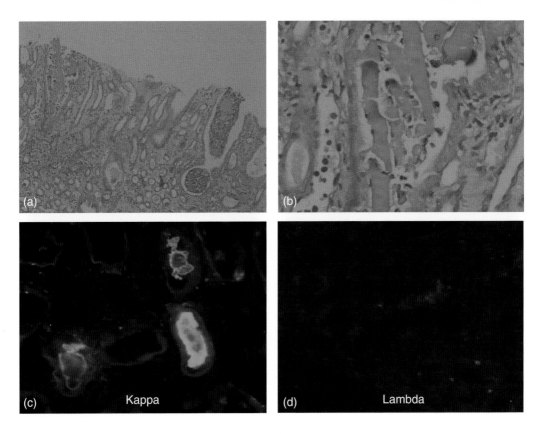

Figure 16.1 Myeloma cast nephropathy. (a) Low-power magnification shows periodic acid–Schiff (PAS)-negative fractured tubular casts. (b) Higher magnification highlights PAS-negative fractured tubular casts with surrounding epithelial cell reaction. Fractured tubular casts are positive for kappa (c) and negative for lambda (d).

series have reported a predominance of lambda isotype and a rare IgD form of myeloma has been associated with renal failure in >90% of cases. It is important to note that light chains in urine are not detected by urinary dipsticks. Interestingly, when light chains from patients with myeloma cast nephropathy are injected into mice, they precipitate in tubules, causing cast nephropathy more frequently when compared to light chains from myeloma patients with normal renal function. This suggests that these light chains causing cast nephropathy are inherently abnormal [6].

Biopsy reveals that the myeloma casts have a hard and fractured appearance and are periodic acid–Schiff (PAS) negative (thus differentiating them from the similar-appearing hyaline casts, which are strongly PAS positive), besides being strongly eosinophilic (Figure 16.1a and b). These casts often also contain rhomboid or needle-shaped crystals. Immunofluorescence typically shows only one type of light chain (Figure 16.1c and d).

Glomeruli are typically spared unless there is associated amyloidosis or light chain deposition disease.

Treatment of Myeloma Cast Nephropathy

Correction of Reversible Factors

These patients often present with significant dehydration and require aggressive hydration with intravenous normal saline. Nephrotoxic medications such as non-steroidal anti-inflammatory drugs (NSAIDs), angiotensin-converting enzyme (ACE) inhibitors, and angiotensin receptor blockers (ARBs) should be ceased. The use of frusemide to promote diuresis should be avoided, as increased distal delivery of sodium (Na^+) and acidic urinary pH can increase binding of free light chains to Tamm–Horsfall protein and thus promote tubular cast formation. Alkalinization of urine with intravenous sodium bicarbonate inhibits cast formation by inhibiting the interaction between the free light chains and Tamm–Horsfall protein [7].

Reducing the Production of Light Chains

Chemotherapy aimed at rapid reduction in the levels of free light chains has resulted in significant improvements in both renal recovery and overall survival [8]. The immediate commencement of high-dose dexamethasone is advised, as the plasma cells are highly responsive to corticosteroids. The first-line agent in the current era is bortezomib, which is a potent proteasome inhibitor. Bortezomib and high-dose dexamethasone are currently thought to be the most effective therapies in the setting of myeloma and AKI. Bortezomib is safe at all levels of kidney function and no glomerular filtration rate (GFR)-dependent dose adjustment is required [9, 10]. In addition to its potent pro-apoptotic effects on monoclonal Ig-producing malignant plasma cells, it is also thought to reduce interstitial inflammation by inhibiting the inflammatory cell signalling cascade triggered by light chain endocytosis in proximal tubules. Due to the latter effect, in clinical practice, improvement in renal function is often seen before the peak effects on plasma cells (which take around 30 days). However, some of the reduction in interstitial inflammation would be attributable to high-dose steroids used concomitantly. Other commonly used drugs include thalidomide (and its derivative lenalidomide) and cyclophosphamide.

Autologous stem cell transplantation (ASCT) following induction chemotherapy with bortezomib/dexamethasone/thalidomide (or lenalidomide) can lead to a response rate of up to 85% with increased survival [11]. The use of melphalan is generally reserved for patients who are not eligible for ASCT due to advanced age (>70 years) and significant comorbidity, as melphalan can adversely affect successful stem cell harvest. A successful ASCT leading to partial or complete remission improves median survival compared to standard chemotherapy by at least 12 months [12]. Unfortunately, myeloma patients with renal failure who probably benefit the most with ASCT are often denied this treatment, as renal failure is generally classed as a contraindication to ASCT due to an increase in toxicity and mortality. However, ASCT has been used to treat patients with serum creatinine of >153 μmol/l (>2 mg/dl) and even in patients with advanced renal failure, including those on dialysis, with good success rates [13, 14]. Therefore, ASCT should be considered as a therapeutic option following chemotherapy in patients with myeloma and renal failure who do not have other significant comorbidities.

Once peripheral stem cell harvest is done, a standard conditioning high-dose treatment regime of melphalan 200 mg/m^2 is used followed by the ASCT. In the current era, the mortality rate of this procedure is <5%.

Extracorporeal Therapies to Remove Light Chains

Plasmapheresis has been used to remove light chains in an attempt to expedite renal recovery, but its utility in the modern era of bortezomib-based chemotherapy remains unproven. A definitive clinical indication for plasmapheresis would be hyperviscosity syndrome. More recently there has been interest in the use of 'high cutoff' dialyser (Gambro HCO 1100), with a pore size large enough to remove the free light chains, but studies have not shown any advantage over conventional dialysis with regard to the recovery of renal function (EuLITE – European Trial of Free Light Chain Removal) [15, 16]. The high cutoff dialysis leads to increased albumin loss by virtue of the larger pore size of the membrane.

Survival of myeloma patients who remain in renal failure is poor, with the reported median survival on dialysis quite dismal [17]. Sepsis is the major cause of mortality and morbidity. There are infrequent reports of kidney transplantation among patients who are in remission and are free from extrarenal manifestations for more than a year.

With regard to dialysis, both haemodialysis and peritoneal dialysis appear to be equally effective.

Amyloid Light Chain Amyloidosis

Amyloidosis is a disorder characterized by extracellular tissue deposition of fibrils composed of low molecular weight subunits of a variety of proteins, many of which circulate as normal constituents of plasma. The deposition of these fibrils in various organs can lead to different clinical presentations [18]. For reasons which are not yet fully understood, soluble proteins undergo conformational changes leading to the generation of insoluble and rigid fibrillary subunits with a predominantly anti-parallel beta-pleated sheet configuration. These fibrils have a characteristic appearance on electron

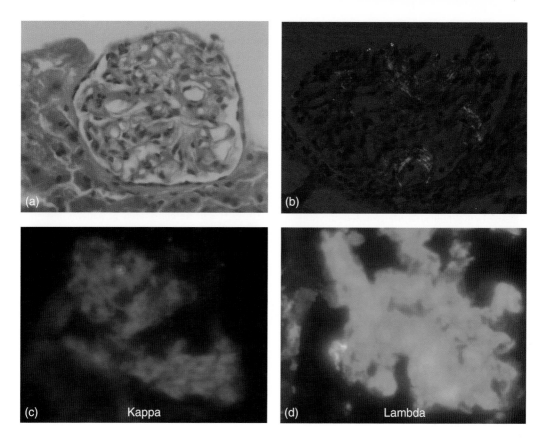

Figure 16.2 Renal Amyloid light chain (AL) amyloidosis. (a) Congophilic material is deposited in glomerular mesangium. (b) Under polarized microscopy the congophilic material shows apple-green birefringence. (c, d) The amyloid deposits show lambda restriction under direct immunofluorescence, thereby indicating primary amyloidosis (AL amyloid, lambda restricted).

microscopy and produce apple-green birefringence under polarized light when stained with Congo red (Figure 16.2).

The two most common types of renal amyloidosis are immunoglobulin-derived amyloidosis, secondary to a monoclonal gammopathy (AL amyloidosis), and secondary or reactive amyloidosis, due to chronic inflammatory conditions (infective or non-infective) where the amyloid deposits are derived from the acute phase reactant – serum amyloid A protein (SAA). Around 20% of patients who present with AL amyloidosis have MM, and the remainder have low-level plasma cell proliferation in the bone marrow of 5–10%. The free light chains that are rendered unstable and prone to self-aggregation form protofilaments that associate into amyloid fibrils. In AL amyloidosis, the clonal plasma cells express lambda light chains much more frequently than kappa.

Clinical Features

Clinical presentations of AL amyloidosis depend upon the affected organ(s). These are the common presenting features:

- Restrictive cardiomyopathy, seen in up to 60% of patients.
- Peripheral neuropathy (20%) and autonomic neuropathy (15%).
- Hepatomegaly, with or without splenomegaly, in around 70%, with liver function tests showing a cholestatic pattern in up to 25%.
- Macroglossia.
- Purpura and other skin manifestations.
- Bleeding diathesis.
- The kidney is the most commonly involved organ in systemic amyloidosis. The renal involvement usually presents with nephrotic

syndrome with or without AKI, or non-nephrotic-range proteinuria [19].

Diagnosis

One should suspect AL amyloidosis in non-diabetic patients with nephrotic syndrome and cardiomyopathy, peripheral neuropathy, autonomic neuropathy, macroglossia, or hepatomegaly. The diagnosis requires demonstration of amyloid deposits in the tissue and a plasma cell dyscrasia.

Choosing a biopsy site for demonstration of amyloid requires consideration:

- Kidney or liver biopsy is positive in over 90% of cases
- Abdominal fat pad aspirate (60–80%)
- Rectal biopsy (50–70%)
- Bone marrow biopsy (50–55%)

According to the International Myeloma Working Group, all four of the following criteria should be fulfilled to diagnose AL amyloidosis:

- *Presence of an amyloid-related systemic syndrome* (e.g. renal, liver, heart, gastrointestinal tract or peripheral nerve involvement): to be included as a diagnostic criterion, the organ damage must be felt to be related to amyloid deposition and not to another common disease, such as diabetes or hypertension.
- *Positive amyloid staining by Congo red in any tissue* (e.g. fat aspirate, bone marrow or organ biopsy) or the presence of amyloid fibrils on electron microscopy: the amyloid deposits are typically negative on methenamine silver stains and stain weakly for PAS. This contrasts with collagen, a major constituent of extracellular matrix and basement membrane, which demonstrates strong positive stain with PAS and silver stains. When stained with Congo red, the amyloid deposits demonstrate an orange-red appearance and apple-green birefringence under polarized light.
- *Evidence that the amyloid is light chain-related*: established by direct examination of the amyloid tissue (e.g. using mass spectrometry-based proteomic analysis).
- *Evidence of a monoclonal plasma cell proliferative disorder*: for instance presence of a serum or urine M protein, abnormal serum free light chain (SFLC) ratio, or clonal plasma cells in the bone marrow.

Management

The management of AL amyloidosis consists of supportive care to treat nephrotic syndrome in the form of ACE inhibitors/ARBs, diuretics, prophylaxis against venous thromboembolism and vaccinations against pneumococcus and *Haemophilus influenzae*. These patients often have cardiac involvement and autonomic neuropathy, and are prone to hypotension, fluctuating blood pressure, and cardiac arrhythmias. Sepsis is a common cause of morbidity and mortality, both due to an immunocompromised state from underlying plasma cell dyscrasia and nephrotic syndrome. Prognosis is poor, with a median survival of 18–24 months.

Specific management consists of chemotherapy and ASCT, which if successful has been shown to prolong the survival significantly to up to 4.5 years [20, 21]. ASCT can be considered in patients less than 70 years of age without significant cardiac involvement [22].

Monitoring response to chemotherapy includes measuring NT-pro-BNP, cardiac troponin T, and SFLCs.

Renal transplantation has been performed in patients with AL amyloidosis with improving results. A retrospective study of 25 patients with AL amyloidosis who underwent kidney transplantation in the UK revealed median graft survival of 5.8 years, with a 5- and 10-year graft survival of 74% and 25%, respectively [23].

Monoclonal Immunoglobulin Deposition Disease

In this disorder, monoclonal immunoglobulins deposit in the glomeruli, leading to proteinuria and renal insufficiency. The commonest form of monoclonal immunoglobulin deposition disease (MIDD) is light chain deposition disease (LCDD), and the predominant light chain in these cases is kappa. MIDD can also be caused by monoclonal heavy chains (HCDD – 20% of cases) or a combination of light and heavy chains (LHCDD – 10% of cases) [24]. Cast nephropathy is uncommon in patients with MIDD and these two lesions generally do not coexist. Most patients with MIDD have >1 g/day of proteinuria and around 40% of patients have nephrotic-range proteinuria. Whilst in patients with MM the predominant extrarenal lesions are skeletal, in MIDD, as with amyloidosis, predominant extrarenal manifestations include cardiac and hepatic involvement [25]. Histologically, MIDD is characterized by the deposition of light chains, heavy chains or both in the glomerular (and often tubular) basement membranes. In contrast to AL amyloidosis, these deposits are Congo red negative and do not form fibrils on electron microscopy. A typical description of MIDD is that of a nodular glomerulosclerosis similar to that seen in diabetic glomerulosclerosis. The glomeruli show acellular, PAS-positive, silver stain, and Congo red-negative nodular deposits. The tubules also often show similar deposits along the basement membrane, leading to ribbon-like thickening.

Treatment of MIDD is similar to that of MM and consists of chemotherapy alone or chemotherapy followed by ASCT. Patients with renal failure secondary to MIDD carry poor prognosis on dialysis, with a median survival of 10–18 months. Kidney transplantation has been performed in these patients, but the recurrence rate is high (around 70%), with the majority of patients losing their grafts due to recurrence within three years [26].

Monoclonal Gammopathy of Renal Significance

MGRS is a term coined recently to describe renal disorders caused by monoclonal immunoglobulin secreted by a non-malignant B cell/premalignant plasma cell clone. These patients have significant renal disease but do not meet the criteria for overt myeloma, though they often satisfy the criteria for MGUS (<3 g/l monoclonal protein and <10% bone marrow plasma cells) or smouldering myeloma (>3 g/l monoclonal protein and/or >10% bone marrow plasma cells but without organ damage).

The renal lesions associated with MGRS can be categorized according to the histological characteristics of the deposits (if present) in the kidney:

- MGRS lesions with organized deposits, further subdivided as:

  (a) MGRS with fibrillary deposits, which includes AL amyloidosis and fibrillary glomerulonephritis. The fibrillary deposits in amyloidosis are Congo red positive, whereas those in fibrillary glomerulonephritis are Congo red negative.
  (b) MGRS lesions with microtubular deposits, which includes monoclonal (type 1) cryoglobulinaemia [27] and immunotactoid glomerulopathy.
  (c) MGRS lesions with crystal inclusions, which includes light chain proximal tubulopathy, crystal-storing histiocytosis, and cryocrystalglobulinaemia.
- MGRS lesions with non-organized deposits: MIDD and monoclonal gammopathy-associated MPGN.

The finding of monoclonal Ig deposits in the kidney should lead to a full haematological evaluation that includes bone marrow examination, tests to identify whole Ig molecules (Immunofixation electrophoresis) and free light chains (SFLC assay), computed tomography (CT) scan of abdomen/pelvis to look for lymphadenopathy (as the underlying disorder could be a non-plasma cell-derived B cell lymphoproliferative disorder).

Although these disorders do not often fulfil the criteria for a haematological malignancy, they do cause significant renal disease, with poor prognosis and a high rate of recurrence following kidney transplantation. Consequently, initiation of efficient chemotherapy is essential to improve the renal prognosis.

Table 16.3 Comparison of serum protein electrophoresis and immunofixation for the detection of monoclonal paraprotein

Serum protein electrophoresis (SPEP)	Immunofixation
Semi-quantitative/*not* qualitative (cannot differentiate immunoglobulin (Ig) from free light chains)	Not quantitative but highly qualitative
False positive in raised polyclonal globulins, haemolytic anaemia, and nephrotic syndrome	Differentiates monoclonal from polyclonal immunoglobulins accurately with very low rates of false positivity
False negative in IgD or IgE myeloma, heavy chain disease	Determines accurately type of Ig/light chain/heavy chain
Sensitivity of about 80%	Combining immunofixation with SPEP increases sensitivity to 93%

Detection of Monoclonal Protein

SFLCs need to be 50 times normal to be detected by serum protein electrophoresis (SPEP) and 15 times normal for detection by immunofixation, though SFLC assay can detect very small rises. Addition of SFLC assay to SPEP and immunofixation increases sensitivity to >97%. The SFLC assay is a quantitative test and, therefore, can be used to monitor response to therapy. The main differences between SPEP and immunofixation for the detection of monoclonal proteins are highlighted in Table 16.3.

In renal impairment, due to non-paraprotein-disorder related conditions, as a consequence of the low GFR, clearance of both kappa and lambda light chains is reduced leading to an increase in serum levels without altering the ratio. A normal reference range of an SFLC ratio of 0.37–3 has been suggested in patients with renal impairment compared to a range of 0.26–1.26 in patients with normal renal function [28].

Acknowledgement

Dr Rajan Duggal, consultant histopathologist, Medanta Hospital, The Medicity, Gurgaon, Haryana, India.

References

1. Palumbo, A. and Anderson, K. (2011). Multiple myeloma. *N. Engl. J. Med.* 364 (11): 1046–1060.
2. Rajkumar, S.V., Dimopoulos, M.A., Palumbo, A. et al. (2014). International Myeloma Working Group updated criteria for the diagnosis of multiple myeloma. *Lancet Oncol.* 15 (12): e538–e548.
3. Palumbo, A., Bringhen, S., Ludwig, H. et al. (2011). Personalized therapy in multiple myeloma according to patient age and vulnerability: a report of the European Myeloma Network (EMN). *Blood* 118 (17): 4519–4529.
4. Heher, E.C., Rennke, H.G., Laubach, J.P., and Richardson, P.G. (2013). Kidney disease and multiple myeloma. *Clin. J. Am. Soc. Nephrol.* 8 (11): 2007–2017.
5. Knudsen, L.M., Hippe, E., Hjorth, M. et al. (1994). Renal function in newly diagnosed multiple myeloma – a demographic study of 1353 patients. The Nordic Myeloma Study Group. *Eur. J. Haematol.* 53 (4): 207–212.
6. Solomon, A., Weiss, D.T., and Kattine, A.A. (1991). Nephrotoxic potential of Bence Jones proteins. *N. Engl. J. Med.* 324 (26): 1845–1851.
7. Durie, B.G., Kyle, R.A., Belch, A. et al. (2003). Myeloma management guidelines: a consensus report from the Scientific Advisors of the International Myeloma Foundation. *Hematol. J.* 4 (6): 379–398.
8. Hutchison, C.A., Cockwell, P., Stringer, S. et al. (2011). Early reduction of serum-free light chains associates with renal recovery in myeloma kidney. *J. Am. Soc. Nephrol.* 22 (6): 1129–1136.
9. San-Miguel, J.F., Richardson, P.G., Sonneveld, P. et al. (2008). Efficacy and safety of bortezomib in patients with renal impairment: results from the APEX phase 3 study. *Leukemia* 22 (4): 842–849.
10. Chanan-Khan, A.A., Kaufman, J.L., Mehta, J. et al. (2007). Activity and safety of bortezomib in multiple myeloma patients with advanced renal failure: a multicenter retrospective study. *Blood* 109 (6): 2604–2606.
11. Korbet, S.M. and Schwartz, M.M. (2006). Multiple myeloma. *J. Am. Soc. Nephrol.* 17 (9): 2533–2545.
12. Child, J.A., Morgan, G.J., Davies, F.E. et al. (2003). High-dose chemotherapy with hematopoietic stem-cell rescue for multiple myeloma. *N. Engl. J. Med.* 348 (19): 1875–1883.
13. Badros, A., Barlogie, B., Siegel, E. et al. (2001). Results of autologous stem cell transplant in multiple myeloma patients with renal failure. *Br. J. Haematol.* 114 (4): 822–829.
14. Lee, C.K., Zangari, M., Barlogie, B. et al. (2004). Dialysis-dependent renal failure in patients with myeloma can be reversed by high-dose myeloablative therapy and autotransplant. *Bone Marrow Transpl.* 33 (8): 823–828.
15. Hutchison, C.A., Cook, M., Heyne, N. et al. (2008). European trial of free light chain removal by extended haemodialysis in cast nephropathy (EuLITE): a randomised control trial. *Trials* 9: 55.
16. Hutchison, C.A., Bradwell, A.R., Cook, M. et al. (2009). Treatment of acute renal failure secondary to multiple myeloma with chemotherapy and extended high cut-off hemodialysis. *Clin. J. Am. Soc. Nephrol.* 4 (4): 745–754.
17. Montseny, J.J., Kleinknecht, D., Meyrier, A. et al. (1998). Long-term outcome according to renal histological lesions in 118 patients with monoclonal gammopathies. *Nephrol. Dial. Transpl.* 13 (6): 1438–1445.
18. Kyle, R.A. and Gertz, M.A. (1990). Systemic amyloidosis. *Crit. Rev. Oncol./Hematol.* 10 (1): 49–87.

19. Kyle, R.A. and Greipp, P.R. (1983). Amyloidosis (AL). Clinical and laboratory features in 229 cases. *Mayo Clin. Proc.* 58 (10): 665–683.

20. Skinner, M., Sanchorawala, V., Seldin, D.C. et al. (2004). High-dose melphalan and autologous stem-cell transplantation in patients with AL amyloidosis: an 8-year study. *Ann. Intern. Med.* 140 (2): 85–93.

21. Goodman, H.J., Gillmore, J.D., Lachmann, H.J. et al. (2006). Outcome of autologous stem cell transplantation for AL amyloidosis in the UK. *Br. J. Haematol.* 134 (4): 417–425.

22. Wechalekar, A.D., Hawkins, P.N., and Gillmore, J.D. (2008). Perspectives in treatment of AL amyloidosis. *Br. J. Haematol.* 140 (4): 365–377.

23. Pinney, J.H., Lachmann, H.J., Bansi, L. et al. (2011). Outcome in renal Al amyloidosis after chemotherapy. *J. Clin. Oncol.* 29 (6): 674–681.

24. Pozzi, C., D'Amico, M., Fogazzi, G.B. et al. (2003). Light chain deposition disease with renal involve-ment: clinical characteristics and prognostic factors. *Am. J. Kidney Dis.* 42 (6): 1154–1163.

25. Lin, J., Markowitz, G.S., Valeri, A.M. et al. (2001). Renal monoclonal immunoglobulin deposition disease: the disease spectrum. *J. Am. Soc. Nephrol.* 12 (7): 1482–1492.

26. Leung, N., Lager, D.J., Gertz, M.A. et al. (2004). Long-term outcome of renal transplantation in light-chain deposition disease. *Am. J. Kidney Dis.* 43 (1): 147–153.

27. Terrier, B., Izzedine, H., Musset, L. et al. (2011). Prevalence and clinical significance of cryofibrin-ogenaemia in patients with renal disorders. *Nephrol. Dial. Transpl.* 26 (11): 3577–3581.

28. Abadie, J.M., van Hoeven, K.H., and Wells, J.M. (2009). Are renal reference intervals required when screening for plasma cell disorders with serum free light chains and serum protein elec-trophoresis? *Am. J. Clin. Pathol.* 131 (2): 166–171.

Questions and Answers

Questions

1. The CRAB criteria for the diagnosis of multiple myeloma does not include:
   a. Hypercalcaemia
   b. Anaemia
   c. Altered free light chain ratio
   d. Renal Insufficiency
   e. Bone lytic lesions

2. Following are true with regards to myeloma cast nephropathy:
   a. The casts form in proximal convoluted tubule
   b. PAS stain is negative for the casts
   c. More likely to be formed in alkaline pH
   d. Endocytosis by proximal tubule is a requirement for formation of myeloma casts
   e. Interaction of paraprotein with Tamm–Horsfall protein results in cast formation

3. Light chain deposition disease:
   a. Histologically mimics which common glomerular disorder?
   b. Often presents with nephrotic syndrome – T/F
   c. The glomerular deposits are Congo red and silver positive – T/F
   d. Recurrence is uncommon following kidney transplantation – T/F

4. Which one of the following treatment modalities is likely to be used in a 50-year-old patient diagnosed with multiple myeloma?
   a. High cutoff haemodialysis with high-dose dexamethasone
   b. Bortezomib and dexamethasone-based chemotherapy followed by peripheral blood stem cell harvest, melphalan conditioning, and autologous stem cell transplantation (ASCT)
   c. Chemotherapy until paraprotein levels drop and plateau, followed by thalidomide maintenance
   d. Melphalan and dexamethasone

5. Which of the following is/are true?
   a. Serum and urine protein electrophoresis are as sensitive as serum free light chain assay (sFLC) for the detection of paraprotein
   b. sFLC could potentially replace urinary immunofixation electrophoresis for the diagnosis of paraproteinemias
   c. Rapid reduction in sFLC levels aids in renal recovery
   d. High cutoff dialysis to remove free light chains is recommended for all patients with multiple myeloma and cast nephropathy
   e. Renal failure is an absolute contraindication for autologous stem cell transplantation (ASC)

6. Amyloidosis can be defined as:
   a. Intracellular deposition of fragments of abnormal proteins derived from microbes
   b. Extracellular deposition of fibrils composed of low molecular weight subunits of a variety of proteins, many of which are normal constituents of plasma
   c. Intracellular deposition of fragments of normal plasma proteins
   d. Intravascular deposition of fragments of normal plasma proteins

Answers

1. c. The Myeloma-defining CRAB consists of hyper**c**alcaemia, **r**enal failure, **a**naemia, and **b**one lesions.

2. b, e. The casts are formed in the thick ascending limb of loop of Henle and distal tubules as the paraproteins are deposited on the Tamm–Horsfall protein. Under microscope, the casts are characteristically PAS negative and eosinophilic with a fragmented appearance. Risk factors for myeloma cast nephropathy include dehydration, loop diuretics, metabolic acidosis, and exposure to radiocontrast agents.

3. a. Diabetic nodular glomerulosclerosis
   b. True
   c. False
   d. False

4. b. Autologous stem cell transplantation (ASCT) following induction chemotherapy with bortezomib/dexamethasone/thalidomide or lenalidomide can lead to a response rate of up to 85% with increased survival in myeloma patients. The use of melphalan is generally reserved for patients who are not eligible for ASCT due to advanced age (>70y) and significant comorbidity, as melphalan can adversely affect successful stem cell harvest. In those needing dialysis, the use of the expensive high cutoff dialysis does not offer any advantage over conventional dialysis and may lead to increased albumin loss.

5. b, c. Serum free light chains need to be 50 times of normal values to be detected by serum protein electrophoresis (SPEP) and 15 times of normal for detection by immunofixation, but sFLC assay can detect very small rises. Renal damage in myeloma is caused by the glomerular filtration of the serum free light chains and therefore a rapid reduction in their number is associated with improved renal prognosis. Renal failure or dialysis is not a contraindication for ASCT in patients with myeloma, and there is in fact evidence of renal recovery following ASCT.

6. b. Amyloidosis is a disorder characterized by extracellular tissue deposition of fibrils composed of low molecular weight subunits of a variety of proteins, many of which circulate as normal constituents of plasma. The various types of amyloidosis include:

   - **AL amyloid**: caused by plasma cell dyscrasia, amyloid fibrils are derived from immunoglobulin light chain
   - **AA amyloidosis**: recurring inflammation in chronic diseases results in production of serum amyloid A (an acute phase reactant like CRP) which forms the amyloid fibrils
   - Less common forms include dialysis-related amyloidosis (beta-2 microglobulin), age-related systemic amyloidosis (transthyretin), heritable amyloidosis (transthyretin), and organ-specific amyloidosis, e.g. Alzheimer's disease.

17

Tubulointerstitial Diseases

Richard J. Quigg and Edwin Anand

Summary

- Acute interstitial nephritis (AIN) is a potentially reversible cause of acute kidney injury (AKI) and in 80% of cases is caused by drugs, with antibiotics being responsible for half of cases
- AIN usually manifests as AKI 7–10 days after drug exposure in the absence of significant proteinuria or haematuria
- Urine sediment in AIN reveals white cells or white cell casts, whilst eosinophils are neither specific nor sensitive for this condition
- The classic presentation of fever, rash, arthralgia, and eosinophilia, which was common in the past with methicillin-induced AIN, is seen in less than 10% of cases nowadays
- Treatment consists of ceasing the offending drug and, if no response is seen in 3–7 days, then 8–10 weeks of oral prednisolone

- Chronic interstitial nephritis is a histological entity characterized by progressive scarring, fibrosis of the tubulointerstitium with tubular atrophy, and macrophage and/or lymphocyte infiltration of the interstitium
- Chronic interstitial nephritis presents with gradual loss of renal function, minimal or no proteinuria, urinary concentration defects, acidification defects, and an anaemia that is out of proportion to the degree of renal dysfunction
- Chronic interstitial nephritis may be due to drugs, heavy metals, environmental toxins, metabolic conditions, and immunological diseases
- Most glomerular and vascular diseases which lead to decline in renal function have associated secondary tubulointerstitial nephritis and the severity of the tubulointerstitial involvement correlates directly with the severity of renal failure

The renal tubulointerstitial diseases are broadly classified as acute interstitial nephritis (AIN) and chronic interstitial diseases. Whilst AIN is often the result of an immunological response to a drug, chronic tubulointerstitial diseases are often caused by non-immunological mechanisms.

Secondary tubulointerstitial nephritis signifies inflammation in the setting of primary glomerular or vascular disease [1, 2]. We now know that most glomerular and vascular diseases that lead to a decline in renal function have associated tubulointerstitial nephritis and that the severity of the tubulointerstitial involvement correlates directly with the severity of renal failure [3–5]. The state of the tubulointerstitium appears to play a key role in most renal diseases.

The tubulointerstitium can be injured by toxins (e.g. heavy metals), crystals (e.g. uric acid), infections, ischaemia or immunological mechanisms (e.g. drugs) [6, 7]. Specialized fibroblasts in the inner cortex and outer medulla of the kidney respond to hypoxia by secreting erythropoietin (which explains an anaemia that is out of proportion to the degree of renal dysfunction in patients with chronic interstitial nephritis) [8]. A different subset of renal fibroblasts is known to lead to interstitial fibrosis in progressive chronic kidney disease (CKD) by producing extracellular matrix. Dendritic cells are also found in large numbers in the interstitium and presumably play a role in the immunological response.

In this chapter, we will limit our discussion to primary tubulointerstitial nephritis, in which the glomeruli and vessels are typically uninvolved.

Acute Interstitial Nephritis

AIN is an acute and often reversible cause of acute kidney injury (AKI) characterized by inflammatory infiltrates in the interstitium. In a biopsy series of patients with AKI, AIN accounted for about 12% of cases [9]. The incidence seems to be on the rise, especially in the elderly. Drugs account for 80% of the causes of AIN [10].

Initially, the vast majority of AIN was related to exposure to beta-lactam antibiotics, particularly methicillin. Nowadays, AIN is seen with a much broader set of drugs – antibiotics, non-steroidal anti-inflammatory drugs (NSAIDs), anti–convulsants, diuretics, proton pump inhibitors and others as mentioned in Table 17.1.

The causes of AIN can be grouped as follows:

- Drugs (with antibiotics responsible for up to 50% of these cases) – 80%.
- Infections – 4–10%.
- Tubulointerstitial nephritis and uveitis (TINU) syndrome – 5–10%.
- Systemic disease including sarcoidosis, Sjögren's syndrome, systemic lupus erythematosus (SLE) and others – 10–20%.

AIN may be seen with some of the classic as well as the newer anti-cancer drugs. Whilst drugs like ifosfamide are well known to cause tubulointerstitial diseases, the tyrosine kinase inhibitors seem to be unique amongst the newer drugs to cause AIN [11].

TINU syndrome is a rare disease seen predominantly in younger people, with the median age being 15 years. Along with interstitial nephritis and uveitis, these patients may have systemic features such as fever, weight loss, malaise, anorexia, and arthralgia.

Immunoglobulin G4-related disease (IgG4-RD) is a recently defined collection of disorders that can lead to AIN. This group is characterized by tissue infiltration with lymphocytes and IgG4 plasma cells, a variable degree of fibrosis, tumour-like swellings in multiple organs and lymphadenopathy.

Table 17.1 Common causes of acute interstitial nephritis

Drugs
Beta-lactam antibiotics (penicillin and cephalosporin)
Sulfonamides, including trimethoprim-sulfamethoxazole
5-aminosalicylate (e.g. mesalazine)
Anti-tuberculosis drugs (rifampicin and ethambutol)
Tetracyclines
Macrolides
Fluoroquinolones
Vancomycin
Non-steroidal anti-inflammatory drugs, including COX2 inhibitors
Proton pump inhibitors and H2 blockers
Antivirals, including acyclovir and indinavir
Loop and thiazide-type diuretics
Allopurinol
Anti-cancer drugs (ifosfamide and tyrosine kinase inhibitors)
Infections
Bacterial: *Streptococci*, *Escherichia coli*, *Mycobacterium tuberculosis*, *Corynebacterium diphtheriae*
Viruses: HIV, hantavirus, cytomegalovirus, Epstein–Barr virus
Systemic diseases
Systemic lupus erythematosus, Sjögren's disease, sarcoidosis, immunoglobulin G4-related disease

AIN in HIV may be related to an immunological response to the infection itself, but it may also be associated with highly active antiretroviral therapy (HAART) or opportunistic infections [12].

Pathogenesis

AIN is an immunologically mediated reaction to an extrarenal antigen, which is classically a drug or less commonly an infectious agent. The immunological nature of drug-induced AIN is supported by the fact that the condition is not dose related and it recurs after exposure to the same drug or a closely related one. On a similar note, AIN secondary to infections can be differentiated from pyelonephritis by the relative absence of neutrophils in the interstitium and the failure to isolate the infective agent from urine or renal parenchyma, suggesting an immunological pathogenesis.

Extrarenal antigens like drugs or infectious agents can cause AIN by three mechanisms:

- Binding to kidney structures and acting as a planted antigen.
- Acting as a hapten and thus modifying the immunogenicity of native renal antigens.
- Mimicking renal antigens and thus causing a cross-reactive immune reaction.

Most forms of AIN are not associated with antibody deposition, suggesting that cell-mediated immunity plays a major role. However, there are a few reports of anti-tubular basement membrane (anti-TBM) antibodies demonstrated in renal biopsies of patients with AIN.

Pathology

On microscopy, AIN is characterized by a normal-appearing glomerulus with rich interstitial infiltration of T lymphocytes and monocytes–macrophages, whilst plasma cells, eosinophils, and a few neutrophils may also be seen (Figure 17.1). Interstitial infiltrates almost always lead to interstitial oedema, which on microscopy gives the appearance of widely separated tubules. Eosinophils in the infiltrate are seen more often with AIN caused by beta-lactam antibiotics in comparison to other drugs. Tubulitis with mononuclear infiltration of TBM and across the tubular cells is occasionally seen. Sparse granulomas may be seen infrequently in AIN secondary to infection, sarcoidosis or Sjögren's disease.

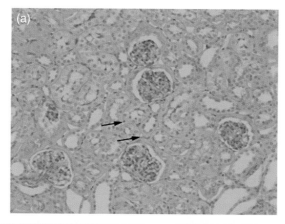

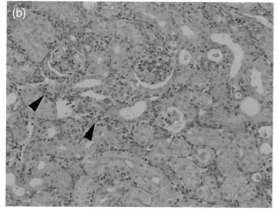
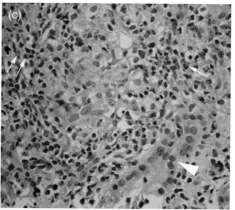

Figure 17.1 Histopathology of acute tubulointerstitial nephritis. (a) Normal renal cortex, showing the 'back-to-back' orientation of tubules. Where the tubular curves separate is the interstitium (black arrows). (b) Early features of experimental acute tubulointerstitial nephritis in mice. The interstitium is now occupied with an inflammatory cell infiltrate (black arrowheads). (c) Acute drug-induced tubulointerstitial nephritis in a human biopsy specimen. There is a dense mononuclear cell infiltrate, scattered eosinophils (white arrows), and significant tubular injury, with tubulitis and infiltrating mononuclear cells (white arrowhead).

Electron microscopy does not show any characteristic findings. Immunofluorescence usually does not show any antibody deposition, except in the rare anti-TBM disease which is marked by IgG deposition along the TBM.

The presence of interstitial fibrosis indicates chronicity.

Clinical Features

The classic extrarenal manifestations of fever, rash, arthralgia, and eosinophilia, which were common in the past with methicillin-induced AIN, are seen in less than 10% of cases now. AIN usually presents as an acute or sometimes gradual loss of renal function in the setting of suspected drug use, with minimum proteinuria (<1 g/day) and absence of hypertension or oedema.

The time to onset from drug exposure is variable and at times difficult to assess, but often manifests after 7–10 days in a typical case. Longer exposure times have been described in the case of NSAIDs. AIN can present abruptly on rechallenge of a drug to which a patient is sensitized.

Diagnosis

The clinical syndrome of acute-onset renal failure in the setting of recent exposure to a drug that is known to cause AIN is often the first clue to diagnosis. The degree of renal failure can vary from mild AKI to AKI requiring dialysis. The classic urinary finding is leucocyturia with white blood cell casts. The presence of a few urinary red blood cells (RBCs) is not uncommon, though dysmorphic RBCs and RBC casts are characteristically not seen. Proteinuria is usually mild (<1 g/day). However, in cases of NSAID-related AIN, nephrotic-range proteinuria may be seen due to a concomitant glomerular process, which is often minimal change disease and occasionally membranous nephropathy.

Eosinophiluria (defined by eosinophils that account for more than 1% of urinary white cells by Hansel stain) is commonly looked for, but its sensitivity as well as specificity is quite low. In a study of 566 biopsy-proven cases of AIN, the sensitivity and specificity of eosinophiluria were 30 and 68%, respectively [12]. Hence, some authors have recommended against routine testing for urine eosinophils in the investigation of suspected AIN [13].

The definitive way to diagnose AIN is a renal biopsy. Often, clinicians choose to diagnose and treat AIN empirically, but if the treating physician is in doubt, a renal biopsy should be performed to ascertain diagnosis. Renal biopsy also provides valuable clues regarding the chronicity and severity of the disease.

Treatment

Prompt withdrawal of the offending drug is obviously the first and the most important step. Immunosuppressive therapy is often employed if there is no subsequent improvement in kidney function by 3–7 days.

Data from many retrospective studies do not show a clear benefit from steroids, although the patients who received steroids in these reports had more severe disease in general [14, 15]. However, steroids seem to be associated with lower rates of progression to CKD in some study series. We suggest using prednisone at a dose of 1 mg/kg and tapering it after 2–4 weeks for a total duration of 8–10 weeks.

In non-drug-related AIN, the treatment is directed to the primary disease, for example the use of cytotoxic agents in lupus nephritis.

Prognosis depends on the duration of drug exposure, which is evident as interstitial fibrosis in cases with longstanding damage. Although renal prognosis was very good with the initial cases of AIN associated with methicillin, the proportion of patients recovering renal function completely is lower in those who develop AIN due to other drugs or causes. About 30% of cases were reported to have developed chronicity during follow-up in a small case series [16].

Chronic Interstitial Diseases

Chronic interstitial nephritis is a histological entity characterized by progressive scarring and fibrosis of the tubulointerstitium, tubular atrophy and macrophage and/or lymphocyte infiltration. The aetiologies are quite varied, including drugs, heavy metals, environmental toxins, connective tissue diseases, radiation injury and metabolic disorders (Table 17.2).

Clinically, these patients present with gradual loss of renal function, minimal or no proteinuria, urinary concentration defects, acidification defects, and an anaemia that is out of proportion to the degree of renal dysfunction (Table 17.3).

Table 17.2 Causes of chronic interstitial nephritis
Drugs
Chronic **lithium** use
Calcineurin inhibitors (cyclosporine, tacrolimus)
Cisplatin
Analgesic nephropathy
Heavy metals
Lead
Cadmium
Environmental
Aristocholic acid nephropathy
Metabolic
Chronic urate nephropathy
Chronic severe **hypokalaemia**
Hypercalcaemia
Hyperoxaluria
Immunological diseases
Sarcoidosis
Sjögren's syndrome
Systemic lupus erythematosus
Antineutrophil cytoplasmic antibody (ANCA)-associated vasculitis
Note: Common causes in **bold text**.

Table 17.3 Common features of chronic tubulointerstitial diseases
Slow loss of glomerular filtration rate (GFR)
Benign urinalysis
Mild or no proteinuria
Concentration defects: polyuria
Acidification defects
Anaemia out of proportion to GFR loss

Drug-Induced Chronic Interstitial Nephritis

Lithium Nephropathy

Renal complications of lithium include chronic interstitial disease and the more common nephrogenic diabetes insipidus.

Lithium use is associated with a nephrogenic diabetes insipidus in as many as 20–40% of chronic users. Patients typically present with polyuria and thirst [17]. Under the influence of anti-diuretic hormone (ADH), aquaporin-2 channels (AQP2) help in water reabsorption in the principal cells of the collecting duct. Lithium enters these principal cells through epithelial sodium channels on the luminal membrane and interferes with the ability of ADH to reabsorb water by the following mechanisms (thus causing diabetes insipidus):

- Lithium reduces AQP2 gene transcription.
- Lithium increases cyclooxygenase-2 and therefore prostaglandin E2 production, which induces lysosomal degradation of AQP2.
- Lithium may lead to initial proliferation of principal cells, which then undergo rapid cell cycle arrest, leading ultimately to a decreased population of principal cells.

Stopping lithium may reverse diabetes insipidus in the early stages. Since lithium is transported into the principal cells through the epithelial sodium channel, amiloride can be used to reduce lithium entry and improve polyuria in cases where lithium cannot be stopped.

Chronic lithium use can lead to tubulointerstitial disease with an associated insidious decline in glomerular filtration rate. The degree of interstitial fibrosis on renal biopsy is directly linked to the duration and cumulative dose of lithium. Cystic changes in the distal tubule are a characteristic finding on biopsy, apart from the usual changes of chronic interstitial nephritis.

Large observational data show that about 20% of long-term lithium users develop mild to moderate CKD [16]. Though most of the patients with CKD induced by lithium use have mild to moderate renal impairment, progression to end-stage renal disease (ESRD) can occur. Such progression occurs after a median of 20 years of exposure or more [18]. There is also evidence that increased awareness and dosing changes have led to a marked decrease in the incidence of ESRD from lithium [19].

Long-term lithium use is also associated with hyperparathyroidism and hypercalcaemia by increasing the threshold for the calcium-sensing mechanism within the parathyroid gland. Chronic hypercalcaemia can also contribute to a mild nephrogenic diabetes insipidus by downregulation of AQP2 water channels.

Analgesic Nephropathy

Analgesic nephropathy was described in Sweden, Belgium, and later Australia in case–control studies of ESRD in patients who were habitually consuming analgesic mixtures often containing phenacetin (which is metabolized to acetaminophen and other metabolites), caffeine, codeine, aspirin, and other agents. The disease was characterized by slow progression, papillary necrosis, a 'bumpy' contour of the kidney and an association with urothelial malignancy. At one time, analgesic nephropathy was blamed to be the cause of as many as 20% of ESRD patients needing dialysis in Australia [20]. This led to the ban on phenacetin being sold as an analgesic medication over the counter in the 1970s and 1980s all over the world. The incidence of analgesic nephropathy has gradually declined over the last few decades.

One must be aware that papillary necrosis is not pathognomonic of analgesic nephropathy and can also be seen in diabetic nephropathy, sickle cell nephropathy, urinary tract obstruction and renal tuberculosis.

The diagnosis of analgesic nephropathy can be suspected by sterile pyuria with non-contrast computed tomography (CT) scan findings of bilateral reduced renal size, 'bumpy' renal contours and papillary calcifications (i.e. small, indented, calcified kidneys) in a patient with a strong history of over-the-counter analgesic use [21].

Treatment consists of stopping analgesic medications. Because of the increased risk of uroepithelial cancers, very close follow-up is necessary.

Chronic Interstitial Nephritis Due to Heavy Metal and Environmental Toxins

Lead Nephropathy

Chronic interstitial nephritis secondary to chronic lead exposure is rarely seen in the developed world today due to occupational controls and removal of lead from paint, gasoline, and other environmental sources.

Lead stored in bones has a half-life of 20–30 years. Lead can reenter the blood stream during periods of increased bone mineral recycling and lead to renal, haematological, musculoskeletal, ocular, immunological, neurological, reproductive, and developmental abnormalities. Lead poisoning causes marked anaemia due to the direct toxic effect of lead on mitochondrial enzyme aminolevunilic acid synthetase (ALAS), which catalyses the first and rate-limiting step in haem synthesis.

Acute exposure to lead causes proximal tubular injury, which can present as proximal (type 2) renal tubular acidosis (RTA) and Fanconi syndrome.

However, the more classic renal effect of lead is chronic interstitial nephritis. These patients are more prone to the development or worsening of gout, hypertension, and increased cardiovascular mortality. Blood lead levels are generally not helpful in diagnosing chronic lead toxicity due to its avid binding to bone. For confirmatory diagnosis, one needs to do a lead mobilization test in which increased 24-hour urinary excretion of lead is demonstrated after injection of the chelating agent calcium ethylenediaminetetraacetic acid (EDTA).

The treatment in acute and chronic lead poisoning consists of a chelating regimen of repeated injections of EDTA salts [22]. A potential adverse effect of chelation therapy is redistribution of lead from bone to the central nervous system and kidney.

Cadmium Nephropathy

Chronic exposure to cadmium can occur from occupational sources like working in factories dealing with production of alloys, glass, galvanizing pigments and nickel-cadmium batteries. Smoking is also a potentially important route of cadmium exposure. Bones and kidneys are the organs chiefly affected by cadmium and the former manifests with multiple fractures and a mixed pattern of osteoporosis and osteomalacia.

Cadmium causes a generalized proximal tubular dysfunction (Fanconi syndrome) or chronic tubulointerstitial nephritis. Specific markers for tubular proteinuria like beta2-microglobulin, alpha-1-microglobulin or retinol-binding protein in the urine indicate proximal tubular dysfunction due to cadmium in the patient with a history of exposure to the metal.

Unlike lead, chelating agents do not effectively clear the body of cadmium that has been deposited.

Aristocholic Nephropathy and Balkan Endemic Nephropathy

Balkan endemic nephropathy has been known for more than 50 years in the rural areas of the Balkans: Serbia, Bosnia and Herzegovina, Croatia, Romania, and Bulgaria. Only recently has it been conclusively proven to be related to inadvertent contamination of wheat grain with aristolochic acid (AA) from the plant *Aristolochia cleanatitis*.

A very similar nephropathy called aristolochic nephropathy was described in the 1990s from Brussels amongst young women who were exposed to AA from a Chinese herb, *Aristolochia fangchi*.

Besides the above geographical areas, exposure to AA and the resultant renal failure has been reported from other countries including China, USA and Australia.

The disease is characterized by severe interstitial fibrosis, progressive renal failure and a very high risk of urothelial malignancy [23]. There is no specific treatment. Given the high incidence of cellular atypia of the genitourinary tract, patients should have annual surveillance for abnormal urinary cytology.

Chronic Interstitial Diseases Due to Connective Tissue Disorders

Sjögren's Syndrome

Renal involvement in the form of chronic interstitial nephritis is known to occur in about 25% of patients with Sjögren's syndrome. Sjögren's syndrome can also lead to distal (type 1) RTA and less commonly nephrogenic diabetes insipidus. Glomerular disease in the form of membranous nephropathy or mesangiocapillary glomerulonephritis is occasionally seen as well [24].

On a renal biopsy, the commonest finding is a brisk lymphoplasmocytic infiltration of the tubulointerstitium and rarely granuloma formation. The autoantibodies anti-Ro (SSA) and anti-La (SSB) are relatively specific for Sjögren's syndrome and their presence can help confirm the diagnosis in the clinical setting of sicca syndrome; that is, dry eyes, dry mouth and parotid enlargement.

Treatment generally includes steroids and sometimes azathioprine in those who become steroid dependent.

Sarcoidosis

Renal biopsy shows occasional tubulointerstitial granulomas in up to 40% of sarcoid patients, but only a minority of them develop CKD [25–27]. The main mechanism of renal damage in sarcoidosis is from hypercalcaemia and hypercalciuria. Nephrocalcinosis and nephrolithiasis are common in the 10–25% of patients who present with renal disease. The condition often presents as urinary concentration or acidification defects.

Whilst ESRD is uncommon in sarcoidosis, when it occurs, it is most often due to hypercalcaemic nephropathy rather than granulomatous nephritis (even though nephrocalcinosis is less common overall than histological evidence of interstitial nephritis).

When renal failure is secondary to biopsy-proven interstitial nephritis in patients with sarcoidosis, corticosteroids are the mainstay of treatment.

Chronic Interstitial Diseases Due to Metabolic Disorders

Chronic Urate Nephropathy

Before the advent of drugs that lower serum uric acid levels, more than 50% of patients with gout had impaired renal function and nearly 100% had evidence of renal disease on biopsy. Chronic urate nephropathy is now thought to be uncommon and some feel that the diagnosis cannot be made on clinical grounds in the absence of a renal biopsy. Others feel that chronic urate nephropathy can be considered in patients who have CKD with hyperuricaemia out of proportion to the degree of renal insufficiency [28]. It must be remembered that almost all of these patients are hypertensive and so it is difficult to be sure of the exact contributory role played by the raised urate in causing CKD here.

It is thought that chronic hyperuricaemia and the resultant uricosuria lead to intratubular sodium urate crystal deposition. The crystals can block the tubules and eventually rupture into the interstitium and cause a granulomatous interstitial nephritis.

Whilst whether lowering of serum uric acid is renoprotective remains controversial, withdrawal of allopurinol from patients with stable CKD can lead to worsening of hypertension and acceleration of kidney dysfunction.

Hypokalaemic Nephropathy

Chronic hypokalaemia causes a mild nephrogenic diabetes insipidus by decreasing the expression of AQP2 in the collecting duct. Potassium (K^+) depletion causes the movement of K^+ from the intracellular to extracellular compartment, which is counterbalanced by the movement of hydrogen (H^+) into the cells (resulting in intracellular acidosis). Hypokalaemia-induced intracellular acidosis in proximal tubular cells causes the cells to try to get rid of the extra H^+ by secreting it into the tubules. However, H^+ secretion by the proximal tubular cells is linked to reabsorption of sodium (Na^+) by the Na^+–H^+ exchanger in the luminal membrane. The resulting Na+ retention produces volume expansion and can modestly elevate blood pressure.

Chronic hypokalaemia for more than a month can produce characteristic vacuolar lesions in the epithelial cells of the proximal tubule and occasionally the distal tubule. These changes are usually reversible with K$^+$ replacement. Prolonged hypokalaemia can lead to irreversible changes, including cystic changes in the medulla accompanied by tubular atrophy and interstitial fibrosis [29].

Hypercalcaemic Nephropathy

Hypercalcaemia can cause both a reversible AKI due to renal vasoconstriction, as well as chronic interstitial nephritis. Chronic hypercalcaemia also leads to mild nephrogenic diabetes insipidus in up to 20% of patients by downregulation of AQP2 water channels [30].

Longstanding hypercalcaemia and hypercalciuria may lead to chronic interstitial nephritis by degeneration and necrosis of the tubular cells, with eventual tubular atrophy and interstitial fibrosis. Histologically, the presence of calcific deposits in the interstitium (nephrocalcinosis) is the most distinctive feature associated with longstanding hypercalcaemia. Clinically, a defect in urinary concentration due to characteristic tubular dysfunction often manifests as polyuria and polydipsia. Macroscopic nephrocalcinosis is often detected on imaging. ESRD is a rare consequence of longstanding hypercalcaemia and when present is almost always associated with nephrocalcinosis.

References

1. Nath, K.A. (1992). Tubulointerstitial changes as a major determinant in the progression of renal damage. *Am. J. Kidney Dis.* 20 (1): 1–17.
2. Eddy, A.A. (1994). Experimental insights into the tubulointerstitial disease accompanying primary glomerular lesions. *J. Am. Soc. Nephrol.* 5 (6): 1273–1287.
3. Risdon, R.A., Sloper, J.C., and De Wardener, H.E. (1968). Relationship between renal function and histological changes found in renal-biopsy specimens from patients with persistent glomerular nephritis. *Lancet* 2 (7564): 363–366.
4. Wehrmann, M., Bohle, A., Held, H. et al. (1990). Long-term prognosis of focal sclerosing glomerulonephritis. An analysis of 250 cases with particular regard to tubulointerstitial changes. *Clin. Nephrol.* 33 (3): 115–122.
5. Schainuck, L.I., Striker, G.E., Cutler, R.E., and Benditt, E.P. (1970). Structural-functional correlations in renal disease. II. The correlations. *Hum. Pathol.* 1: 631–641.
6. Kaissling, B. and Le Hir, M. (2008). The renal cortical interstitium: morphological and functional aspects. *Histochem. Cell Biol.* 130 (2): 247–262.
7. Kurts, C. (2006). Dendritic cells: not just another cell type in the kidney, but a complex immune sentinel network. *Kidney Int.* 70 (3): 412–414.
8. Pan, X., Suzuki, N., Hirano, I. et al. (2011). Isolation and characterization of renal erythropoietin-producing cells from genetically produced anemia mice. *PLoS One* 6 (10): e25839.
9. Goicoechea, M., Rivera, F., and Lopez-Gomez, J.M. (2013). Increased prevalence of acute tubulointerstitial nephritis. *Nephrol. Dial. Transplant.* 28 (1): 112–115.
10. Appel, G.B. (2008). The treatment of acute interstitial nephritis: More data at last. *Kidney Int.* 73 (8): 905–907.
11. Airy, M., Raghavan, R., Truong, L.D., and Eknoyan, G. (2013). Tubulointerstitial nephritis and cancer chemotherapy: update on a neglected clinical entity. *Nephrol. Dial. Transplant.* 28 (10): 2502–2509.
12. Muriithi, A.K., Nasr, S.H., and Leung, N. (2013). Utility of urine eosinophils in the diagnosis of acute interstitial nephritis. *Clin. J. Am. Soc. Nephrol.* 8 (11): 1857–1862.
13. Perazella, M.A. and Bomback, A.S. (2013). Urinary eosinophils in AIN: farewell to an old biomarker? *Clin. J. Am. Soc. Nephrol.* 8 (11): 1841–1843.
14. Clarkson, M.R., Giblin, L., O'Connell, F.P. et al. (2004). Acute interstitial nephritis: clinical features and response to corticosteroid therapy. *Nephrol. Dial. Transplant.* 19 (11): 2778–2783.
15. Gonzalez, E., Gutiérrez, E., Galeano, C. et al. (2008). Early steroid treatment improves the recovery of renal function in patients with drug-induced acute interstitial nephritis. *Kidney Int.* 73 (8): 940–946.
16. Chen, D., Luo, C., Tang, Z. et al. (2012). Delayed renal function recovery from drug-induced acute interstitial nephritis. *Am. J. Med. Sci.* 343 (1): 36–39.
17. Boton, R., Gaviria, M., and Batlle, D.C. (1987). Prevalence, pathogenesis, and treatment of renal dysfunction associated with chronic lithium therapy. *Am. J. Kidney Dis.* 10 (5): 329–345.
18. Aiff, H., Attman, P.O., Aurell, M. et al. (2014). End-stage renal disease associated with prophylactic lithium treatment. *Eur. Neuropsychopharmacol.* 24 (4): 540–544.
19. Aiff, H., Attman, P.O., Aurell, M. et al. (2014). The impact of modern treatment principles may have

eliminated lithium-induced renal failure. *J. Psychopharmacol.* 28 (2): 151–154.

20. Chang, S.H., Mathew, T.H., and McDonald, S.P. (2008). Analgesic nephropathy and renal replacement therapy in Australia: trends, comorbidities and outcomes. *Clin. J. Am. Soc. Nephrol.* 3 (3): 768–776.

21. De Broe, M.E. and Elseviers, M.M. (2009). Over-the-counter analgesic use. *J. Am. Soc. Nephrol.* 20 (10): 2098–2103.

22. Evans, M. and Elinder, C.G. (2011). Chronic renal failure from lead: myth or evidence-based fact? *Kidney Int.* 79 (3): 272–279.

23. De Broe, M.E. (2012). Chinese herbs nephropathy and Balkan endemic nephropathy: toward a single entity, aristolochic acid nephropathy. *Kidney Int.* 81 (6): 513–515.

24. Bossini, N., Savoldi, S., Franceschini, F. et al. (2001). Clinical and morphological features of kidney involvement in primary Sjogren's syndrome. *Nephrol. Dial. Transplant.* 16 (12): 232.

25. Hilderson, I., Van Laecke, S., Wauters, A. et al. (2014). Treatment of renal sarcoidosis: is there a guideline? Overview of the different treatment options. *Nephrol. Dial. Transplant.* 29 (10): 1841–1847.

26. Shah, R., Shidham, G., Agarwal, A. et al. (2011). Diagnostic utility of kidney biopsy in patients with sarcoidosis and acute kidney injury. *Int J Nephrol Renovasc Dis* 4: 131–136.

27. Casella, F.J. and Allon, M. (1993). The kidney in sarcoidosis. *J. Am. Soc. Nephrol.* 3 (9): 1555–1562.

28. Murray, T. and Goldberg, M. (1975). Chronic interstitial nephritis: etiologic factors. *Ann. Intern. Med.* 82 (4): 453–459.

29. Torres, V.E., Young, W.F. Jr., Offord, K.P., and Hattery, R.R. (1990). Association of hypokalemia, aldosteronism, and renal cysts. *N. Engl. J. Med.* 322 (6): 345–351.

30. Earm, J.H., Christensen, B.M., Frøkiaer, J. et al. (1998). Decreased aquaporin-2 expression and apical plasma membrane delivery in kidney collecting ducts of polyuric hypercalcemic rats. *J. Am. Soc. Nephrol.* 9 (12): 2181.

Questions and Answers

Questions

1. A 55-year-old female was recently diagnosed with Crohn's disease and started on sulfasalazine for maintenance treatment. Two weeks later she develops an exfoliative rash which was treated with prednisone. Her creatinine was found to have increased from a baseline of 65 μmol/l (ref. range 45–90) to 145 μmol/l.

   What initial tests would provide clues towards AIN?
   What is the utility of urine eosinophils?
   How would you manage her renal failure?

2. A 62-year-old male with bipolar disorder is referred for evaluation of chronic renal failure. He has been on lithium for the past 15 years, which in general provides good control of his symptoms. His serum creatinine is 166 μmol/l (ref. range 45–90). He has no family history of renal illness and he does not have hypertension or diabetes mellitus.

   What initial clues would help in making a diagnosis of lithium nephropathy?
   What electrolyte disorder can co-occur?

3. A 55-year-old male, who has been working as a smelter at a mine is being evaluated for progressive renal failure. Other notable problems in his history include recurrent gout and difficult to control hypertension. His uric acid level is 12.0 mg/dl (ref. range 4.0–8.5 mg/dl) and creatinine is 145 μmol/l (ref. range 45–90). Blood lead levels were normal on two separate occasions. He does not have proteinuria.

   Could this be lead nephropathy?
   How would you prove the diagnosis?

4. A 63-year-old African American female presents with progressive renal failure with minimum proteinuria for the past three years. She also has a chronic dry cough for many years. Chest X-ray shows mediastinal widening and a CT of the chest shows interstitial disease in addition to diffuse hilar and mediastinal adenopathy. She has had two episodes of symptomatic renal calculi in the past year.

   What disease can explain her pulmonary and renal processes?

5. A 35-year-old office secretary presents with a mild renal impairment that has started a year ago. She also has dry eyes and mouth. A year ago, she had an episode of a salivary calculus.

   What is the aetiology of her renal failure?
   What other disorder can you see in routine chemistry?

6. A 50-year-old Bulgarian female is admitted with severe renal failure needing dialysis. She says that she knows several people in her neighbourhood with the same condition.

   Given her demographics, what is a likely diagnosis?
   What other associated urological condition can be present?

Answers

1. The patient has acute interstitial nephritis (AIN) from sulfasalazine. The onset of the renal failure soon after the initiation of the sulfasalazine drug and the rash provide clues to the diagnosis. AIN typically presents within one to two weeks after exposure to a culprit drug, but the duration may be prolonged with PPIs. The urinalysis often shows leucocyturia and WBC casts. Proteinuria is minimal and microscopic haematuria is not uncommon. Eosinophiluria is neither sensitive nor specific in making a diagnosis of AIN. A renal biopsy would confirm the diagnosis. The biopsy would show a brisk infiltration of the interstitium with lymphocytes and it is common to see eosinophils in the infiltrate. Cessation of the offending drug is the most important step. Treatment with an oral steroid is reasonable if the kidney function does not improve within three to seven days of ceasing the medication.

2. The prolonged exposure to lithium and the slow progression of renal failure are clues to lithium nephrotoxicity. Lithium nephrotoxicity occurs after an average of 20 years of exposure to lithium in about 20% of patients. The renal failure is usually mild with GFR in the range of 45–60 ml/min. Absence of significant proteinuria (>1 g/24 hours) or haematuria also supports the diagnosis. In addition, many patients on lithium have nephrogenic diabetic insipidus (NDI) with significant polyuria which may lead to serum sodium concentration in the higher end of normal or frank hypernatraemia. The disease is reversible in the early stages, but a small proportion of patients progress to ESRD. Amiloride is known to cause some alleviation of NDI by reducing lithium entry into the principal cells of the collecting duct.

3. Lead nephropathy is a possible diagnosis in this patient. The history of occupational exposure to lead, hyperuricaemia, and recurrent gout are clues to the diagnosis. Lead exposure can occur from many sources like paint (houses and industrial paints from before 1980s), smelting yards, soil in places where there has been significant lead contamination, water pipes, and soldering material. Lead content in gasoline has been generally regulated. However, lead continues to be a significant cause of concern among workers and children in the developing world. Chronic lead exposure leads to accumulation of the heavy metal in the bone. Blood levels are often normal. Mobilizing the lead using calcium ethylenediaminetetraacetic acid (EDTA) and then measuring 24 urine lead levels confirm the diagnosis of lead overload. A prominent microcytic anaemia is common due to the toxic effect of lead on RBCs.

4. The presence of mediastinal and hilar adenopathy, progressive renal failure with minimum proteinuria, and history of nephrocalcinosis suggest sarcoidosis. Renal involvement is characterized by a chronic interstitial nephritis and sarcoid granulomas are sometimes seen on biopsy. Co-existing hypercalcaemia is often the cause of renal failure. Early disease responds well to steroids, but progression to ESRD can happen. Renal calculi are very common in sarcoid renal disease.

5. The patient has dry eyes and mouth which makes Sjögren's syndrome a strong possibility. Renal failure in Sjögren's syndrome is due to chronic interstitial nephritis. Often these patients have a distal (type 1) renal tubular acidosis, leading to normal anion gap metabolic acidosis and hypokalaemia.

6. The patient has aristolochic acid nephropathy. The disease is endemic in the Balkans and is a result of contamination of the wheat crop with the plant *Aristolochia cleanatitis,* which has a toxin called aristolochic acid that causes progressive interstitial fibrosis. Progression to renal failure is common. Aristolochic acid nephropathy is also characteristically seen in Chinese herbal nephropathy. There is a high incidence of cellular atypia of the genitourinary tract and patients should have regular surveillance with urine sent for cytology at least once a year.

18

Maintenance Haemodialysis

Lukas Kairaitis

Summary

- Haemodialysis (HD) is a process whereby the solute composition of blood is altered by exposing it to another solution (dialysate) through a semipermeable membrane
- Solutes like urea and creatinine from the blood are removed by diffusion as well as convection when these solutes are dragged along with water molecules across the semipermeable membrane into the dialysate
- For patients with end-stage kidney disease, maintenance HD is provided on an intermittent basis, with treatments usually given three or four times a week

- While both arteriovenous access and chronic HD access catheters (central venous catheters) are the two types of vascular access used for maintenance HD, the former is associated with much lower morbidity and mortality and hence should be the modality of choice
- Hypotension and cramps are the commonest intradialytic complications during HD
- Interdialytic complications include fluid overload, hyperkalaemia, and thrombosis of a HD catheter or arteriovenous access
- Dialysis disequilibrium syndrome manifests with neurological symptoms of varying severity and is usually seen when patients have a rapid reduction in their urea levels due to urgent HD

On a global level, haemodialysis (HD) provides life-sustaining treatment for millions of sufferers of acute and chronic kidney failure. However, despite decades of refinement, it remains a technically complicated treatment that places unique physiological stress on the patient. Haemodialysis is limited in its effectiveness due to its intermittent nature and its inability to substantially replace lost kidney function.

For patients with end-stage renal disease (ESRD), maintenance HD is provided on an intermittent basis, with treatments given in a range of frequencies (from daily to weekly, but usually three or four times a week). Maintenance HD treatment programmes incorporate varying degrees of machine complexity and differing degrees of dialyser reuse. The frequency of treatment offered depends partly on resource availability, but to a large degree is related to the substantial cost and the degree to which this cost is met by the patient and/or the health system or insurance provider. For facility-based HD, the variability in cost of treatment delivery is largely related to labour costs and the extent of reuse of dialysis consumables. In parts of the world, the way in which HD is provided is also influenced by local variations in the way in which different treatments influence reimbursement of dialysis providers and supervising physicians.

Physiology of Dialysis

HD is a process whereby the solute composition of a solution (blood in this case) is altered by exposing it to a second solution (dialysis fluid, i.e. dialysate) through a semipermeable membrane. The semipermeable membrane in this case is the lining of the hollow tubes in the dialysis filter through which blood flows, whilst the dialysis fluid flows in an opposite direction outside of these tubes (Figure 18.1).

Solutes pass from blood to dialysate across the semipermeable membrane by two mechanisms [1]:

- *Diffusion*: the net movement of molecules from a region of high concentration to a region of low concentration. This movement is the outcome of random movement, and so smaller molecules moving at a higher velocity will collide with the semipermeable membrane more often, hence their rate of diffusion will be higher. In comparison, larger molecules, though they can fit into the membrane pores, diffuse across the membrane slowly because they move at a slower velocity and hence collide with the membrane less frequently.
- *Hydrostatic ultrafiltration (convective transport)*: water molecules are much smaller than the pores in the semipermeable dialysis membranes. Ultrafiltration occurs when water is forced across the membrane from the blood to the dialysate side by the generation of a positive hydrostatic pressure across the membrane, called transmembrane pressure (TMP). Solutes which are smaller than the pores on the membrane are effectively dragged across the membrane with the water. This is an example of convective transport.

In HD, diffusion is the predominant mechanism for solute removal. As already discussed, diffusive transport depends on the speed of random molecular motion and this speed is inversely proportional to molecular weight. Therefore, larger molecules, even when they are small enough to cross through the pores on the semipermeable membrane, are not removed adequately during HD.

Most solutes are removed by diffusive clearance from the blood to the dialysate side of the membrane. However, some solutes such as bicarbonate move from the dialysate to the blood side (in this case to assist with the correction of acidosis).

Haemofiltration and Haemodiafiltration

Haemofiltration uses convective movement, which is akin to a wave of water carrying all particles, irrespective of their size, if they are small enough to cross through the pores on the semipermeable membrane. Understandably, larger molecules are cleared much better by haemofiltration in comparison to HD. Haemofiltration is used in many of the slow, continuous renal replacement therapies used in the Intensive Care Unit (ICU) setting. In continuous haemofiltration used in the ICU setting, no dialysis fluid (dialysate) is used. Instead, a large volume of replacement fluid (25–50l/day) is infused into either the inflow or outflow blood line and both this replacement fluid and excess fluid in the patient are removed by ultrafiltration. The chief role of haemofiltration-based slow dialysis therapies is in the sick and hypotensive patient in ICU, who cannot withstand the rapid solute and fluid shifts that occur in conventional HD.

Haemodiafiltration (HDF), which can be done in outpatient dialysis centres, utilizes convective in combination with diffusive clearance; that is, it is essentially a combination of HD and haemofiltration. Compared with conventional HD, HDF allows increased clearance of higher molecular weight molecules and is believed to be associated with better clinical outcomes. HDF requires the infusion of significant amounts (usually 15–30 l per session) of infusate to replace the ultrafiltrate. It is technically more challenging and expensive than conventional HD.

Patient Selection for Maintenance Haemodialysis

Initiating maintenance HD places unique physiological stress on the body. Although HD prolongs the life of patients with ESRD, it exposes the patient to significant treatment-related morbidity and inconvenience. In addition, HD is a relatively expensive treatment that can potentially deprive the individual and medical system of economic resources.

For multiple reasons, the life expectancy of a patient on maintenance HD is reduced. For patients with considerable vascular and age-related pathology, the survival benefit of dialysis when compare to a conservative (i.e. non-dialytic) treatment pathway may only be measured in months (with a significant component of this increased survival being spent undergoing treatment) [2].

It is therefore recommended that, whenever possible, a maintenance dialysis programme should offer appropriate education to patients with progressive chronic kidney disease (CKD) at risk of terminal uraemia about the risks and benefits of future dialysis treatment. This serves partly to facilitate adequate preparation for treatment in patients planned for dialysis (e.g. timely vascular access creation), but also helps to minimize the difficult discussions that eventuate when a patient presents with life-threatening complications of uraemia, but is unprepared for the possibility that life-sustaining dialysis treatment may not be regarded as appropriate.

In a patient with established CKD at risk of terminal uraemia, there are no strong evidence-based sources to advise on when a decision for or against future dialysis treatment should be made. Part of the difficulty here relates to the cause of an individual patient's CKD and how rapidly their glomerular filtration rate is expected to decline. In general, however, a patient chosen as suitable for future HD needs sufficient time for the creation of permanent vascular access (thereby avoiding the need for a HD catheter, with the associated risks of life-threatening infection). A conservative recommendation therefore is that patients should have appropriate education and counselling at least 12 months before a need to start dialysis is anticipated [3].

Access for Haemodialysis

Arteriovenous (AV) access and chronic HD access catheters (central venous catheters) are the two types of vascular access used for maintenance HD. The Kidney Disease Outcomes Quality Initiative (KDOQI) guidelines recommend that AV fistulas should be used in more than 65% of prevalent patients, whilst chronic HD access catheters (more than three months in the absence of a maturing permanent access) should be used in less than 10% of prevalent patients who do not have a contraindication for permanent AV access [2, 3].

Arteriovenous Access

An AV fistula is formed by subcutaneous anastomosis of an artery to an adjacent native vein, allowing blood flow directly from the artery to vein. Formation of the AV fistula increases blood flow in the artery and thus the AV fistula by up to 10 times, which over six to eight weeks usually makes the vein dilated and arterialized (more muscular), enabling it to undergo venepuncture repeatedly for ongoing dialysis. Conceptually an AV graft is similar, but the distance between the artery and the vein is bridged by a tube made of prosthetic material. Whilst one must wait for up to six weeks for the vein in an AV fistula to mature enough to be used for dialysis, AV grafts can be used within one to three weeks of creation. However, AV grafts are more prone to stenosis and infections compared to fistulas, though they are superior to central venous catheters.

Central Haemodialysis Access Catheters

These are most often used when an immediate need for HD arises, for instance in acute kidney injury (AKI), thrombosed HD access or poisoning. The rate of infectious complications with catheters is significantly more than with AV fistulas. They are of two types, as follows:

- Non-tunnelled HD catheters are the preferred catheter for immediate HD vascular access when dialysis is likely to be needed only in the short term.
- Tunnelled catheters are preferred when dialysis is likely to be used for more than a week.

Anatomy of a Typical Haemodialysis Session

HD can be considered to have three sequential sections: the arterial blood line, which pumps blood from the access (AV fistula or dialysis catheter) to the dialyser; the dialyser, where the actual process of diffusion and/or ultrafiltration occurs; and the venous blood line, through which the purified blood is returned to the patient (Figure 18.1).

Extraction of Blood into the Dialysis Circuit via the Arterial Line

The arterial line is connected either to a needle placed in the HD vascular access or the arterial limb of a central venous HD catheter.

A peristaltic pump is used to draw blood into and through the dialysis circuit; the resistance to this flow is monitored by the arterial pressure monitor, which

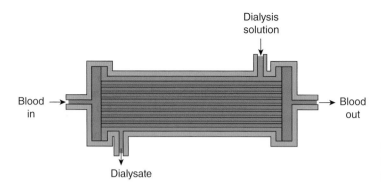

Figure 18.1 Blood and dialysis solution flow pathways through a hollow-fibre dialyser.

triggers an alarm and stops the blood pump if high resistance is found.

An anticoagulant is added to the arterial line, as either a heparin infusion or a bolus of low molecular weight heparin. The purpose of this is to prevent thrombosis of the dialysis filter and lines. A bag of saline is also attached to the arterial line. This is used to flush the dialyser in the case of clots or streaks occuring as well as to enable a fluid bolus to be given to the patient if needed (such as in the case of intra-dialytic hypotension- see below).

Passage of Blood through the Dialyser (Haemodialysis Filter)

Blood from the arterial line enters the arterial end of the dialysis filter. From here, blood then passes through the multitude of hollow tubular fibres of the dialysis filter to the venous end of the filter (Figure 18.2). These hollow fibres are constituted from the semipermeable membrane material through which the actual processes of diffusion and convection occur. Blood and the dialysate solution flow in opposite directions in the dialyser, with blood flowing inside the hollow tubes and the dialysate fluid outside them. The dialysate flow rates are generally set at 1.5–2 times the blood flow rates, with usual flow rates being 300–500 ml/min for blood and 500–800 ml/min for dialysate.

The pore size of the membrane determines the molecular size of solutes that can pass between the blood and dialysate compartments

Diffusive transfer of solutes enables the removal of toxins from the blood side of the membrane to the dialysate. Some solutes (such as bicarbonate) diffuse in the opposite direction from the dialysate to the blood side of the membrane.

Removal of Fluid from the Blood Compartment in the Dialyser Blood

A higher pressure on the blood compartment compared to the dialysate side of the membrane favours the filtration of plasma solutes and water from the blood side into the dialysate (the difference between the pressure in the blood and dialysate compartment is referred to as the TMP). This movement of fluid is termed ultrafiltration and contributes to solute removal (solutes that are small enough to pass through the membrane are removed in equal concentration to the amount of water that is removed from the plasma by ultrafiltration).

The extent of ultrafiltration is normally determined by the TMP, and in most dialysis machines is measured in real time by flow or volumetric sensors, which adjust the TMP continuously to obtain the ultrafiltration target specified by the user at the beginning of the treatment, as part of the dialysis prescription.

Due to ultrafiltration, the volume of blood returned to the patient is less than that entering the dialysis circuit and this results in a contraction of the blood volume of the patient. Due to the removal of solutes, it also has a lower osmolality than the blood entering the filter. This change in osmolality can contribute to contraction of blood volume in the patient (and hypotension), as discussed subsequently.

Return of Treated Blood to the Patient

Blood is returned to the patient via the venous line into the venous needle of the dialysis access or the venous limb of the central venous catheter. The resistance to this return of blood is monitored by the venous pressure monitor.

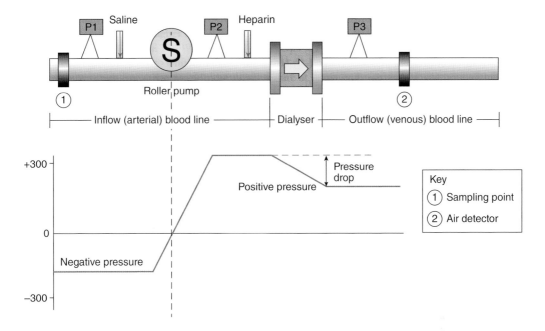

Figure 18.2 Various components of the haemodialysis circuit (P1, P2 and P3 are pre-pump, post-pump and venous pressure monitors, respectively).

Increased resistance to the return of blood above predetermined levels triggers a venous pressure alarm, which stops the blood pump. Increased venous pressure is multifactorial, but is usually related to the dialysis access (e.g. needle placement against the vessel wall, high-flow access with high vessel pressure or thrombosed catheter lumen).

In some circumstances (mainly due to low flow in the dialysis access), the treated blood is drawn back up into the arterial line or needle ('access recirculation') rather than returning to the systemic circulation. This results in a reduction in the effectiveness of treatment. Low blood flow in the dialysis access may be due to venous stenosis, intra-access stenosis or arterial inflow stenosis.

Sawtoothing, the Inevitable Consequence of an Intermittent Treatment

Due the intermittent nature of HD, solutes and fluids are removed from the patient during the treatment and gradually accumulate between treatments.

If plotted over time, the profile of solutes and fluids will assume a 'sawtooth' pattern (Figure 18.3). This pattern highlights the significant differences between

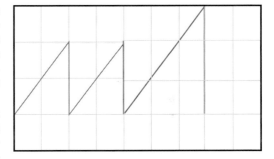

Figure 18.3 Modification to the 'sawtooth' pattern in patients undergoing thrice weekly haemodialysis. This treatment pattern is characterised by two short and one long interdialytic period. Solute and fluid accumulation is at its greatest level at the end of the longest interdialytic period.

the short period of solute and fluid removal (typically 3–5 hours) and the much longer period of reaccumulation (typically 48–72 hours). Both phases of removal and accumulation can be associated with adverse effects on the patient.

A further subtle variation in this pattern is seen in patients on thrice-weekly HD. These patients typically have two shorter interdialytic periods of two days and one longer interdialytic period of three days (the 'long break'). In these patients, there is a higher peak of fluid and electrolyte accumulation after their long break, at which time they are at greatest risk of toxicity from solute and fluid accumulation.

This pattern of removal and accumulation is important when considering the complications that can occur either during the rapid removal phase (*intradialytic consequences*) or the accumulation phase (*interdialytic consequences*).

Because of this sawtooth pattern, biochemical markers measured in the patient will vary significantly over time. By convention, biochemical markers in thrice-weekly HD patients are assessed before the start of their mid-week treatment; although their interpretation must also take into consideration that higher values (and potential toxicity) for these markers (e.g. potassium) are likely to be experienced by the patients after their long break.

Physicians involved in the care of HD patients should be aware of this pattern when assessing both the fluid state and biochemical results of their patients, particularly when altering components of their dialysis prescription (see later).

The sawtooth pattern is also thought to be the cause for the increased risk of sudden death of HD patients experienced at the end of their long break.

Haemodialysis-Associated Complications

Haemodialysis-associated complications can be grouped into intradialytic or interdialytic complications.

Intradialytic Complications

- Hypotension – 25–55% of treatments
- Cramps – 5–20%
- Nausea and vomiting – 5–15%
- Headache – 5%
- Chest pain – 2–5%
- Back pain – 2–5%
- Itching – 5%
- Fever and chills – <1%

Intradialytic Hypotension

Intradialytic hypotension refers to the development of symptomatic hypotension during dialysis. It is characterized by symptoms of light-headedness, abdominal cramping, nausea or palpitations and, in severe cases, loss of consciousness.

The main cause of intradialytic hypotension is a reduction of the effective circulating blood volume, usually related to a mismatch between the amount of fluid removed from the circulation and the extent of plasma refilling [4].

There are several possible explanations for the development of intradialytic hypotension (Table 18.1):

- Extent of ultrafiltration is too high.
- Rate of ultrafiltration is too fast.
- Rate of plasma refilling is too slow.
- 'Reverse plasma refill' occurs.
- Mechanisms to maintain blood pressure during dialysis are impaired (usually due to diminished cardiac reserve or autonomic neuropathy).

In most patients on maintenance HD, there is insufficient urinary volume from residual renal function to prevent an accumulation of fluid in the patient between dialysis sessions, following the sawtooth pattern described earlier. Excess fluid gain leads to zealous attempts to remove fluid by ultrafiltration, which at times precipitates hypotension.

The maximum rate of ultrafiltration and how it is tolerated by the patient is individually determined. Minimizing fluid accumulation between dialysis sessions requires adherence to recommendations for dietary salt and fluid restriction, and occasionally the use of high-dose loop diuretics in patients with a degree of residual urine output.

Extent of Ultrafiltration Is Too High

In the situation where the ultrafiltration target is too high, the patient will reach a point during their HD session where they become effectively hypovolaemic. The hypotension that results in these patients is typically manifest in the later stages of their HD session.

The commonest cause of this is when the patient's target (or dry) weight has been inaccurately determined to be lower than its true level (i.e. the patient's actual dry weight has increased over time). Common causes for this include increased appetite following correction of uraemia in a patient starting dialysis and weight gain following a period of illness-associated weight loss.

Rate of Ultrafiltration Is Too Fast

From a physiological perspective, maintaining adequate circulating blood volume during a patient's HD session requires significant intercompartmental fluid shifts for plasma refill to occur to prevent hypotension.

Table 18.1 Assess for the underlying cause and treat appropriately

Possible cause	Suggested by	Possible solutions
Dry or target weight is set too low (ultrafiltration target is set too high)	Hypotension occurs late in treatment Recent downward adjustment of dry or target weight	Reassess dry or target weight
Ultrafiltration rate is set too high	Ultrafiltration rate is greater than 10 ml/kg/h or 1 l/h	Increase dialysis duration Minimize interdialytic weight gain by salt and fluid restriction Consider high-dose loop diuretic therapy if significant urine volume
Underlying cardiac insufficiency	History or clinical findings of cardiac disease Blood pressure may be low at the beginning of dialysis	Treat underlying cause if possible Consider whether access flow is contributing to cardiac dysfunction Consider high-dose diuretics if residual urine output present Increase dialysis frequency or duration to increase fluid removal Reduce dialysate temperature reduction to 35–36° (induces vasoconstriction) Use of vasoconstrictor treatment (e.g. midodrine or caffeine) during dialysis Use isolated ultrafiltration at initiation of dialysis to minimize osmotic shifts contributing to contraction of plasma volume (reverse plasma refill) Consider change to peritoneal dialysis if appropriate
Excessive or inappropriate antihypertensive therapy	Interdialytic hypotension Low blood pressure at the beginning of dialysis	Review current dose or requirement for antihypertensive therapy by reviewing weekly blood pressure profile
Impaired rate of plasma refill	Low serum albumin level	Treat or reverse underlying cause if possible Prime dialysis circuit with 20% concentrated albumin solution at start of dialysis
Diversion of blood to gastrointestinal tract due to meal during dialysis treatment	Hypotension associated with eating	Avoid meals during dialysis

Clearly, in an individual patient, if the rate of ultrafiltration is set too high, it will exceed the rate of plasma refill and result in the development of hypotension. The maximal rate of tolerated ultrafiltration will vary from patient to patient and is partly dependent on cardiovascular and oncotic factors. In most patients without significant cardiac impairment or disordered plasma refill, a rough rule of thumb for the maximum rate of tolerated ultrafiltration is 10 ml/kg/h.

Rate of Plasma Refill Is Too Slow

During a dialysis treatment in which ultrafiltration occurs, haemodynamic stability is partly dependent on the patient's ability to 'refill' and maintain effective circulating blood volume by intercompartmental fluid shifts. Movement of fluid between compartments is partly related to factors influencing perfusion (i.e. cardiac output) and oncotic factors in the circulation (particularly the serum albumin level).

Some patients with a low serum albumin level who develop hypotension during dialysis will benefit from the infusion of concentrated albumin given during their HD to improve plasma refill and enable appropriate ultrafiltration.

Reverse Plasma Refill

Reverse plasma refill refers to the situation whereby fluid moves out of the plasma compartment when dialysed blood is returned to the patient. This is typically experienced at the start of an HD session when, due to solute removal, the returned blood has a lower osmolality (i.e. contains more water than the blood drawn into the dialysis circuit). The reduced osmolality of the blood returned after dialysis causes extracellular water to move into the cells, which decreases the extracellular volume (i.e. reverse plasma refill).

This phenomenon is typically evident at the commencement of HD, due to the higher solute concentration in the circulation enabling a greater osmotic difference between the circulating blood and the blood returned to the patient. This phenomenon is more likely when the pre-dialysis urea, glucose or sodium (contributors of plasma osmolality) is excessively high.

Mechanisms to Preserve Cardiac Output and Blood Pressure Are Impaired

In some patients, preexisting disease or treatment limits their ability to maintain adequate cardiac output during ultrafiltration. These include:

- *Underlying cardiac failure*: these patients may be excessively sensitive to minor changes in effective circulating blood volume and mismatches between ultrafiltration and plasma refill.
- *Medication that limits cardiovascular responses*: including the use of antihypertensive therapy or beta-blocker (anti-arrhythmic) therapy.
- *Autonomic neuropathy*: common in diabetics.
- *High-volume AV access*: which limits the ability of the patient to adjust non-access cardiac output at the expense of access flow.

Immediate Management of the Patient with Intradialytic Hypotension

- Lie patient flat or in the Trendelenburg position, where the body is laid flat on the back with the feet higher than the head by 15–30°; administer oxygen if unconscious.
- Turn off machine ultrafiltration.
- Infuse 200–500 ml of normal saline via arterial line (or fluid replacement bolus in patients on HDF).
- Consider whether the hypotension is unrelated to the dialysis treatment itself, e.g. due to sepsis, blood loss, myocardial infarction or pulmonary embolus.

Muscle Cramps

The pathogenesis of muscle cramps is believed to involve hypotension, hypovolaemia (excessive fluid removal), need for a high ultrafiltration rate (due to excess water intake in the interdialytic period) and use of low-sodium dialysis solution. All these factors cause vasoconstriction, resulting in muscle hypoperfusion, leading in turn to impairment of muscle relaxation. Although often associated with hypotension, muscle cramps tend to persist after resolution of the hypotension. The use of pre-dialysis quinine is sometimes useful for muscle cramps. Some people suggest carnitine supplementation, 5–10 mg of oxazepam pre-dialysis or prazosin, though hypotension may complicate therapy with the latter.

One needs to be aware though that sometimes hypocalcaemia, hypokalaemia or hypomagnesaemia may be the causative factor for cramps [5].

Chest Pain

Chest pain in a patient being dialysed may be associated with hypotension or dialysis disequilibrium syndrome (DDS; discussed later). In the absence of these two conditions, angina should always be considered given the high incidence of coronary artery disease in patients with ESRD. Other rarer causes of chest pain in this setting include haemolysis and air embolism. Air embolism causing chest pain in the setting of dialysis is extremely rare now due to the presence of air detectors in HD machines.

Haemolysis

Haemolysis usually presents with chest pain or tightness, back pain and dyspnoea [6]. Signs include portwine appearance of the blood in the venous line, pink discoloration of plasma in centrifuged specimens, a rapidly falling haematocrit and sometimes a dramatic deepening of skin coloration. Causes include:

- Overheated dialysis solution.
- Hypotonic dialysis solution.
- Dialysis solution contamination with formaldehyde, bleach, chloramine, fluoride or nitrates from the water supply and copper from copper tubing or piping.
- Blood line obstruction or narrowing due to kinks.

If not detected early, haemolysis can lead to severe hyperkalaemia due to release of potassium from the damaged erythrocytes. Management consists of stopping dialysis immediately, clamping the blood lines (to prevent return of blood and avoid increasing the risk of hyperkalaemia) and preparing to treat hyperkalaemia and the potentially severe anaemia.

Intradialytic Sepsis

Fevers during dialysis should always be presumed to be due to infection of the dialysis access, particularly if the patient is receiving dialysis through an HD catheter (unless there is an obvious source of infection, e.g. florid pharyngitis or infective gastroenteritis) [7]. Other possible causes include:

- Bacterial or viral infection unrelated to the dialysis access.
- Bacterial contamination of the dialysis circuit or membrane (the latter is more common due to membrane reuse).
- Endotoxin or bacterial contamination of the water supply used for dialysate production.
- Membrane reactions (uncommon and rare, usually associated with symptoms of histamine release).

Immediate Management

- Assess oxygenation and blood pressure, administer oxygen and treat hypotension if present.
- Obtain blood cultures from the arterial line of the HD circuit. A full blood count including white cell count is also recommended.
- In most cases with a significant fever, inpatient assessment and treatment are usually required.

Further Assessment

- Take a history from the patient to determine if an infective process was initiated prior to the dialysis session.
- Examine the vascular access for signs of cellulitis, exit site infection or purulent discharge from an HD catheter.
- Examine the patient for other potential sources of infection (especially respiratory, urinary tract or skin sources).
- Perform a chest X-ray.

Initial Antibiotic Treatment

- Unless an alternative source of infection is identified, assume that the infection is related to the vascular access.
- Administer empiric Gram-positive and Gram-negative cover depending on the type of access and the patient's colonization status for multi-resistant organisms (MROs).
- Sample initial antibiotic regimes include:

  o Cephazolin 1.5 g daily and a stat dose of 80 mg gentamicin for a patient not known to be colonized with MROs.
  o Vancomycin 1 g stat and a stat dose of 80 mg gentamicin for a patient colonized with multi-resistant *staphylococcus aureus* (MRSA).
  o Linezolid 600 mg twice daily and a stat dose of 80 mg gentamicin for a patient colonized with vancomycin-resistant enterococcus (VRE).

Further Management

- Tailor the antibiotic choice and duration depending on the culture results.
- For patients with a temporary (non-tunnelled) HD catheter, organize for immediate removal.
- For patients with a permanent (tunnelled) HD catheter, organize for removal if the infection has not been adequately controlled within 48 hours.

In a patient with an infected AV graft, there is a high risk of persistent or necrotic perforation unless the infected graft material is surgically removed.

Interdialytic Complications

- Fluid overload
- Hyperkalaemia
- Thrombosis of a haemodialysis catheter or AV access

Apart from those mentioned, a potential complication associated with overly aggressive lowering of urea due to urgent HD in the AKI patient is DDS, discussed later.

Fluid Overload Due to Dry or Target Weight Being Too High

In this situation, the patient has fluid overload present at the end of their dialysis session. The presence of pre-existing fluid overload (even when mild and relatively asymptomatic) means that the patient is more likely to develop symptoms of excess fluid overload prior to their next scheduled treatment.

Clues to this being present are:

- Symptoms or signs of fluid overload that persist at the end of a dialysis session despite the patient achieving their dry or target weight.
- Recent acute or intercurrent illness associated with weight loss that has not been associated with a downward adjustment of the dry or target weight.
- A recent upward adjustment of dry weight.

In this situation the management is to reduce the target or dry weight and reassess the patient after a short period to determine if the dry weight needs to be further adjusted. The degree of dry weight reduction required is variable from patient to patient and has to take into account how severe the symptoms are. For patients with milder manifestations of fluid overload in this situation the degree of fluid overload is typically 40–100 mL/kg. Reducing the dry weight in sequential dialysis sessions by 1 kg with weekly reassessment is a conservative recommendation. Significant complications of fluid overload either indicate a greater extent of fluid overload (100 mL/kg or above) or more moderate degrees of fluid overload in a patient with underlying cardiac insufficiency. Management of these patients should address the cause of their underlying cardiac disease if possible as well as consideration of other contributory factors (e.g. anaemia, excessive arteriovenous access flow).

Assessment for a Possible Cause of Interdialytic Fluid Overload

Review dialysis treatment chart:

- Has the patient been compliant with the prescribed dialysis regime and treatment time? (Missed or shortened dialysis sessions place the patient at risk of fluid overload due to less fluid being removed over a period of time).

- Is the current targeted dry weight being achieved during treatments?
- Has the dry weight been recently adjusted upward?
- What is the dialysate sodium? Is sodium profiling being used to prevent intradialytic hypotension?

What is the interdialytic weight gain? As mentioned above the tolerated ultrafiltration rate for an individual patient may vary, however, most guidelines recommend limiting the ultrafiltration rate to 10 mL/kg per hour or 1 L per hour. Depending on the prescribed dialysis duration, this places limits on the ability of each haemodialysis treatment to achieve the target or dry weight. Excessive interdialytic weight gain is usually linked either to excessive salt and fluid intake by the patient or excessive thirst due to prescribed medication. An alternative cause is increased thirst as a result of sodium transfer to the patient during their haemodialysis session.

Fluid Overload Due to Excessive Interdialytic Weight Gain

In some patients, the reason for fluid overload is due to excessive intake of salt and fluid between dialysis sessions. As mentioned, there are limitations placed on the extent of fluid that can be removed in an individual patient, dependent upon:

- The duration of each dialysis session and the maximum hourly ultrafiltration rate tolerated by the patient.
- The number of dialysis sessions performed over a period (e.g. treatments per week).

In a patient with interdialytic fluid overload, a review of their dialysis treatment chart (which typically includes details about measured weights pre- and post-dialysis) will usually show an inability of the patient to achieve their prescribed dry or target weight.

Excessive interdialytic fluid and sodium intake can be determined by several patient-related factors, including:

- Excessive dietary salt intake (which is a determinant of thirst).
- Medications which induce thirst, e.g. antidepressant medications.
- Poorly controlled blood sugar levels.
- Cardiac dysfunction associated with reduced perfusion.

An additional contributor to thirst is diffusive sodium transfer into the patient occurring during their dialysis treatment related to the difference between dialysate sodium (typically 140 mM, titratable between 125–155 mmol/L) and plasma sodium. The degree of sodium transfer can be increased by the use of 'sodium profiling'. Sodium profiling refers to the use of higher than physiological levels of dialysate sodium in an attempt to prevent intradialytic hypotension. Although effective in this regard it has fallen out of favour due to the resultant sodium transfer that occurs leading to increased interdialytic weight gain.

Fluid Overload as a Consequence of a Long Interdialytic Period

As mentioned, fluid overload is most common during a thrice-weekly treatment plan during the long break. The risk of fluid overload is further increased in patients receiving maintenance treatment less often than thrice weekly or patients who are non-adherent with scheduled sessions. In addition, patients who shorten their treatment sessions voluntarily are at risk of fluid overload, since they rarely achieve their prescribed target or dry weight.

Treatments to Minimize Interdialytic Fluid Overload

The initial management of the patient with fluid overload depends on the timing (with relation to scheduled HD treatments) and severity of the clinical manifestations.

Patients who have severe hypoxaemia typically require hospitalization and resuscitation with oxygen and may require positive pressure airway ventilation. These patients may also require urgent unscheduled HD if they cannot safely wait until their next scheduled dialysis session. Alternative causes of acute respiratory distress need to be excluded (particularly myocardial ischaemia or arrhythmia).

Milder degrees of fluid overload can often be managed without hospitalization; however, the patient requires further assessment as detailed to determine the underlying cause. Interventions that may help with reducing recurrence of fluid overload include:

- Downward adjustment of target or dry weight with frequent reassessment.
- Dietary counselling on sodium and fluid intake.
- Use of high-dose oral loop diuretic treatments in patients with residual urine output.
- Downward adjustment of the dialysate sodium level (guided by the measured pre-dialysis sodium level).
- Increasing the frequency or duration of dialysis (thereby increasing the ultrafiltration potential).

- Treating underlying cardiac disease.
- Restricting HD access flow if measured more than 2 l/min, or when the access flow to cardiac output ratio exceeds 30%.
- Considering a change to peritoneal dialysis.

Hyperkalaemia

Potassium can pose a significant risk of toxicity due to its accumulation in the interdialytic period. As would be expected, the risk is greatest after the longest interdialytic period, particularly if there have been missed dialysis sessions.

Symptomatic hyperkalaemia in a patient without fatal arrhythmia is usually manifest as muscle weakness and may be associated with bradycardia, hypotension and classical electrocardiogram (ECG) changes. These patients require urgent resuscitation as per local practice, with intravenous calcium given as soon as intravenous access can be safely obtained. Stabilization of cardiac effects is mandatory before HD can be commenced; other measures to shift potassium into cells, including insulin/dextrose and bicarbonate injection, should also be continued until the patient is stable.

Any patient with hyperkalaemia on routine testing should be evaluated for a possible cause. This is because by convention, routine biochemical testing for a patient on maintenance thrice-weekly haemodialysis is performed prior to the *mid-week* haemodialysis session. Hyperkalaemia on these tests will underestimate the degree of hyperkalaemia after the longer interdialytic break for a thrice-weekly treatment schedule. In most patients found to have hyperkalaemia on routine testing, the results of the test are only made apparent after the patient has commenced HD, so in effect part of the treatment has already begun.

In simplistic terms, pre-dialysis hyperkalaemia is related to either inadequate removal or excessive accumulation. Each is discussed separately [8].

Inadequate Removal

Determinants of potassium removal during dialysis include:

- The intensity of the delivered dialysis treatment (e.g. hours/week). The extent of dialysis not only determines the degree of potassium removal, but also whether the metabolic acidosis of uraemia has been corrected. Correction of acidosis during dialysis facilitates potassium removal from the body by shifting potassium out of cells.

- Dialysate potassium levels.
- Extent of recirculation within the dialysis access:
  - Reversal of blood lines for a haemodialysis catheter
  - Poor access flow.
- Cardiopulmonary recirculation, which occurs when a significant component of cardiac output is diverted back to the vascular access instead of returning to the systemic circulation. Cardiopulmonary recirculation is more common when there is reduced cardiac function and worsened when AV access flow exceeds more than 2 l/min or represents more than 30% of cardiac output [9].

Excessive Accumulation

Serum potassium levels increase inexorably between HD sessions along the sawtooth profile already described. The main factors that contribute to excessive accumulation are dietary sources of potassium and medications that increase potassium.

Medications associated with hyperkalaemia include potassium-containing supplements and agents that block the renin–angiotensin system – that is, angiotensin-converting enzyme inhibitors and angiotensin receptor blockers – and aldosterone antagonists like spironolactone.

Dietary sources of potassium are multiple, and on a global scale there is significant variability of 'culprit' foods that should be restricted in the diet of patients with hyperkalaemia. The assistance of a dietician is invaluable in identifying high-potassium sources in the diet and recommending substitute foods.

Suggested Approach to the Patient with Interdialytic Hyperkalaemia

Evaluate for Cause

- Review previous results and serum bicarbonate levels. Incomplete correction of uraemia-associated acidosis is a key to an inadequate dialysis dose, as mentioned.
- Check dialysate potassium (typically 1–3 mM, can be reduced if necessary).
- Take a medication and dietary history.
- Check for non-adherence to dialysis schedule or prescribed treatment times.
- In the absence of a clear cause, assess for access recirculation, cardiac disease or excessive flow in an AV access.

Treatment

Patients with significant or life-threatening hyperkalaemia typically require multiple interventions to bring their potassium back to a safe level. Possible interventions include:

- Review diet and modify to exclude high-potassium food sources.
- Reduce dialysate potassium level.
- Increase delivered dialysis dose (frequency, treatment time).
- Remove or reduce dose of medications contributing to hyperkalaemia.
- Prescribe potassium-binding resins. These resins are effective but expensive. A typical dosing for Calcium Resonium® is 15 g three times daily during periods of hyperkalaemia. The long-term safety of regular Resonium use as an alternative to other interventions is questionable due to cost and side effects (particularly constipation).
- Treat access dysfunction (low- or high-flow states) if present.
- Consider switch to peritoneal dialysis if feasible. Hyperkalaemia is much less common in peritoneal dialysis patients due to greater removal.

Access Thrombosis

Thrombosis of an HD catheter or AV access presents a management challenge, mainly because there are potentially conflicting demands to maintain the stability of the patient with dialysis whilst safely managing the clotted access. A patient presenting with a clotted access may potentially require urgent HD before access patency can be restored. The requirement for acute dialysis and temporary access is dependent upon both the biochemical and fluid status of the patient as well as the anticipated delay before intervention on the clotted access.

Initial assessment of the patient presenting with access thrombosis should therefore involve a fluid state and biochemical assessment to determine whether dialysis can be safely delayed until the access can be declotted. Depending on local practice, the patient may need to be fasted if operative correction is typically used.

For patients with a permanent HD catheter, luminal patency can often be restored though the use of a thrombolytic agent such as recombinant tissue plasminogen activator (rTPA). A typical protocol for rTPA use involves locking the blocked lumen with a solution of 1 mg/ml rTPA (volume administered is determined by the luminal volume). The patency of the lumen is then assessed at regular time points.

If catheter patency is not established, then catheter exchange or endovascular techniques can be performed.

For patients dialysing with an AV fistula or graft, the main risks for access thrombosis are reduced access flow, hypotension and raised haematocrit secondary to erythropoietin usage. Thrombosis is more common in an AV graft than in an AV fistula. Flow-based fistula surveillance programmes have been shown to reduce the incidence of access thrombosis. In these programmes, reduced fistula or graft flow detected with prospective monitoring can reduce subsequent thrombosis when a reversible cause (typically a stenosis within the access) is identified and corrected [10].

Options for treatment of a clotted AV access include open surgical or endovascular techniques. Clot removal is usually attempted with a combination of mechanical and thrombolytic techniques. Thrombectomy of an AV access should always involve an assessment during the intervention as to the underlying cause, with a stenotic lesion identified in most cases.

Dialysis Disequilibrium Syndrome

DDS manifests with neurological symptoms of varying severity that affect dialysis patients, particularly when they are first started on HD [11]. It is thought that rapid solute removal lowers the extracellular osmolality, leading to water shift from extracellular to intracellular compartment, causing cerebral oedema manifesting as DDS.

Clinically, the condition is most commonly seen when patients with very high urea levels have a rapid reduction in their urea levels due to urgent HD.

Symptoms of DDS include headache, nausea, confusion and blurring of vision. It may in severe cases be complicated by seizures or even coma.

DDS can be prevented by:

- Identifying situations where it is more likely to occur, i.e. patients undergoing their first HD treatment or recommencing treatment after multiple missed treatments, or significantly elevated predialysis urea levels, e.g. greater than 50 mmol/l.
- Initiating dialysis in such situations with a low-clearance filter (i.e. small surface area dialyser).
- At the commencement of maintenance dialysis, initial treatment should utilize several short durations, e.g. two hours of dialysis at a relatively low blood flow rate of 150–250 ml/min on a daily or second-daily basis. If the patient shows no signs of dialysis disequilibrium, then blood flow rate can

be increased by 50 ml/min per treatment (up to 300–400 ml/min), and the duration of dialysis can be increased in 30-minute increments.
- If urgent fluid removal is required, isolated ultrafiltration can be used to prevent dialysis disequilibrium, as the fluid removed in this situation has the same osmolality as the patient.

If DDS occurs, treatment is generally supportive and one must determine whether dialysis should be ceased or modified. Generally, it is recommended to cease the treatment and consider recommencement of treatment with a lower-clearance filter and slower blood flow rates the following day.

Elements of the Basic Haemodialysis Prescription

Prescribing maintenance HD for an individual patient is influenced partly by local resource availability, the degree of residual renal function and whether/how the cost of treatment is met by the patient or service provider.

The basic components of the dialysis prescription are:

- Dialysis dose (principally determined by treatment time and frequency)
- Target or dry weight
- Type and dose of anticoagulation
- Dialysate concentrations of sodium, potassium and calcium

Dialysis Dosing

The major determinants of the delivered dose of dialysis are the treatment time and frequency of treatment. Lesser determinants are the filter characteristics (permeability and surface area), blood and dialysate flow rates.

Although shorter treatment times can be modified to give equivalent removal of simple solutes such as urea (assessed by Kt/V), it has been unequivocally shown that longer dialysis treatment times are independently associated with decreased mortality at equivalent levels of urea removal [12]. Longer treatment times allow for greater removal of larger molecular weight solutes, increase the achievable ultrafiltration and minimize post-dialysis symptoms.

Table 18.2 Commonly prescribed levels of dialysate electrolytes and variations that may be performed in specific circumstances

Electrolyte	Commonly prescribed level	Alteration	Potential benefit	Potential risk
Sodium	137–140 mmol/l	Increase to 140–145 mmol/l	Improved haemodynamic stability and less intradialytic cramps	Sodium loading of patient increases interdialytic thirst and weight gain
		Reduce to 130–135 mmol/l	Minimizes sodium transfer and reduces interdialytic thirst and weight gain	Increased intradialytic cramping
		'Ramped' sodium (high at start, low at end – 'sodium profiling')	Improved haemodynamic stability and fewer intradialytic cramps	Sodium loading of patient increases interdialytic thirst and weight gain
Dialysate potassium	2–3 mmol/l	Reduce to 1 mmol/l	Greater potential extent of potassium removal in patients with hyperkalaemia	Risk of precipitating atrial arrhythmias during dialysis
Dialysate calcium	1.5 mmol/l	Reduce to 0.9–1.2 mmol/l	Reduced calcium in patients with hypercalcaemia Stimulation of parathyroid hormone production in patients with suppressed parathyroid hormone and low bone turnover	Increased risk of cardiac arrhythmia and intradialytic hypotension
		Increase to 1.7–1.9 mmol/l	Treatment of patients with hypocalcaemia post-parathyroidectomy	Risk of precipitating hypercalcaemia with ongoing use

Similarly, increased dialysis frequency has been shown to have favourable impacts on patient outcomes, as exemplified by the positive results of the recent Frequent Haemodialysis Network trial [13].

Determining the treatment time and frequency for an individual patient is a difficult decision for the dialysis prescriber. On one hand, there are benefits from more frequent or longer treatments, as described. On the other hand, shorter or less frequent treatment times increase resource availability for other patients. Patient acceptance of long or short treatment times is variable. At the end of the day, a compromise needs to be reached between the patient and the dialysis provider regarding the acceptability of a treatment plan and its impact on the health and finances of the individual and the dialysis provider. A reasonable goal for a dialysis treatment plan is to provide dialysis thrice-weekly with a minimum duration of four hours, ideally with the goal of being able to offer longer or more frequent treatments. The use of shorter or less frequent treatments is a less ideal solution, but one that is often influenced by local resource availability.

Target or Dry Weight

As already discussed, part of the prescription for dialysis requires an estimation of the dry or target weight of the patient. Repeat clinical assessment of the patient's fluid status remains the major tool for determining the dry weight, and dialysis prescribers should become familiar with the physical examination findings of volume overload and depletion.

A number of tools may assist in determination of the dry or target weight including the use of bio impedance measurements and 'relative blood volume' measurements. A detailed description of these measures is beyond the scope of this chapter. Although these measures have not been validated extensively, they may assist in dry weight changes in patients who tolerate ultrafiltration poorly or present with fluid overload, particularly if fluid status examination is difficult to interpret.

Although it is relatively easy to identify the need to adjust the dry or target weight in patients experiencing volume overload or hypotension, monitoring the fluid status in stable patients is also difficult at times. The sawtooth pattern of fluid accumulation and removal means that physical examination of fluid status needs to take into consideration the timing of the patient's last and next dialysis sessions.

Anticoagulation for Haemodialysis

Without systemic anticoagulation, there is an increased risk of clotting of the extracorporeal circuit [14]. Partial clotting ('streaking') of the dialysis filter reduces the membrane surface area for dialysis; complete clotting of the circuit resulting in a need to discard the filter and blood lines can equate to the loss of several hundred millilitres of blood.

In special situations (e.g. in an actively bleeding patient or when the patient is scheduled for surgery following dialysis), anticoagulant-free dialysis can be performed. This requires close monitoring of the dialysis filter and lines for signs of clotting and frequent flushes of the circuit with saline.

Anticoagulation for HD is normally provided using either a single shot of low molecular weight heparin or an infusion of unfractionated heparin. Most dialysis machines incorporate a syringe driver designed to administer a heparin infusion at a prescribed rate. The general principle for heparin prescribing is to use the minimum dose required to prevent streaking and facilitate haemostasis after removal of the dialysis cannula.

Dialysate Sodium, Potassium and Calcium

As already detailed, the dialysate solution is prepared continuously by the HD machine by dilution of pre-packaged concentrates containing sodium, bicarbonate, potassium, calcium and magnesium. Different concentrations of potassium and calcium are achieved by using different specific formulations of acid concentrate (Table 18.2) [15]. The sodium level of the dialysate can be varied in real time by the dialysis machine by altering the proportioning of the sodium bicarbonate concentrate. The sodium level of the dialysate is estimated continuously by measuring the conductivity (which is largely determined by sodium as the predominant cation).

References

1. Hall, N.A. and Fox, A.J. (2006). Renal replacement therapies in critical care. *Cont. Educ. Anaest. Crit. Care Pain* 6 (5): 197–202. https://doi.org/10.1093/bjaceaccp/mkl038.

2. Chandna, S.M., Da Silva-Gane, M., Marshall, C. et al. (2011). Survival of elderly patients with stage 5 CKD: comparison of conservative management and renal replacement therapy. *Nephrol. Dial. Transplant.* 26 (5): 1608–1614.

3. Kidney Disease: Improving Global Outcomes (KDIGO) CKD Work Group (2013). KDIGO 2012 clinical practice guideline for the evaluation and management of chronic kidney disease. *Kidney Int.* 3: 1–150.

4. Palmer, B.F. and Henrich, W.L. (2008). Recent Advances in the Prevention and Management of Intradialytic Hypotension. *JASN* 19 (1): 8–11. https://doi.org/10.1681/ASN.2007091006.

5. Lynch, P.G., Abate, M., Suh, H., and Nand, K. (2014). Magnesium and Muscle Cramps in End Stage Renal Disease Patients on Chronic Hemodialysis. *Wadhwa Adv. Nephrol*: Article ID 681969. http://dx.doi.org/10.1155/2014/681969.

6. Tharmaraj, D. and Kerr, P.G. (2017). Haemolysis in haemodialysis. *Nephrology (Carlton).* 22 (11): 838.

7. Lata, C., Girard, L., Parkins, M., and James, M.T. (2016). Catheter-related bloodstream infection in end-stage kidney disease: a Canadian narrative review. *Can. J. Kidney Health Dis.* 3: 24. https://doi.org/10.1186/s40697-016-0115-8.

8. Pani, A., Floris, M., Rosner, M.H., and Ronco, C. (2014). Hyperkalemia in hemodialysis patients. *Semin. Dial.* 27 (6): 571–576. https://doi.org/10.1111/sdi.12272.

9. Basile, C., Lomonte, C., Vernaglione, L. et al. (2008). The relationship between the flow of arteriovenous fistula and cardiac output in haemodialysis patients. *Nephrol. Dial. Transplant.* 23 (1): 282–287.

10. National Kidney Foundation (2006). KDOQI clinical practice guidelines and clinical practice recommendations for 2006 updates: hemodialysis adequacy, peritoneal dialysis adequacy and vascular access. *Am. J. Kidney Dis.* 48: S1–S322.

11. Arieff, A.I. (1994). Dialysis disequilibrium syndrome: current concepts on pathogenesis and prevention. *Kidney Int.* 45 (3): 629.

12. Saran, R., Bragg-Gresham, J.L., Levin, N.W. et al. (2006). Longer treatment time and slower ultrafiltration in hemodialysis: associations with reduced mortality in the DOPPS. *Kidney Int.* 69 (7): 1222–1228.

13. FHN Trial Group, Chertow, G.M., Levin, N.W. et al. (2010). In-center hemodialysis six times per week versus three times per week. *N. Engl. J. Med.* 363 (24): 2287–2300.

14. Suranyi, M. and Chow, J.S. (2010). Review: anticoagulation for haemodialysis. *Nephrology (Carlton).* J15 (4): 386–392. https://doi.org/10.1111/j.1440-1797.2010.01298.x.

15. Pun, P.H. and Middleton, J.P. (2017). Dialysate potassium, dialysate magnesium, and hemodialysis risk. *JASN* 28 (12): 3441–3451. https://doi.org/10.1681/ASN.2017060640.

Questions and Answers

Questions

1. Which of the following is not a potential complication following formation of a brachiocephalic arteriovenous fistula?
   a. Increased blood supply to the ipsilateral hand
   b. Increased heart rate
   c. Oedema of the ipsilateral hand
   d. Increased cardiopulmonary recirculation
   e. Increased blood flow in the brachial artery

2. A 72 year-old patient with cardiac failure due to valvular heart disease is on maintenance dialysis. However, his haemodialysis is complicated by symptomatic hypotension. To reduce this, the dialysis nursing staff modify his treatment so that no fluid is removed by ultrafiltration during the initial hour of treatment. Despite this change, symptomatic hypotension occurs. Which of the following is likely to explain this phenomenon?
   a. Myocardial stunning causing a reduction in contractility during dialysis
   b. 'Reverse plasma refill' resulting in a contraction of circulating blood volume
   c. Peripheral vasodilation in response to thermal transfer
   d. Augmented vascular access flow contributing to high output cardiac failure
   e. Elevated pre-dialysis potassium levels influencing myocardial contractility

3. Which of the following is the most effective way of increasing the delivered dose of haemodialysis?
   a. Increase the size of the filter by 25%
   b. Increase blood flow by 25%
   c. Increase dialysate flow by 50%
   d. Increase delivered dialysis time by 25%

4. Which of the following is not a potential cause of pre-dialysis hyperkalaemia?
   a. Recent commencement of metoprolol
   b. Increased intake of potato chips
   c. Significant mitral stenosis associated with dyspnoea
   d. Loss of bicarbonate from a high output ileostomy
   e. Shortened treatment time by the patient

5. Which of the following describes the solute movements that occur during haemodialysis?
   a. Diffusion of solutes down a concentration gradient from the blood to the dialysate side of the membrane
   b. Diffusion of solutes down a concentration gradient from the dialysate to the blood side of the dialysis membrane
   c. Convective clearance of solutes due to filtration across the dialysis membrane from the blood to the dialysate side
   d. All the above

6. Which of the following is true regarding dialysis vascular access?
   a. Cuffed and tunnelled haemodialysis catheters have a similar infection rate to non-cuffed dialysis catheters
   b. Arteriovenous fistulae are more prone to thrombosis at low flow rates than arteriovenous grafts
   c. High-flow upper arm arteriovenous fistulae can contribute to ineffective treatment due to recirculation
   d. Arteriovenous grafts are the preferred form of vascular access in most chronic haemodialysis patients
   e. When a stenosis occurs in a forearm radiocephalic fistula, it typically occurs in the outflow segment

7. What proportion of renal function/clearance is replaced by a 'conventional' model of haemodialysis (three sessions of four hours per week)?
   a. 5%
   b. 10%
   c. 15%
   d. 20%
   e. More than 20%

8. Which of the following is true regarding fluid overload in a haemodialysis patient?
   a. Dependent pitting oedema is always a sign of intravascular fluid overload and should be managed with increased dialysis fluid removal
   b. Can usually be managed acutely with high-dose loop diuretic therapy
   c. Relates directly to dietary potassium intake
   d. A reduced serum albumin level increases the risk of intradialytic hypotension

Answers

1. a. Placement of a brachiocephalic AV fistula can reduce perfusion of the more distal extremity because of shunting (steal) of arterial blood flow into the fistula. Symptomatic steal occurs in up to 20% of patients receiving an upper extremity access with severe manifestations requiring intervention in 4%. If the fistula flow becomes excessive or a venous outflow obstruction is present (for example, in the setting of central venous stenosis following a haemodialysis catheter), then venous oedema of the arm can occur with the possible finding of multiple collateral channels over the shoulder. Arteriovenous access diverts blood from the systemic circulation and facilitates cardiopulmonary recirculation which can reduce the efficiency of dialysis and contribute to systemic symptoms of cardiac insufficiency. If fistula flow is excessive, the heart rate is increased in response to the diversion of blood into the fistula; a reduction in heart rate following temporary fistula occlusion is a sign of cardiac compromise because of fistula flow. Formation of the AV fistula increases blood flow in the artery and thus the AV fistula by up to 10 times, which over a period makes the vein dilated and arterialized (more muscular) enabling it to undergo venepuncture repeatedly for ongoing dialysis.

2. b. Ultrafiltration is facilitated by a difference in transmembrane pressure and controlled by ultrafiltration controllers in most modern dialysis machines. Even when ultrafiltration is minimal or zero, the circulating blood volume of the patient can contract by reverse plasma refill. This phenomenon occurs when the osmolality of the blood returning to the patient from the dialysis circuit has a relative excess of water (lower tonicity) due to solute removal. Answer c is incorrect if the dialysate is at a normal temperature (lowering dialysate temperature can induce vasoconstriction which may help to reduce intradialytic hypotension). Answer d is incorrect as although excessive vascular access flow may contribute to cardiac decompensation, access flow typically falls during dialysis.

3. d. Although many studies quoting dialysis dose suggest that urea removal measures (kt/v for example) can be achieved by shorter dialysis duration times and higher filter sizes, this measure only estimates small solute clearance and is affected significantly by post dialysis rebound. Middle molecule clearance is more effectively increased by changing the dialysis duration.

4. a. Potato chips are a dietary source of potassium. Metabolic acidosis due to bicarbonate loss (e.g. from high output ileostomy) causes shift of potassium from the cells and contributes to hyperkalaemia. Significant cardiac failure reduces the efficiency of dialysis due to cardiopulmonary recirculation and poor control of uraemic acidosis. Missed or shortened dialysis sessions are associated with reduced potassium removal and a risk of hyperkalaemia.

5. d. Most solutes are removed by diffusive clearance from the blood to the dialysate side of the membrane; however, some solutes such as bicarbonate move from the dialysate to the blood side (in this case to assist with the correction of acidosis). Convective clearance refers to the removal of solutes and water by filtration assisted by a higher hydrostatic pressure on the blood side of the membrane (transmembrane pressure); this excludes solutes of higher molecular weight based on the pore size of the membrane.

6. c. In the setting of high flow fistulae, although 'access recirculation' (caused by mixing of blood between needling sites) is unusual, cardiopulmonary recirculation is common if the fistula flow comprises a significant proportion of cardiac output (in rough terms, if basal fistula flow is 40% of cardiac output, then 40% of the dialysed blood returning to the heart is recirculated back to the fistula). Non-cuffed haemodialysis catheters have a very high infection rate which is the reason why short-term use is recommended in clinical practice guidelines such as KDOQI. Arteriovenous fistulae are much less prone to thrombosis than arteriovenous grafts and can remain patent at low flow rates. They are the preferred form of vascular access in most long-term patients due to higher patency and lower risks of infection. As opposed to AV grafts or upper arm fistulae, limiting stenosis of radiocephalic AV fistulae are most commonly in the *inflow* segment and increase the risk of 'access' recirculation and thrombosis (even though unlike AV grafts they can remain patent at very low flow rates).

7. b. Due to the intermittent nature of haemodialysis (in this case given for approximately 7% of the week) it is impossible for haemodialysis to replace a significant proportion of renal function or clearance, even if the dialysis machine provides more effective clearance of solutes from the blood during the treatment itself.

8. d. Dependent oedema may sometimes reflect local venous hypertension, low serum albumin, or the use of calcium antagonist therapy and may not respond to removal of fluid from the intravascular compartment during dialysis. Acute fluid overload in a dialysis patient may respond to high-dose loop diuretic therapy in the setting of significant residual urinary volume; however, that is the exception rather than the usual. Dietary sodium rather than potassium intake is a major determinant of interdialytic thirst and the risk of fluid overload. Removal of fluid during dialysis from the intravascular compartment requires subsequent 'plasma refilling' to maintain cardiac output. Mobilization of extravascular fluid is reduced in patients with a low albumin level and increases the risk of intradialytic hypotension.

19

Peritoneal Dialysis: Principles, Indications, and Common Complications

Sarah So and Kamal Sud

Summary

- Peritoneal dialysis (PD) is a cost-effective dialysis modality that can be used to treat patients with both acute kidney injury and end-stage kidney failure. It uses the semipermeable peritoneal membrane through which both diffusion and ultrafiltration (UF) occur
- Sterile pre-prepared hyperosmotic PD fluid is exchanged several times a day through a PD catheter to achieve adequate solute clearances and fluid removal
- PD exchanges can be conducted either manually or using an automated cycler to suit patients' needs, as well as peritoneal membrane transport characteristics
- Peritoneal membrane transport characteristics of individual patients can be measured and determine the relative effectiveness of solute clearance and UF; those with a more permeable membrane have good solute clearances but poor UF while those with less permeable membrane have relatively poor solute clearances but good UF
- Glucose is the standard osmotic agent used in PD fluids to achieve UF and fluids with different concentrations of glucose can be prescribed to achieve the desired volume of UF. High concentrations of glucose are, however, associated with adverse metabolic effects in patients, and lead to the production of glucose degradation products (GDPs) that are injurious to the PD membrane
- Icodextrin is a polymaltose glucose macromolecule polymer that can be used as a glucose-sparing agent in the long dwell of PD exchange to achieve good UF
- Low GDP–neutral pH PD fluids are associated with preservation of urine output and residual renal function, as well as lower incidence of inflow pain
- PD-related peritonitis is a major cause of technique failure as well as mortality that is best treated with intermittent dosing of antibiotics administered intraperitoneally

Lecture Notes Nephrology: A Comprehensive Guide to Renal Medicine, First Edition. Edited by Surjit Tarafdar.
© 2020 John Wiley & Sons Ltd. Published 2020 by John Wiley & Sons Ltd.

- PD has some advantages over haemodialysis (HD), including maintaining residual renal function and promoting independent lifestyle and ability to travel
- Although PD shows an initial survival advantage compared to HD, the long-term survival rate is similar for the two modalities

Peritoneal dialysis (PD) is one of the two major dialysis modalities that can be used in patients with renal failure, both from acute kidney injury (AKI) as well as in those with end-stage renal disease (ESRD). In patients with AKI, PD is used in settings where renal replacement therapies requiring extracorporeal circulation are either not possible or unsuitable, such as in children and neonates [1, 2] or in resource-constrained settings [3]. In these settings, PD is generally employed as an intermittent therapy using a temporary PD catheter. In the developed world, PD is primarily used in patients with ESRD as a chronic (and often continuous) treatment using a permanent PD catheter. In the latter group, PD, together with intermittent haemodialysis (HD) and kidney transplantation, is an important modality to maintain health and sustain life.

Principles of Peritoneal Dialysis

PD utilizes the semipermeable peritoneal membrane that lines the peritoneal cavity for dialysis. The peritoneal membrane has a surface area roughly equal to the body surface area and ranges between 1 and $2\,m^2$ in adults [4]. The visceral peritoneum that lines the gastrointestinal tract and other viscera in the abdomen accounts for 80% of this surface area, whilst the rest of peritoneal membrane (parietal peritoneum) lines the walls of the abdominal cavity. The peritoneal membrane derives its blood supply from the superior mesenteric, lumbar, intercostal, and epigastric arteries (between 50 and $100\,ml/min$), whilst venous blood drains into the portal vein and the inferior vena cava [5]. Lymphatic drainage mainly occurs via stomata in the diaphragmatic peritoneum into the right lymphatic duct.

The semipermeable peritoneal membrane allows both diffusion and ultrafiltration (UF) – the two key components of dialysis therapy. Diffusion is a process that allows movement of solutes across a semipermeable membrane along their *concentration* gradients, whereas UF involves movement of solvent across the semipermeable membrane along a *pressure* gradient [6].

As opposed to HD, where UF is promoted mainly by a hydrostatic pressure gradient across the semipermeable membrane, UF in PD is primarily promoted by an osmotic pressure gradient created by the hyperosmotic PD fluid instilled in the peritoneal cavity [5]. These two processes can only occur when the semipermeable peritoneal membrane separates the blood compartment and dialysis fluid. To improve the efficiency of these processes, the peritoneal membrane has to be continuously exposed to both the blood compartment and the dialysis fluid [4]. The latter is achieved by repeatedly exchanging the prescribed PD fluid in the peritoneal cavity though a PD catheter, the tip of which sits in the most dependent area of the peritoneal cavity – the pouch of Douglas.

The peritoneal membrane is lined by a single-layered mesothelium, under which the interstitium contains peritoneal capillaries and lymphatics interspersed in a collagenous matrix. Most of the resistance to the diffusion of solutes occurs at the level of capillary endothelium and capillary basement membrane, with interstitium and the peritoneal mesothelial layer producing trivial resistance [5, 7]. Factors that influence solute transport and diffusion include the concentration gradient of the solute across the peritoneal semipermeable membrane; the effective surface area of the peritoneal membrane that comes into contact with the dialysis fluid (which can be increased by increasing the volume of dialysis fluid in the peritoneal cavity); the molecular weight of solutes – with small molecular weight solutes diffusing more rapidly and vice versa; and, to a lesser extent, by the peritoneal membrane blood flow rates [6].

Conversely, peritoneal UF depends on an osmotic pressure gradient that is exerted mostly by using a high concentration of glucose in the PD fluids. Since the concentration gradient of glucose dissipates as glucose readily diffuses from the peritoneal cavity into the blood compartment, UF is maximal at the beginning of the PD fluid dwell and decreases with ongoing dwell time [4]. UF can therefore be maximized either by using shorter dwell times and/or by using osmotic agents that diffuse poorly (such as icodextrin), so that the osmotic gradient can be maintained over a longer time. Shorter dwell times also promote UF by reducing the net volume of fluid that can be absorbed back from the peritoneal cavity. Peritoneal fluid absorption occurs constantly via the lymphatics at a rate of approximately 1–2 ml/min [7]. This rate can be increased by higher intraperitoneal hydrostatic pressures, typically by larger volumes of PD fluid in the peritoneal cavity, and also modulated by posture, with higher pressures in a supine position promoting fluid reabsorption. Other factors that affect UF include the inherent hydraulic conductance of the peritoneal membrane, determined by the density of small and ultra-small pores in the peritoneal capillaries; and the hydrostatic pressure gradient – where higher pressures in the peritoneal capillaries (compared to intraperitoneal pressures) and lower oncotic pressures, as in hypoalbuminaemia, favour UF [4].

The movement of water and solute molecules across the peritoneum in PD occurs through pores of three different sizes: large, small, and ultra-small pores. The large pores, which are 10–20 nm and make up <0.01% of the total pores, are formed by clefts between the endothelial cells and account for <10% of the total solute removal. The much more numerous small pores, which range from 4 to 6 nm in diameter, are also formed by clefts between the endothelial cells. The small pores account for >90% of solute removal and 50% of water removal as well. The ultra-small pores, which are composed mainly of aquaporin-1 (AQP1) and are 0.4–0.6 nm, are transcellular channels that help with osmotically mediated water transport only. These channels are responsible for approximately 50% of water movement [4, 5]. Water transport across the AQP1s is free of electrolytes, as opposed to that occurring via the paracellular pathways, accounting for the sieving coefficient of 50% for sodium. AQP1 is therefore a potential therapeutic target for promoting UF in patients on PD [5].

Diffusion and UF are intimately related to the patient's individual peritoneal membrane characteristics. These characteristics can be measured in clinical practice by the Peritoneal Equilibration Test (PET) [4]. This measures the equilibration ratios between dialysate and plasma (D/P) creatinine over time on a standardized PD exchange, but can also measure these ratios for other solutes such as urea and sodium. Concentrations of these solutes during an exchange are dependent on both diffusion and UF, so the equilibration ratios measure the net effect of both these processes. A standardized PET utilizes an exchange with 2L of 2.5% dextrose-containing PD fluid, with samples taken at 0, 2, and 4 hours into the exchange. These results are plotted on a graph to indicate the individual's peritoneal membrane characteristics. These are classified into four categories: high, high-

average, low-average, and low transport status. During the PET, net UF during the standardized exchange is also assessed, with the ratio of dialysate glucose at 4 hours to the dialysate glucose at time 0 (D/D_0), as an indicator of net glucose absorption during an exchange [7].

Individuals with high peritoneal membrane transport status achieve more rapid and complete equilibration of solutes because of their higher peritoneal membrane permeability, leading to better solute clearances [5]. However, they also have more rapid diffusion of glucose from the dialysate into the blood compartment, which causes rapid loss of the osmotic gradient, which in turn leads to compromised UF volumes. Therefore, individuals with a high transport status do better with short dwell times to maximize UF, without appreciable loss in solute clearances. On the other hand, individuals with low peritoneal membrane transport status, who have slow and incomplete equilibration of solutes, have poorer solute clearances but better UF, as their osmotic gradient is maintained for longer because of the slower absorption of dialysate glucose. These patients do better with longer dwell times and higher dwell volumes to maximize diffusion, without an appreciable loss of UF.

Delivery of Peritoneal Dialysis

Despite the relatively complex physiology and principles, the actual delivery of PD is quite simple and requires minimal apparatus or expertise. In patients with AKI requiring short-term PD, a stiff PD catheter is typically inserted blindly and percutaneously under a local anaesthetic using the Seldinger technique [4, 8]. This is especially useful for rapidly initiating dialysis in a resource-constrained setting [9].

In patients with ESRD requiring chronic PD, the more pliable silicone or polyurethane PD catheter is inserted either surgically, laparoscopically or percutaneously, depending on the availability of local expertise. These catheters have numerous side holes and are either straight or coiled at the peritoneal end [10, 11]. The prototype Tenckhoff catheter usually has two Dacron cuffs. The distal cuff is anchored to the rectus sheath and the catheter is brought out though a subcutaneous tunnel, with the proximal cuff in the subcutaneous tissues approximately 2 cm below the exit site (Figure 19.1). The Dacron cuffs provoke a local inflammatory reaction with granulation and fibrosis, so that the distal cuff assists in fixing the catheter and the proximal cuff prevents pericatheter

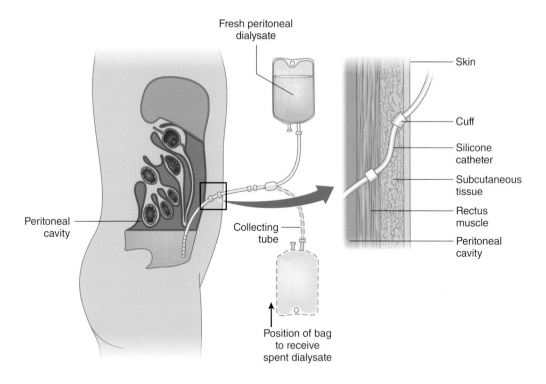

Figure 19.1 Delivery of peritoneal dialysis (PD) and position of PD catheter.

migration of bacteria into the subcutaneous tunnel and the peritoneum [4]. A number of modifications to the prototype have been made over the years, including a single cuff, a swan-neck bend between the two Dacron cuffs and a coiled intraperitoneal segment or a disc at the end of the intraperitoneal segment. A recent systematic review and meta-analysis examined the influence of PD catheter types on catheter survival rates and found no differences in straight versus swan-neck and single versus double-cuffed catheters [11]. However, catheter survivals were better with catheters with a straight intraperitoneal segment, compared to a coiled intraperitoneal segment [11]. The stiff PD catheters inserted percutaneously for short-term PD have purse-string sutures at the exit site to prevent pericatheter leakage of PD fluid and can be used immediately for conducting PD exchanges. The Tenckhoff catheters for chronic PD are typically left in place for at least two weeks, to allow healing of the surgical sites and prevent pericatheter leakage before PD exchanges can be commenced [7].

Once PD is initiated, hyperosmotic sterile fluids are exchanged within the peritoneal cavity using the twin-bag and Y-set systems, which have been shown to reduce the risk of peritonitis [12]. Standard PD fluids contain sterile water with electrolytes, lactate

(which is converted to bicarbonate in vivo to act as a buffer to treat uraemic acidosis) and glucose (which acts as an osmotic agent to promote UF) [4]. Heat sterilization of the dextrose-based PD fluid leads to the formation of advanced glycation end products and glucose degradation products (GDPs), which can have deleterious effects on the peritoneal membrane with long-term exposure [4]. GDPs play a critical role in protein glycosylation, resulting in mesothelial cell death, neoangiogenesis, and peritoneal membrane inflammation, which can compromise peritoneal membrane integrity [13]. Glucose absorption during PD also leads to adverse metabolic effects, including weight gain, insulin resistance, hyperlipidaemia, and worsening glycaemic control in diabetics [4]. The latter effects could be minimized by using PD fluids with non-glucose osmotic agents such as icodextrin and amino acids.

Non-Glucose-Containing Peritoneal Dialysis Fluids

Icodextrin is a mixture of relatively inert, high molecular weight polymaltose glucose macromolecule polymers [14] that induce transcapillary UF across the peritoneal membrane by exerting a colloidal osmotic pressure. Icodextrin molecules are less permeable than glucose and therefore remain in the peritoneal cavity for long periods, enabling UF to occur over a longer time. For this reason, icodextrin is used in long nocturnal dwells in patients on continuous ambulatory peritoneal dialysis (CAPD) or the long-day dwells in automated peritoneal dialysis (APD). A 7.5% icodextrin-containing PD fluid provides the equivalent UF volume to a 4.25% dextrose PD fluid bag and provides no more UF than glucose for short dwells.

Use of icodextrin has been found to significantly reduce episodes of uncontrolled fluid overload compared to glucose exchanges in a large recent meta-analysis [13]. In addition, carbohydrate load per exchange is lower than with conventional dextrose-containing solutions, and therefore icodextrin is associated with a more favourable metabolic profile in both diabetic and non-diabetic patients [14, 15]. However, one of the icodextrin metabolites – maltose – may interfere with blood glucose readings from certain glucometers, as some glucometers are not specific for glucose and will read maltose as glucose, giving a spuriously elevated reading. Glucometers that use glucose dehydrogenase with pyrroloquinoline quinone (GDH-PQQ) as the reagent are therefore contraindicated in patients using icodextrin, but glucometers that use glucose oxidase, glucose dehydrogenase or flavin adenin dinucleotide reagents are safe [7]. Further, icodextrin also interferes in the measurement of amylase concentrations – amylase levels may be falsely low in patients on icodextrin-containing PD fluids who develop acute pancreatitis – leaving clinicians to depend on elevations in lipase and lactose dehydrogenase (LDH) levels to make this diagnosis [5].

Since conventional PD leads to loss of protein and amino acids into the dialysate, amino acid-based PD solutions have been developed to address this issue. These solutions contain a mixture of nine essential and six non-essential amino acids in a total concentration of 1.1%, but do not contain any glucose [7]. Since amino acids are also osmotically active, they confer the same osmotic properties and UF as dextrose 1.5% PD solutions. The use of amino-acid-containing PD fluids is limited to one exchange per day, as more frequent use can worsen metabolic acidosis and urea levels [7]. Although amino acid-based PD solutions have been documented to improve the nutritional parameters in malnourished patients on PD, there is no effect on mortality [16].

Newer Low Glucose Degradation Product, Neutral pH Solutions

Newer, 'biocompatible' dialysis solutions, with a neutral pH and lower GDP content, are thought to be more biocompatible than the conventional PD fluids

with a high GDP content [13]. These solutions minimize the generation of GDPs during heat sterilization by storing the PD solutions in multichamber bags, whereby the glucose component is separated from other electrolytes [7]. Immediately before use, the contents of the chambers are mixed, yielding a final solution with a neutral pH (6.8–7.3) and a low GDP content. A recent meta-analysis [13] reported that low-GDP PD solutions were associated with preservation of residual renal function and less inflow pain compared to conventional solutions, without any differences in technique and patient survival.

Mode of Delivery of Peritoneal Dialysis

PD can be delivered in several different regimens, either manually, or with the use of a mechanized device to conduct exchanges.

Continuous Ambulatory Peritoneal Dialysis

In CAPD, dialysis exchanges are conducted manually, by either the patient or a carer. A typical CAPD prescription consists of four exchanges a day – with fluid of the previous exchange drained first, and then fresh PD fluid instilled into the peritoneal cavity. Each fresh aliquot of PD fluid is kept inside the peritoneal cavity typically for four and six hours before it is drained at the time of the next exchange [4]. Most patients on CAPD will have a long nocturnal dwell where the PD fluid stays in the peritoneal cavity overnight (Figure 19.2). Adjustments to the PD prescription can be made by changing either dwell volumes or dwell times to optimize solute clearance and UF, although increasing manual exchanges to more than four per day is generally not tolerated by patients in the long term [7]. CAPD is ideally suited to patients with low or low-average peritoneal membrane transport status, who would benefit from the longer dwells for enhancing solute clearances, whilst also maintaining UF.

Automated Peritoneal Dialysis

Automated peritoneal dialysis (APD) refers to all forms of PD that employ a mechanized device (PD cycler) to assist in performing the exchanges. Typically, patients use the cycler to perform PD exchanges at night whilst they are asleep. Different regimens within APD include continuous cyclic PD (CCPD), nocturnal intermittent PD (NIPD), and tidal

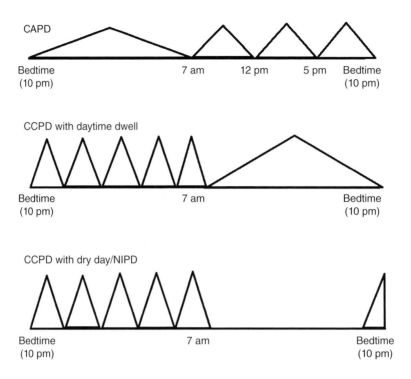

CAPD

Bedtime (10 pm) · 7 am · 12 pm · 5 pm · Bedtime (10 pm)

CCPD with daytime dwell

Bedtime (10 pm) · 7 am · Bedtime (10 pm)

CCPD with dry day/NIPD

Bedtime (10 pm) · 7 am · Bedtime (10 pm)

Figure 19.2 Common peritoneal dialysis (PD) regimens. CAPD, continuous ambulatory PD; CCPD, continuous cyclic PD; NIPD, nocturnal intermittent PD.

PD (TPD); and the cyclers can be programmed to deliver any of these dialysis regimens (Figure 19.2). Further, the cyclers can also be programmed to deliver particular dwell volumes, fill, dwell, and drain times per cycle, in addition to a last fill option for any additional daytime exchanges or dwells [4].

CCPD is a continuous automated PD regimen, which is essentially a reversal of CAPD. At bedtime, the patient connects up to the cycler machine, which drains and refills the abdomen three or more times during the night. After the last cycle during the night, the machine is programmed to deliver a final exchange of dialysate for a long daytime dwell. The patient carries PD solution in their peritoneal cavity throughout the day, and can perform a daytime exchange manually, if indicated. A typical starting volume is 10 or 12L daily, with a typical cycler time being 8–10 hours [4, 7].

NIPD is similar to CCPD, however, instead of having a daytime dwell, patients have a 'dry day', that is, there is no PD fluid in the abdomen during the day time. Because of the absence of a long-duration dwell, clearances are lower on NIPD, which may not be as much of an issue in patients with significant residual renal function or high or high-average peritoneal membrane transport status (Figure 19.2).

TPD is a regimen that maintains a volume of dialysate in the peritoneal cavity at all times. After an initial fill of the peritoneal cavity, only a portion of dialysate is drained and replaced by fresh dialysate (tidal volume), leaving a 'reserve volume' in the peritoneal cavity. TPD is useful in patients who have slow drainage or pain whilst draining PD fluid – 'drain pain' [5, 7].

The increased convenience of APD makes it more suitable for patients who have work commitments during the day; it can also be offered to patients getting burnt out from CAPD. APD is ideally suited for patients with a high or high-average peritoneal membrane transport status, since multiple short dwells during the night maximize UF volumes whilst maintaining solute clearances.

Peritoneal Dialysis Adequacy

The term 'adequacy' is often used to refer to the quantity of clearance of solutes delivered by dialysis. However, this term can also be used in a broader sense to reflect the impact of dialysis on improving patients' symptoms and enhancing well-being. Conventionally, adequacy as a measure of solute clearances is assessed by calculating the clearance of urea, a small molecular weight solute, and is represented as Kt/V_{urea} [17]. Kt/V is the clearance of urea (K) multiplied by the duration of the dialysis treatment (t, in minutes) divided by the volume of distribution of urea in the body (V, in ml), which is approximately equal to the total body water, corrected for volume lost during UF. Kt/V measurements are obtained by the 'adequacy test', which calculates the urea clearance in dialysate effluent and urine collected over 24 hours, normalized to the estimated volume of distribution of urea, as shown in Table 19.1.

Current guidelines from the International Society of Peritoneal Dialysis (ISPD) [18] aim for a target Kt/V_{urea} of at least 1.7, which is a composite of urea clearance from PD and residual renal function. Randomized controlled trials did not find any statistically significant difference in survival of patients randomized to higher Kt/V targets [19, 20]. In addition to Kt/V targets, some guidelines, including the Australian CARI Guidelines, advocate aiming for a weekly creatinine clearance (CrCl) of at least 50 L/week normalized to 1.73 m² body surface area [18]. One must be mindful that in addition to free glomerular filtration, while urea is reabsorbed by the tubules, a variable amount of creatinine is actually secreted. Consequently, preserved tubular function in those with residual renal function increases the total creatinine clearance and decreases urea clearance. Therefore, in these patients, CrCl overestimates and urea clearance (Kt/V) underestimates renal solute clearance. Current guidelines recommend performing adequacy test within six weeks of commencing PD and then six monthly [18].

Table 19.1 Calculation of Kt and V

Kt calculation

Kt (total Kt) = peritoneal Kt + renal Kt

Peritoneal Kt = 24-hour dialysate urea nitrogen content/serum urea nitrogen

Renal Kt = 24-hour urine urea nitrogen content/serum urea nitrogen

V calculation (by Watson formula)

V = 2.447 − (0.09516 × age, years) + (0.1704 × height, cm) + (0.3362 × weight, kg) in males

V = −2.097 + (0.1069 × height, cm) + (0.2466 × weight, kg) in females

Source: Adapted from Daugirdas et al. [4].

Complications of Peritoneal Dialysis

PD can be associated with several complications that can be divided into three categories: mechanical, infective, and other complications. Mechanical complications generally occur within the first few weeks or months of starting PD.

Mechanical Complications

Pericatheter Leaks

Pericatheter leak refers to leakage of dialysis fluid around the catheter exit site. This complication is usually related to catheter implantation technique, timing of initiation of dialysis, and strength of tissues in the anterior abdominal wall. When dialysis is initiated, subcutaneous leakage may occur at the catheter exit site, appearing as fluid through the incision or through the exit site itself. Delaying dialysis initiation (typically for 14 days after catheter placement) reduces the risk of developing a leak. In patients on steroids (associated with poor wound healing) or those with thin anterior abdominal walls, a longer interval between catheter placement and commencement of PD could mitigate the risk of a leak. However, if there is soakage of dressing over the exit site, a PD fluid leak can be confirmed by a positive glucose dipstick indicating high glucose concentration. Temporarily discontinuing dialysis for one to three weeks usually results in spontaneous cessation of an early leak [4, 5, 7].

Genital Oedema

Genital oedema in patients on PD could occur because of PD fluid travelling down the patent processus vaginalis to the tunica vaginalis, resulting in hydrocoele. Genital oedema could also occur due to a defect in the anterior abdominal wall, often around the PD catheter tract, from where the dialysis fluid tracks inferiorly, leading to oedema of the foreskin and scrotum or mons pubis. The defect can be diagnosed with a dye-assisted computed tomography (CT) scan, whereby Omnipaque dye is added to a bag of dialysate and then instilled in the peritoneal cavity. An alternative is nuclear medicine study with radioactive isotope added to the PD bag. Treatment involves temporary cessation of PD and surgical repair. At times, APD with low-volume dwells with the patient in a supine position (to reduce intra-abdominal pressures) can be used in the interim whilst surgery is being planned [4, 5].

Hydrothorax

Because of raised intra-abdominal pressure, the dialysate can also travel from the peritoneal cavity into the pleural cavity through a congenital or acquired defect in the hemidiaphragm. These defects are more common on the right side and patients present with a large and rapidly accumulating pleural effusion within days or weeks of commencement of PD. Thoracentesis can be performed for diagnosis and/or to relieve symptoms. The fluid is typically a transudate with a high glucose content. In addition, absence of albumin in the pleural fluid is another indicator of the pleural effusion being a result of a dialysate leak. Radionuclide scanning with technetium may be used to confirm the site of leakage. Initial treatment involves temporary cessation of PD and possible thoracentesis for symptomatic relief. Definitive treatment requires either pleurodesis or surgical repair of defects in the hemidiaphragm [4].

Delayed Fill or Drain Times

Although slow fill or drain times can be due to a multitude of reasons, constipation remains the most important contributor to poor flows. If the colon is distended with stool, this reduces the space within the peritoneal cavity or impinges on the catheter itself, preventing adequate fluid movement to and from the PD catheter. Patients on PD should aim to open their bowels daily. Other causes include catheter malposition, omental wrapping or a kink in the PD catheter. An abdominal X-ray is often useful to ascertain whether there is residual stool after laxative administration or the need for more laxatives.

In addition, an abdominal X-ray can document if a PD catheter is in the correct position within the pelvis and can pick up any kinks within the catheter [7]. A kink in the catheter or fibrin blocking the PD catheter will often cause both delayed filling and drainage times, whereas constipation, omental wrapping or malpositioning of the PD catheter will only lead to prolonged drain times [5]. If the catheter has migrated out of the pelvis and laxative therapy has not resolved the issue, the catheter can be repositioned either laparoscopically or via stiff-wire manipulation under fluoroscopy by an interventional radiologist [4, 7]. Redundant omentum occluding the distal catheter and its side holes can be confirmed on abdominal imaging with iodinated contrast injected into the catheter fluoroscopically, and surgical intervention with

omentopexy or omentectomy is generally required to reestablish catheter function. If fibrin is noted, heparin can be added to the dialysate (typically 1000 units per 2 l bag) or catheter flows can also be restored by forceful flushing of the catheter with saline. If these approaches are not successful, thrombolytics (i.e. urokinase 10 000 IU/mL suspended in normal saline administered in a volume enough to fill the catheter lumen) can be used to disrupt the fibrin clots [7].

Infusion Pain

Patients may complain of a painful sensation during the infusion of PD fluid. This often occurs in patients newly commenced on PD and is usually transient, spontaneously disappearing over several weeks. Persistent infusion pain can be due to several causes. If pain is due to the acidic pH of standard solutions (pH 5.2–5.5) from the lactate buffer, this can be eliminated by using neutral pH solutions (pH 7.0–7.4). A forceful stream of dialysate may also cause pain and is best treated by slowing the infusion rate. In addition, catheter malposition with the tip against the abdominal wall can produce inflow pain, for which catheter repositioning would be the only alternative to relieve symptoms [7].

Outflow Pain

Outflow pain is more common in new patients initiating PD. As the intraperitoneal structures siphon up to the catheter tip during the drain, the catheter contacts the sensitive parietal peritoneum. Constipation can also cause or contribute to the severity of these symptoms. Outflow pain often resolves with time or with treatment of constipation. If persistent, the use of TPD regimens with the characteristic incomplete drainage (discussed above), can minimize this symptom [7].

Hernias

The instillation of dialysis fluid in the peritoneal cavity is accompanied by an increase in intra-abdominal pressure that predisposes patients to developing hernias. Furthermore, actions such as coughing, bending or straining at stool transiently increase intra-abdominal pressure. It has been suggested that up to 10–20% of patients on PD develop hernia at some time. Pericatheter hernias need to be distinguished from pericatheter haematomas, seromas, or abscesses, and ultrasonography is often useful. Delineation of a hernia can be further aided by dye-assisted CT scan, whereby Omnipaque dye is added to a bag of dialysate and then instilled into the peritoneal cavity. The CT scan is then performed after a two-hour period of patient ambulation.

Once detected, hernias should be repaired surgically to reduce the risk of incarceration or strangulation of the bowel. After surgical repair, the intra-abdominal pressure must be minimized to facilitate wound healing, for which patients may occasionally need to cease PD temporarily and transition onto HD for a period of up to four to six weeks [4, 5]. Most of the times PD can be resumed within several days of the herniotomy, using low-volume, supine, rapid cycling PD with reinstitution of original PD regimen slowly over two to four weeks.

Infective Complications

Patients on PD can present with infections at the catheter exit site, along the catheter tunnel and/or with peritonitis. As PD is usually a home-based therapy, it is important that patients are educated about the symptoms and signs of infection and advised to seek medical attention early.

Exit-Site Infections

Patients are trained to perform exit-site care daily, wherein the exit site is cleaned with soap and water, rinsed and dried, followed by topical application of an antibiotic cream or ointment [7, 21]. The exit site is then covered with dry gauze, and the catheter is immobilized with a dressing to help avoid mechanical trauma. Many ointments and creams have been trialled for prevention of exit-site infections. Daily application of mupirocin cream or ointment has been shown to be effective in preventing exit-site infections caused by *Staphylococcus aureus* [21, 22]. Other interventions include eradication of nasal carriage of *Staph. aureus*, topical application of medicated honey or topical gentamicin cream [23, 24].

An exit-site infection is defined as the presence of purulent discharge, with or without erythema of the skin at the catheter–epidermal interface [21]. Patients are trained to inspect their exit sites daily for any evidence of infection. Common pathogens associated with exit-site infections include *Staph. aureus* and *Pseudomonas aeruginosa*. Initial empirical oral antibiotics should cover Gram-positive organisms, particularly *Staph. aureus*, and include dicloxacillin/flucloxacillin or first-generation cephalosporins for two weeks. If *Pseudomonas spp.* are the causative organism, infections can be difficult to eradicate despite using oral fluoroquinolones with or without aminoglycosides or ceftazidime and therapy should continue for at least four weeks [7, 21].

Tunnel Infections

An exit-site infection can extend along the catheter track within the abdominal wall and result in 'tunnel' infection. Patients typically present with erythema, tenderness on palpation of the catheter's subcutaneous track, and boggy induration of the area, often with a coexisting exit-site infection or peritonitis [21]. In addition, ultrasound can pick up fluid collection lining the tunnel. Tunnel infections are best treated with intraperitoneal or intravenous antibiotics for at least three weeks and, in a case of concomitant peritonitis, the PD catheter often needs to be removed.

Peritoneal Dialysis Peritonitis

Prevention

PD peritonitis is a common complication of PD, and is associated with significant morbidity, including death and hospitalization. In Australia, it is also the most common reason for technique failure, causing patients to change from PD to HD [25, 26]. Patient education is key to preventing peritonitis. Most episodes of peritonitis are due to touch contamination with some break in proper technique [7]. The concept of 'flush before fill' – drainage of a small amount of dialysate from the new PD bag into the drain bag first, to flush away any contaminating bacteria from the line, before infusion of new dialysate into the peritoneal cavity – helps in reducing peritonitis rates [27]. There is high-quality evidence to suggest that prevention of exit-site infections with topical antibiotic creams or ointments, prophylactic antibiotics at the time of PD catheter insertion and improvements in connectology with the use of Y-sets have led to a reduction in peritonitis rates [28, 29]. Gastrointestinal issues including constipation and enteritis may also increase the risk, because of translocation of bacteria across the bowel walls [7].

Pathways of Infection

PD peritonitis can be caused through the intraluminal (or touch contamination during exchanges) and periluminal (or extension from exit-site or tunnel infection) contamination; transvisceral migration from bowel source or rarely the haematogenous route [4, 7]. Peritonitis from the intraluminal route occurs most commonly because of errors in technique during making or breaking a transfer set-to-bag connection or catheter-to-transfer set connection, allowing bacteria to gain access to the peritoneal cavity via the catheter lumen. Typical organisms involved are coagulase-negative *Staphylococcus*, *Staph. aureus* or diptheroids [7]. Alternatively, bacteria present on the skin surface can enter the peritoneal cavity via the peritoneal catheter tract–pericatheter route and the organisms typically involved are *Staph. aureus* or *Pseudomonas aeruginosa*. In addition, peritonitis may occur through the bowel route in patients with enteritis, constipation or from instrumentation of the colon, such as with a colonoscopy, wherein bacteria of intestinal origin migrate across the bowel wall into the peritoneal cavity. Typical organisms involved are Gram-negative bacteria, such as *Escherichia coli*, *Klebsiella spp.*, and anaerobic bacilli. Rarely, peritonitis may occur due to bacteria seeding the peritoneum from a distant site through the haematogenous route, where typical bacteria implicated are *Streptococci* and *Staphylococci* [4].

Diagnosis

Patients present with abdominal pain which is often diffuse, along with cloudy dialysate effluent. They may also be febrile, or have nausea, vomiting, and general malaise. Patients should be educated regarding these symptoms to avoid delays in administration of intraperitoneal antibiotics. The absolute peritoneal fluid cell count in CAPD patients is usually <50 and often <10 cells/mm³ and peritoneal fluid generally becomes cloudy when the cell count exceeds 50–100/mm³. However, PD fluid can also appear cloudy from fibrin, blood, fluid being drained after a prolonged dwell period or, rarely, malignancy or chyle [7]. Therefore, for confirmation of PD-related peritonitis, the drained fluid should be sent for Gram stain, total and differential cell counts, and cultures.

For diagnosis of PD-related peritonitis, the ISPD recommends that at least two of the following three findings should be present [27]:

- Clinical features consistent with peritonitis, e.g. abdominal pain and/or cloudy dialysis effluent.
- Dialysis effluent white cell count >100/µL or >0.1 × 10⁹/L (after dwell time of at least 2 hours), with >50% of cells being neutrophils/polymorphonuclear cells.
- Demonstration of bacteria in the peritoneal effluent by Gram stain or culture.

Management

Patients on PD presenting with cloudy effluent should always be presumed to have peritonitis and be treated empirically until the diagnosis can be confirmed or excluded. Most centres have established protocols for the empirical antibiotic management of PD peritonitis based on their local microbiological profiles. These will include coverage for both Gram-positive organisms, such as a first-generation cephalosporin or vancomycin, and Gram-negative organisms, such as an aminoglycoside [27]. Unless patients have systemic signs of sepsis, intraperitoneal dosing has been found to be superior to the intravenous route, as it leads to rapid intraperitoneal therapeutic drug levels. In addition, dosing antibiotics in a single dwell is as effective as continuous dosing in all PD dwells, leading to ease of administration of antibiotics. A PD dwell containing antibiotics should dwell for at least six hours for antibiotics to be effective. Although patients are treated empirically, the dialysate culture results are still vital to determine whether alterations in antibiotics are warranted. Patients are treated for a period of two to four weeks, with length of treatment varying depending on organisms. Coagulase-negative *Staphylococci* can be treated for two weeks, whereas peritonitis due to *Staph. aureus* or *Enterococci* should be treated for three weeks. If *Pseudomonas* or *Stenotrephomonas* is the causative organism, patients should be treated with two effective agents for three to four weeks. Antifungal prophylaxis with oral nystatin or fluconazole should be commenced when patients on PD receive antibiotics to prevent fungal peritonitis [27].

Indications for Peritoneal Dialysis Catheter Removal

With effective treatment, patients should begin to demonstrate clinical improvement within 12–48 hours, and the total cell count and neutrophil percentage in the peritoneal fluid should start to decrease. Catheter removal should be considered in patients with refractory PD peritonitis, defined as PD peritonitis that is not responding to intraperitoneal antibiotics after five days. In addition, catheter removal is also indicated in patients with recurrent or relapsing peritonitis and those with polymicrobial infections, which indicate a bowel perforation. Other indications for catheter removal include fungal and tubercular peritonitis [4, 27].

Encapsulating Peritoneal Sclerosis

Encapsulating peritoneal sclerosis (EPS) is a rare but devastating complication of patients on long-term PD that ultimately results in a fibrotic cocoon encapsulating the small bowel. Its prevalence varies between 0.4 and 8.9% of patients and is associated with a 50% mortality within 12 months of diagnosis [30]. EPS is noted to develop over two phases. The early inflammatory phase is associated with vague abdominal discomfort and a change to a rapid membrane transport status. The inflammatory phase can then progress to a sclerosing phase, where a fibrotic cocoon slowly encapsulates the small bowel. The patient will generally lose weight, experience nausea and vomiting, and suffer recurrent bowel obstructions [7].

Abdominal imaging is helpful for diagnosis in the sclerosing phase, which demonstrates cocooning of the bowel, in conjunction with generalized thickening, tethering, enhancement, and calcification of the peritoneal membrane.

In the inflammatory stage, corticosteroids are the treatment of choice, while in the fibrotic stage, tamoxifen may be beneficial. In practice, distinguishing between these stages may be difficult and both are often used. In patients with established abdominal cocoon and recurrent bowel obstructions, surgery may be necessary. Patients are often transitioned to HD permanently and may require nutritional support with parenteral nutrition [7, 31].

Advantages of Peritoneal Dialysis over Haemodialysis

Residual renal function is an important factor in reducing mortality amongst patients with ESRD [5]. Beyond its contribution to small solute removal, residual renal function is also associated with a reduction in blood pressure and left ventricular hypertrophy, increased sodium removal, larger molecular weight solute clearances and maintenance of metabolic and endocrine function [32]. Multiple studies have demonstrated that residual renal function is maintained longer in patients on PD compared to those commenced on HD [19, 33–35]. Furthermore, as PD is primarily a home-based therapy, it gives patients greater flexibility with their lifestyle and saves them from visiting the hospital regularly, as in HD. Patients on PD find it easier to travel compared to those on HD. The rate of invasive-access interventions is also reduced in patients receiving PD compared to HD, partially because PD catheters are less likely to experience primary failure [36]. Patients on PD have shown more satisfaction with their care compared with patients on HD [37]. Finally, from a government financial perspective, PD is significantly more cost-effective than HD [38–40].

Contraindications and Barriers to Peritoneal Dialysis

Factors that affect an individual's eligibility for PD can be divided into contraindications and barriers. Contraindications are factors that absolutely disqualify the patient from PD, whilst barriers are factors that are associated with difficulties that can be potentially overcome if there is sufficient support available to the patient [41].

Examples of contraindications to PD include morbid obesity, large abdominal wall hernias, active diverticulitis, large abdominal aortic aneurysms, multiple previous major abdominal surgeries, and multiple abdominal wall ostomies and conduits or ventriculo-peritoneal shunts. Barriers to PD could be physical, cognitive, and psychosocial – examples of physical barriers include poor strength or dexterity, impaired vision or poor hygiene. Cognitive barriers include history of non-adherence, psychiatric illness or dementia; and psychosocial barriers include unsuitable place of residence (poor hygiene).

Assessment of PD eligibility is therefore quite complex and requires major inputs from a social worker or a PD nurse in a multidisciplinary environment. Family support or provision of paid carers (assisted PD) can often increase eligibility for PD significantly in patients with barriers to self-care [42].

Patient Survival

Studies attempting to compare mortality between patients with ESRD receiving HD and PD have shown conflicting results. The ideal study design, which should be a large randomized controlled trial, has not been possible to date because of low enrolment, partly driven by patients' preferences for one dialysis modality or the other [43]. Most mortality data is therefore drawn from observational studies, which are inevitably affected by residual confounding from possible differences in baseline characteristics amongst patients who choose PD over HD.

A meta-analysis of several large studies and recent studies [44, 45] suggests that overall, there is no significant difference in survival between patients receiving PD and HD. Data from the Australian and New Zealand Dialysis and Transplantation Registry (ANZDATA) from 2016 demonstrate that for patients on PD in Australia, one-year survival is 96% and three-year survival is 79% [25]. For patients on HD in Australia, one-year survival is 91% and three-year survival is around 70% [46]. PD tends to be associated with an initial observed survival advantage compared to HD in multiple studies [47–49]. In one study, the reduced mortality risk was present for up to three years after PD initiation [47]. This effect may be due to a selection bias, as patients referred late to therapy or those who are acutely unwell are more likely to be initiated on HD through a vascular catheter, which is associated with poorer outcomes. However, literature does seem to highlight certain differences within select subgroups of patients. Survival tends to differ depending on the age of the patient and whether they have diabetes mellitus, with PD generally being associated with equivalent or better survival amongst patients without DM and in younger patients [44, 48, 50]. The survival advantage found with PD also reduces with a longer time on dialysis [49], indicating the need to proactively transition long-term patients to HD if they are not doing well on PD.

Technique Survival

Technique survival refers to the length of time a patient remains on PD before transferring to HD, after censoring for death or transplantation. Technique survival varies considerably in different countries [5]. Technique survival at one year in patients newly commenced on PD can be up to 80% [26], with the most common causes of transfer to HD being infectious complications and mechanical catheter related complications. Non-diabetics and patients on APD, as opposed to CAPD, have a significantly higher rate of technique survival at one year [51].

References

1. Ponce, D., Balbi, A.L., and Amerling, R. (2012). Advances in peritoneal dialysis in acute kidney injury. *Blood Purif.* 34 (2): 107–116.
2. Kohli, H.S., Bhalla, D., Sud, K. et al. (1999). Acute peritoneal dialysis in neonates: comparison of two types of peritoneal access. *Pediatr. Nephrol.* 13 (3): 241–244.
3. Mishra, O.P., Gupta, A.K., Pooniya, V. et al. (2012). Peritoneal dialysis in children with acute kidney injury: a developing country experience. *Perit. Dial. Int.* 32 (4): 431–436.
4. Daugirdas, J.T., Blake, P.G., and Ing, T.S. (2015). *Handbook of Dialysis*. USA: Wolters Kluwer.
5. Khanna, R. and Krediet, R.T. (2009). *Nolph and Gokal's Textbook of Peritoneal Dialysis*, 3e. USA: Springer.
6. Ronco, C. and Clark, W. (2001). Factors affecting hemodialysis and peritoneal dialysis efficiency. *Seminars in Dialysis*: 257–262.
7. Guest, S. (2010). *Handbook of Peritoneal Dialysis*. Scotts Valley, CA: CreateSpace.
8. Tullavardhana, T., Akranurakkul, P., Ungkitphaiboon, W., and Songtish, D. (2016). Surgical versus percutaneous techniques for peritoneal dialysis catheter placement: a meta-analysis of the outcomes. *Ann. Med. Surg.* 10: 11–18.
9. Kohli, H.S., Barkataky, A., Kumar, R.S. et al. (1997). Peritoneal dialysis for acute renal failure in infants: a comparison of three types of peritoneal access. *Ren. Fail.* 19 (1): 165–170.
10. Stylianou, K.G. and Daphnis, E.K. (2014). Selecting the optimal peritoneal dialysis catheter. *Kidney Int.* 85 (4): 741–743.
11. Hagen, S.M., Lafranca, J.A., JN, I.J., and Dor, F.J. (2014). A systematic review and meta-analysis of the influence of peritoneal dialysis catheter type on complication rate and catheter survival. *Kidney Int.* 85 (4): 920–932.
12. Campbell, D.J., Johnson, D.W., Mudge, D.W. et al. (2015). Prevention of peritoneal dialysis-related infections. *Nephrol. Dial. Transpl.* 30 (9): 1461–1472.
13. Cho, Y., Johnson, D.W., Craig, J.C. et al. (2014). Biocompatible dialysis fluids for peritoneal dialysis. *Cochrane Database Systematic Rev* (3): Cd007554. https://doi.org/10.1002/14651858.
14. Szeto, C.C. and Johnson, D.W. (2017). Low GDP solution and glucose-sparing strategies for peritoneal dialysis. *Sem. Nephrol.* 37 (1): 30–42.
15. Frampton, J.E. and Plosker, G.L. (2003). Icodextrin: a review of its use in peritoneal dialysis. *Drugs* 63 (19): 2079–2105.
16. Li, F.K., Chan, L.Y., Woo, J.C. et al. (2003). A 3-year, prospective, randomized, controlled study on amino acid dialysate in patients on CAPD. *Am. J. Kidney Dis.* 42 (1): 173–183.
17. Lerma, E.V. and Weir, M.R. (2017). *Henrich's Principles and Practice of Dialysis*, 5e. Beijing: Wolters Kluwer.
18. Lo, W.K., Bargman, J.M., Burkart, J. et al. (2006). Guideline on targets for solute and fluid removal in adult patients on chronic peritoneal dialysis. *Perit. Dial. Int.* 26 (5): 520–522.
19. Paniagua, R., Amato, D., Vonesh, E. et al. (2002). Effects of increased peritoneal clearances on mortality rates in peritoneal dialysis: ADEMEX, a prospective, randomized, controlled trial. *J. Am. Soc. Nephrol.* 13 (5): 1307–1320.
20. Lo, W.K., Ho, Y.W., Li, C.S. et al. (2003). Effect of Kt/V on survival and clinical outcome in CAPD patients in a randomized prospective study. *Kidney Int.* 64 (2): 649–656.
21. Szeto, C.C., Li, P.K., Johnson, D.W. et al. (2017). ISPD catheter-related infection recommendations: 2017 update. *Perit. Dial. Int.* 37 (2): 141–154.
22. Xu, G., Tu, W., and Xu, C. (2010). Mupirocin for preventing exit-site infection and peritonitis in

patients undergoing peritoneal dialysis. *Nephrol. Dial. Transpl.* 25 (2): 587–592.

23. Chu, K.H., Choy, W.Y., Cheung, C.C. et al. (2008). A prospective study of the efficacy of local application of gentamicin versus mupirocin in the prevention of peritoneal dialysis catheter-related infections. *Perit. Dial. Int.* 28 (5): 505–508.

24. Johnson, D.W., van Eps, C., Mudge, D.W. et al. (2005). Randomized, controlled trial of topical exit-site application of honey (Medihoney) versus mupirocin for the prevention of catheter-associated infections in hemodialysis patients. *J. Am. Soc. Nephrol.* 16 (5): 1456–1462.

25. Australia and New Zealand Dialysis and Transplantation Registry (2017). *ANZDATA Registry: 39th Report.* Chapter 5: Peritoneal Dialysis. Adelaide: ANZDATA.

26. Mujais, S. and Story, K. (2006). Peritoneal dialysis in the US: evaluation of outcomes in contemporary cohorts. *Kidney Int. Suppl.* (103): S21–S26.

27. Li, P.K., Szeto, C.C., Piraino, B. et al. (2016). ISPD peritonitis recommendations: 2016 update on prevention and treatment. *Perit. Dial. Int.* 36 (5): 481–508.

28. Strippoli, G.F., Tong, A., Johnson, D. et al. (2004). Catheter-related interventions to prevent peritonitis in peritoneal dialysis: a systematic review of randomized, controlled trials. *J. Am. Soc. Nephrol.* 15 (10): 2735–2746.

29. Campbell, D., Mudge, D.W., Craig, J.C. et al. (2017). Antimicrobial agents for preventing peritonitis in peritoneal dialysis patients. *Cochrane Database Syst. Rev* (4): Cd004679. https://doi.org/10.1002/14651858.CD004679.pub3.

30. Balasubramaniam, G., Brown, E.A., Davenport, A. et al. (2009). The Pan-Thames EPS study: treatment and outcomes of encapsulating peritoneal sclerosis. *Nephrol. Dial. Transpl.* 24 (10): 3209–3215.

31. Brown, E.A., Bargman, J., van Biesen, W. et al. (2017). Length of time on peritoneal dialysis and encapsulating peritoneal sclerosis – position paper for ISPD: 2017 update. *Perit. Dial. Int.* 37 (4): 362–374.

32. Wang, A.Y. and Lai, K.N. (2006). The importance of residual renal function in dialysis patients. *Kidney Int.* 69 (10): 1726–1732.

33. Jansen, M.A., Hart, A.A., Korevaar, J.C. et al. (2002). Predictors of the rate of decline of residual renal function in incident dialysis patients. *Kidney Int.* 62 (3): 1046–1053.

34. Termorshuizen, F., Korevaar, J.C., Dekker, F.W. et al. (2003). The relative importance of residual renal function compared with peritoneal clearance for patient survival and quality of life: an analysis of the Netherlands Cooperative Study on the Adequacy of Dialysis (NECOSAD)-2. *Am. J. Kidney Dis.* 41 (6): 1293–1302.

35. Marron, B., Remon, C., Perez-Fontan, M. et al. (2008). Benefits of preserving residual renal function in peritoneal dialysis. *Kidney Int. Suppl.* (108): S42–S51.

36. Oliver, M.J., Verrelli, M., Zacharias, J.M. et al. (2012). Choosing peritoneal dialysis reduces the risk of invasive access interventions. *Nephrol. Dial. Transpl.* 27 (2): 810–816.

37. Rubin, H.R., Fink, N.E., Plantinga, L.C. et al. (2004). Patient ratings of dialysis care with peritoneal dialysis vs hemodialysis. *J. Am. Med. Assoc.* 291 (6): 697–703.

38. Ghaffari, A., Kalantar-Zadeh, K., Lee, J. et al. (2013). PD first: peritoneal dialysis as the default transition to dialysis therapy. *Sem. Dial.* 26 (6): 706–713.

39. Eriksson, J.K., Neovius, M., Jacobson, S.H. et al. (2016). Healthcare costs in chronic kidney disease and renal replacement therapy: a population-based cohort study in Sweden. *BMJ Open* 6 (10): e012062.

40. De Vecchi, A.F., Dratwa, M., and Wiedemann, M.E. (1999). Healthcare systems and end-stage renal disease (ESRD) therapies – an international review: costs and reimbursement/funding of ESRD therapies. *Nephrol. Dial. Transpl.* 14 (Suppl 6): 31–41.

41. Blake, P.G., Quinn, R.R., and Oliver, M.J. (2013). Peritoneal dialysis and the process of modality selection. *Perit. Dial. Int.* 33 (3): 233–241.

42. Oliver, M.J., Garg, A.X., Blake, P.G. et al. (2010). Impact of contraindications, barriers to self-care and support on incident peritoneal dialysis utilization. *Nephrol. Dial. Transpl.* 25 (8): 2737–2744.

43. Korevaar, J.C., Feith, G.W., Dekker, F.W. et al. (2003). Effect of starting with hemodialysis compared with peritoneal dialysis in patients new on dialysis treatment: a randomized controlled trial. *Kidney Int.* 64 (6): 2222–2228.

44. Vonesh, E.F., Snyder, J.J., Foley, R.N., and Collins, A.J. (2006). Mortality studies comparing peritoneal dialysis and hemodialysis: what do they tell us? *Kidney Int. Suppl.* 103: S3–S11.

45. Mehrotra, R., Chiu, Y.W., Kalantar-Zadeh, K. et al. (2011). Similar outcomes with hemodialysis and peritoneal dialysis in patients with end-stage renal disease. *Arch. Int. Med.* 171 (2): 110–118.

46. Australia and New Zealand Dialysis and Transplantation Registry (2017). *ANZDATA Registry: 39th Report.* Chapter 4: Haemodialysis. Adelaide: ANZDATA.

47. Kumar, V.A., Sidell, M.A., Jones, J.P., and Vonesh, E.F. (2014). Survival of propensity matched incident peritoneal and hemodialysis patients in a United States health care system. *Kidney Int.* 86 (5): 1016–1022.

48. Heaf, J.G. and Wehberg, S. (2014). Relative survival of peritoneal dialysis and haemodialysis patients: effect of cohort and mode of dialysis initiation. *PLoS One* 9 (3): e90119.

49. Liem, Y.S., Wong, J.B., Hunink, M.G. et al. (2007). Comparison of hemodialysis and peritoneal dialysis survival in the Netherlands. *Kidney Int.* 71 (2): 153–158.

50. Yeates, K., Zhu, N., Vonesh, E. et al. (2012). Hemodialysis and peritoneal dialysis are associated with similar outcomes for end-stage renal disease treatment in Canada. *Nephrol. Dial. Transpl.* 27 (9): 3568–3575.

51. Guo, A. and Mujais, S. (2003). Patient and technique survival on peritoneal dialysis in the United States: evaluation in large incident cohorts. *Kidney Int. Suppl.* 88: S3–S12.

Questions and Answers

Questions

1. Which of the following statements pertaining to the principles of peritoneal dialysis is TRUE?
   a. Solute removal is achieved by the movement of solutes down a pressure gradient
   b. Solute removal is achieved by diffusion
   c. Ultrafiltration is achieved by movement of solvent across the concentration gradient
   d. Ultrafiltration is achieved by diffusion

2. Which of the following is NOT a factor influencing solute transport in peritoneal dialysis?
   a. Concentration gradient of the solute across the peritoneal membrane
   b. Effective surface area of the peritoneal membrane
   c. Patient position while performing peritoneal dialysis exchanges
   d. Molecular weight of the solutes

3. Which of the following does NOT significantly influence ultrafiltration in peritoneal dialysis?
   a. Increasing volume of dwell
   b. Reducing dwell times
   c. Using larger molecular weight agents in the peritoneal dialysis fluid, such as icodextrin
   d. Changing glucose concentration of the peritoneal dialysis fluids

4. Which of the following statements regarding peritoneal membrane transport status is TRUE?
   a. Individuals with low peritoneal membrane transport status should ideally be managed with automated PD
   b. Individuals with high peritoneal membrane transport status have better ultrafiltration compared to low membrane transport status
   c. Individuals with high membrane transport status should have longer dwell times
   d. Individuals with low membrane transport status have poorer solute clearances compared to high membrane transport status

5. Which of the following is NOT a risk factor for peritonitis?
   a. Use of a twin-bag and Y-set giving system
   b. Having a pet cat
   c. Living far away from a peritoneal dialysis unit
   d. Recent colonoscopy

6. Which of the following is NOT true regarding 'biocompatible' dialysis solutions?
   a. Biocompatible dialysis solutes have been designed with lower glucose degradation product content
   b. Biocompatible solutions may possibly have a renoprotective benefit
   c. Biocompatible solutions can improve patient survival
   d. Biocompatible solutions can potentially worsen uraemia

7. Which dialysis regimen is MOST preferred for a patient with pain on drainage of dialysate?
   a. Nocturnal intermittent peritoneal dialysis
   b. Continuous ambulatory peritoneal dialysis
   c. Continuous cyclic peritoneal dialysis with a day dwell.
   d. Tidal peritoneal dialysis

8. Mr. X, a 60 year-old gentleman, has been commenced on peritoneal dialysis two weeks ago. He presents with increasing scrotal oedema, but no tenderness, erythema, or penile discharge. What is the MOST appropriate next test to perform?
   a. Dye-assisted CT scan
   b. CT scan without contrast
   c. Scrotal ultrasound
   d. Abdomen X-ray

9. Mr. X's CT scan demonstrated a hernia, which was successfully repaired surgically. He has now been restarted on peritoneal dialysis for two months, but then presents with abdominal pain, a low-grade temperature, and cloudy dialysate. What is the BEST next course of action?

a. Administer intravenous antibiotics immediately
b. Take blood cultures
c. Send peritoneal dialysate effluent for a cell count, differential, and cultures and administer intraperitoneal antibiotics
d. Change the peritoneal dialysis catheter

10. Mr. X responds to the intraperitoneal antibiotics and is discharged home at Day 5 with no abdominal pain, afebrile, and with clear dialysate. Unfortunately, he re-presents two weeks later with more abdominal pain and cloudy dialysate again. In this clinical context, what is the MOST CONCERNING differential diagnosis?

a. Relapse of PD peritonitis
b. Fungal peritonitis
c. Bowel perforation
d. Chyloperitoneum

Answers

1. b. Removal of solutes in peritoneal dialysis is achieved by the process of diffusion – the movement of solutes across the semipermeable membrane down a concentration gradient, from an area of higher concentration to lower concentration.

2. c. Patient position does not influence solute transport in peritoneal dialysis.

3. a. Increasing volume of the dwell primarily will increase solute clearance, rather than increasing ultrafiltration, as ultrafiltration depends on the osmotic pressure gradient. The osmotic pressure gradient can be increased by using icodextrin or higher concentration glucose dialysate. Because over time, the glucose diffuses from the peritoneal cavity into the blood component, the osmotic pressure gradient is usually maximal at the beginning of a dwell (for conventional glucose-based dialysis solutions), and the ultrafiltration rate is maximal at the beginning of a dwell. Therefore, shortening dwell times will increase the amount of ultrafiltration achieved.

4. d. Individuals with low membrane transport status have slow and incomplete equilibration of solutes across the peritoneal membrane, and therefore they clear the solutes more poorly. On the other hand, they have better ultrafiltration because their osmotic gradient is maintained for longer because of slower absorption of dialysate glucose. These individuals are better managed with longer dwells, with CAPD, as this allows more time for equilibration of solutes across the membrane and subsequent solute removal.

5. a. Use of a twin-bag and Y-set giving system has been shown to reduce risk of PD peritonitis.

6. c. Biocompatible solutions have not been shown to improve patient survival, although they have been shown to significantly delay time to anuria, suggesting a possible renoprotective benefit. Certain biocompatible solutions, with amino acids as the osmotic agent, may worsen uraemia and metabolic acidosis as the increased absorption of amino acids leads to increased nitrogenous waste breakdown systemically.

7. d. Tidal peritoneal dialysis can minimize pain on drainage of peritoneal dialysis solution, as patients usually experience pain right at the end of the drain. Tidal peritoneal dialysis only drains a portion of dialysate and leaves a 'reserve volume' in the peritoneal cavity, thereby reducing the pain associated with the end of the drain.

8. a. In this man, the main differential diagnoses would be a leak via the patent processus vaginalis or in the abdominal wall, or a hernia. A dye-assisted CT scan can help distinguish between these differentials. Omnipaque dye is added to a bag of dialysate and then instilled into the peritoneal cavity. The scan is then performed after a two-hour period of ambulation. If the patient has a leak, then the route of leakage can be elucidated on CT with the assistance of the dye. A nuclear medicine study, with a radioactive isotope being added to the peritoneal dialysis bag is another option.

9. c. In a patient with peritoneal dialysis presenting with cloudy dialysate, the provisional diagnosis should be PD peritonitis until proven otherwise. The most appropriate course of action would be to confirm this diagnosis by sending the peritoneal dialysis effluent for a cell count, differential, and cultures. A white cell count $>100/mm^3$, with >50% of cells neutrophils is diagnostic of PD peritonitis. The patient should be given intraperitoneal antibiotics immediately, without waiting first for the cell count for confirmation, as untreated peritonitis can lead to significant mortality and morbidity.

10. b. Fungal peritonitis is a dreaded complication with high rates of hospitalization, catheter removal, transfer to haemodialysis, and death (27). Preceding bacterial peritonitis is a significant risk factor for development of fungal peritonitis (52, 53). It is for this reason that oral antifungal agents are administered at the time of PD peritonitis antibiotic treatment.

20

Renal Transplantation

Stephen McDonald, Robert Carroll, and Philip Clayton

Summary

- Kidney transplantation is the preferred method of renal replacement therapy
- Kidneys are utilized for transplantation from both living and deceased donors
- In addition to the surgical considerations surrounding retrieval of the organ and transplantation, recipients of kidney transplants require extensive medical oversight, with management of therapeutic immunosuppression and associated issues
- Compared with dialysis, recipients of kidney transplants have lower mortality and better quality of life
- However, the mortality rates amongst recipients are still substantially higher than the general population. In particular, rates of cardiovascular disease, malignancy- and infection-related deaths are substantially higher

Kidney transplantation had been discussed and considered for many years, but it was not until the 1950s that concerted surgical efforts began, with minimal success other than isolated reports of transplants between identical twins [1]. The key factors underlying the evolution of kidney transplantation were the development of dialysis therapy and therapeutic immunosuppression. The availability of dialysis allowed patients to be supported and prevented uraemic death whilst awaiting transplantation. Further, developments in immunosuppression were vital to successful allografts – transplants between non-genetically identical individuals. In the 1960s the number of transplants performed throughout the world progressively increased, with immunosuppression largely based on azathioprine (and other antiproliferative agents) and corticosteroids. Subsequent important elements to therapeutic immunosuppression were the development of antibody preparations, with earlier poly- and monoclonal preparations directed against T cells, and then more recent agents against a variety of cellular targets.

Graft and patient survival gradually improved over time but remained (by modern standards) modest until the mid-1980s, when traditional dual therapy of an antiproliferative agent and steroids was coupled with cyclosporine (a calcineurin inhibitor, CNI) which led to a marked reduction in rates of early graft loss. Following this, there has been the progressive introduction of a range of other immunosuppressive drugs, including alternative CNIs (tacrolimus), other antiproliferative agents (mycophenolate), and newer classes of maintenance immunosuppressives.

Immunobiology of Kidney Transplantation

There are four different types of transplant grafts:

- *Syngeneic*: between genetically identical individuals (such as in identical twins)

Lecture Notes Nephrology: A Comprehensive Guide to Renal Medicine, First Edition. Edited by Surjit Tarafdar.
© 2020 John Wiley & Sons Ltd. Published 2020 by John Wiley & Sons Ltd.

Table 20.1 Type and distribution of major histocompatibility complex (MHC) I and II proteins

	Human leucocyte antigen	Expression	Peptides processed	Cell interactions
MHC I	A	All nucleated cells	Intracellular, e.g. viral, tumour	CD8$^+$ T cells
	B			
	C			
MHC II	DR	Antigen-presenting cells only, i.e. dendritic cell, macrophages, and B-lymphocytes	Extracellular, e.g. bacterial products	CD4$^+$ T cells
	DQ			
	DP			

- *Allogeneic*: between genetically different individuals of the same species (most common solid organ transplants are allografts)
- *Autologous*: from an individual back to the same individual (e.g. autologous bone marrow)
- *Xenogeneic*: between individuals of different species

The genes that determine the acceptance or rejection of tissue grafts reside in a locus on chromosome 6 and are called major histocompatibility complex (MHC) or human leucocyte antigen (HLA) in humans. The protein products of these genes from the donor tissue are called MHC I or II and activate T cells in the recipient, causing the recipient's immune system to reject the graft.

Syngeneic transplant, where organs are transplanted between identical twins who have identical MHC, are readily accepted, whilst an allogeneic transplant (allograft), where organs are transplanted between MHC antigen-mismatched individuals, are inevitably rejected without the requisite use of immunosuppressive agents.

Major Histocompatibility Complex

The MHC proteins can be divided into two main classes, MHC I and MHC II. Class I MHC molecules are expressed on all nucleated cells, whilst class II are expressed only on antigen-presenting cells (APC), such as dendritic cells (DC), macrophages and B-lymphocytes (Table 20.1). MHC I binds peptides derived from proteins within the cytoplasm of cells, such as viral and tumour proteins, whereas MHC II binds extracellular peptides, such as bacterial products (internalized via phagocytosis by the APCs). The

protein-bound MHC classes I and II are then recognized and bind to CD8$^+$ and CD4$^+$ T cells, respectively, leading to T cell activation.

Immune Cells (T Cells, B Cells, and Antigen-Presenting Cells)

Immune cells can be broadly categorized into effector cells (T cells, B cells, and natural killer or NK cells) and APC (DC, macrophages, and B-lymphocytes).

T cells are derived from the thymus and are distinguished from other lymphocytes like B cells and NK cells by the characteristic T cell receptor (TCR; with co-receptor CD3) on their cell surface. The TCR can only bind and recognize antigens which are bound to MHC proteins. The surface antigens CD4 and CD8 distinguish T cells into two major subsets: T-helper cells and cytotoxic T cells, respectively. Whilst T-helper cells (CD4$^+$) can only recognize antigens bound to MHC II complexes, cytotoxic T cells (CD8$^+$) recognize antigens bound to the MHC I complex.

The other important subset of T cells is regulatory T cells (Treg), which maintain tolerance to self-antigens by downregulating the induction and proliferation of other T cells, thus preventing excessive self-immunity. Treg cells express CD4, CD25, and FOXP3, with a subset that express CD17.

NK cells are innate immune cells that recognize foreign bodies in the absence of MHC or antibodies, thus allowing for a much faster immune reaction. This is important, as viruses can prevent the expression of viral peptides on MHC to prevent being killed by CD8 T cells. NK cells provide rapid responses to viral-infected cells, acting at around three days after infection, and they play a role in antagonizing tumour cells.

B cells originate in bone marrow and have two main roles: to serve as precursors of antibody-producing plasma cells and as APCs that present MHC II-bound antigens to T cells.

B cells characteristically express the surface receptor CD20 (which can be lysed by the monoclonal anti-CD20 antibody rituximab). From the bone marrow, B cells migrate to lymphoid organs such as spleen and lymph nodes for final maturation. The B cells in the lymphoid organs can produce immunoglobulins (Ig) M and D only. B cells internalize and degrade foreign antigens and present the peptide–MHC II complex on their surfaces to follicular T-helper cells. These follicular T-helper cells express CD40L (CD 154), which serves as a necessary co-stimulatory factor for B cell activation by binding to the B cell surface receptor CD40. This leads to B cell proliferation and Ig class switching, whereby the B cells become capable of producing IgG, IgA, and IgE (rather than just IgM and IgD). The B cells thus mature into antibody-secreting plasma cells, which then travel to the bone marrow.

Memory B cells or plasma cells downregulate CD20 and are less susceptible to rituximab compared to pre-plasma cell stages of B cell development.

T Cell Stimulation

The specificity of the immune response is determined by the interaction between the TCR of a T cell and the MHC–peptide complex on the APC. However, this interaction is not enough to sustain the immune response and needs additional co-stimulation between the two cells through accessory molecules. These accessory molecules play two roles. First, they provide extra adhesive strength to keep the T cell and APC in contact and thus allow the TCR more time to attach to the MHC–peptide complex on the APC; leukocyte factor antigen 1 (LFA-1) on the T cells binding to intercellular adhesion molecule (ICAM) on the APCs is probably the best example of this. The second role of accessory molecules is to cooperate with the TCR-initiated process of ongoing T cell activation; without this role played by the accessory molecules, the initial interaction between the TCR and MHC–peptide would fail to initiate ongoing T cell activation. Probably the most potent second signals ensuring ongoing T cell clonal expansion are between CD28 on the T cell and its ligands B7-1 and B7-2 (CD 80 and 86, respectively) on the APCs. Belatacept has been used

to prevent rejection in kidney transplantation, as it binds to the co-stimulatory CD80 and CD86, preventing activation of T cells which would inevitably contribute to graft rejection [2]. CD80 and CD86 also regulate the T cell response by binding to the cytotoxic T-lymphocyte antigen-4 (CTLA-4), which inhibits T cell proliferation.

Alternatively, APCs can express negative co-stimulatory signals, such as PD-1, or in some cases not provide co-stimulation via CD40 and CD80. This can induce the development of Treg, anergic or unresponsive T cells [3]. Treg can suppress immune responses, as discussed earlier, and have been used as cellular therapy to prevent rejection in experimental models [4].

Activation Pathways and Immunosuppression

Within minutes of TCR engagement with MHC, ZAP 70, which is an associated protein of the TCR, is phosphorylated. This in turn leads to phosphorylation and activation of phospholipase CΥ1 (PLC Υ1). Activated PLC catalyses phosphatidylinositol 4, 5-bisphosphate (PIP_2) into inositol 1,4,5 triphosphate (IP_3) and diacylglycerol. IP_3 raises intracellular calcium ions (Ca^{2+}), which upon binding to calmodulin activate the phosphatase calcineurin. Calcineurin dephosphorylates nuclear factor of activated T cells (NFAT), allowing it to translocate from the cytoplasm to the nucleus. Within the nucleus, NFAT leads to multiple effects, the chief for our interest being the transcription of interleukin 2 (IL-2), a major T cell growth factor (Figure 20.1). The CNI drugs cyclosporine and tacrolimus bind to intracellular proteins cyclophilin and FKBP, respectively, leading to the inhibition of calcineurin and thus inhibit the transcription of IL-2. Without IL-2, further proliferation of T cells is inhibited.

Cell survival and/or proliferation in virtually all cells are dependent on the mammalian target of rapamycin (mTOR) pathway. Both sirolimus and everolimus bind to mTOR complex 1, which causes inhibition of the process. This has a multitude of effects on all cells, but most importantly inhibits T cell proliferation.

Both these group of drugs together with steroids and other antiproliferative agents such as azathioprine and mycophenolate can be used to downregulate recipient immune cells' effector function and therefore prevent allograft rejection [5].

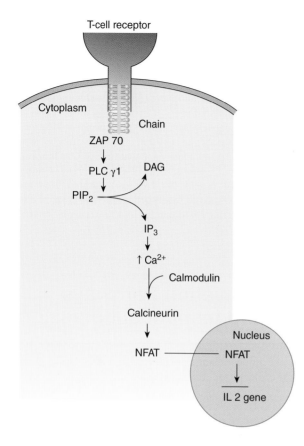

Figure 20.1 Calcineurin pathway: activation of T cell receptor (TCR) leads to interleukin 2 (IL2) production via this pathway. DAG, diacylglycerol; IP3, inositol 1,4,5 triphosphate; NFAT, nuclear factor of activated T cells; PIP2, phosphatidylinositol 4, 5-bisphosphate; PLC ϒ1, phospholipase Cϒ1.

Mechanisms of Allorecognition

T cell recognition of the donor antigen (allorecognition) is the key event in the process of allograft rejection. The following two distinct but not completely mutually exclusive pathways are involved in this process (Figure 20.2):

- *Direct pathway*: in the direct pathway the recipient's T cells recognize donor MHCs bound to donor APCs. Whilst these MHCs may have bound peptide antigens (which may be fragments of donor MHC proteins or enzymes from metabolic pathways etc.), quite often these MHCs do not have any bound peptides. This is a unique situation in the world of immunity; direct recognition of intact surface MHC molecules (without any bound peptides) by T cells has not been demonstrated anywhere outside of alloimmunity. The direct pathway of allorecognition distinguishes

(a) Direct antigen presentation

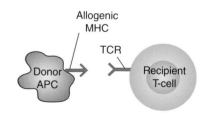

(b) Indirect antigen presentation

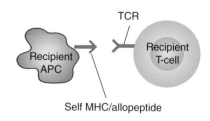

Figure 20.2 Direct and indirect pathways of antigen presentation to recipient T cells after renal transplantation. APC: antigen-presenting cell; MHC: major histocompatibility complex; TCR: T cell receptor.

alloimmunity from ordinary immunity to micro-organisms.

- *Indirect pathway*: in the indirect pathway, donor MHC molecules are shed from their cell surface, taken up by the recipient's APCs, processed and presented as peptides bound to MHC on the surface of the host APCs to T cells.

Recipient Selection

The fundamental principle of recipient selection for transplantation is patient safety. Recipients must be fit enough to have a reasonable chance of surviving the kidney transplant operation, and to have a reasonable long-term post-transplant prognosis. Furthermore, given the need for long-term immunosuppression to prevent rejection, recipients must be free from infection or malignancy and must be able to comply with their medication regimen. Given these considerations, the major contraindications for transplantation are shown in Table 20.2.

Assessment for transplantation is ideally undertaken prior to the commencement of dialysis, to allow consideration of potential preemptive transplantation from living donors. In general, patients being wait-listed for a deceased donor kidney transplant must be fitter than those being assessed for living donor kidney transplantation. This is because deceased donor transplantation is an emergency operation allowing less control over perioperative management, and additional comorbidities commonly develop during the delay between wait-listing and transplantation. Patients are reassessed intermittently and removed from the list should they be found to be no longer fit for transplantation.

Table 20.2 Major contraindications to kidney transplantation

Severe cardiac disease
Severe peripheral vascular disease
Active or recent cancer
Active infection
Consistent non-compliance with therapy
Refractory psychiatric disease

Live and Deceased Donors and Donor Selection

Transplants from living kidney donors are associated with better outcomes for a number of reasons, including better kidney function, shorter ischaemic time and greater ability to plan perioperative management. Thus, when possible, it is generally preferable from an individual perspective to receive a graft from a living rather than from a deceased donor. Also, every living donor reduces the demand on the deceased donor pool. Living donors are generally related to the recipient genetically (e.g. parent or sibling) or emotionally (e.g. spouse or friend). However, unrelated living donation can also occur from a non-directed anonymous donor or via a paired kidney exchange programme. In such a programme, two or more recipients with immunologically incompatible donors exchange kidneys that are immunologically compatible to facilitate transplantation.

Deceased donors are classified into 2 groups:

- *Standard criteria donor (SCD)*: the SCD is a donor who is under 50 years of age and has suffered brain death from any number of causes, including traumatic injuries or medical problems such as a stroke.
- *Expanded criteria donor (ECD)*: the ECD is any donor over the age of 60 years, or a donor over the age of 50 with two of the following: a history of hypertension, a creatinine greater than or equal to 1.5 mg/dl (132 µmol/L), or death resulting from a stroke. In some jurisdictions, ECD kidneys are offered to recipients on a separate list. In that situation, whilst ECD decreases the amount of time a person waits for transplant, the chances of earlier transplant loss are greater with ECD (an SCD graft has a two-year survival rate of 88% versus 80% for ECD). Candidates accepting ECD are usually older patients, have failing dialysis access or are intolerant of dialysis.

Deceased donors may have suffered brain death (donation after brain death, DBD) or circulatory failure following withdrawal of cardiorespiratory support (donation after circulatory death, DCD). Although the risk for delayed graft function (DGF) is more in DCD compared to DBD transplant, they have similar long-term outcomes [6].

Donation after Brain Death

DBD describes a donor who has primary brain death, but whose cardiac circulation and respiration remain intact or are maintained by medical measures, including mechanical ventilation or drugs. A DBD could be an ECD or SCD, depending on which criteria are fulfilled.

Donation after Circulatory Death

Previously termed non-heart beating donor or donation after cardiac death, DCD refers to the donor who does not meet the criteria for brain death, but in whom cardiac standstill or cessation of cardiac function occurred before the organs were procured. The cessation of cardiac function could have occurred spontaneously or been initiated deliberately. DCD can be either "controlled" or "uncontrolled":

- *Controlled DCD*: a donor whose life support will be withdrawn and whose family has given written consent for organ donation in the controlled environment of the operating room.
- *Uncontrolled DCD*: A donor who expires in the emergency room or elsewhere in the hospital before consent for organ donation is obtained, and catheters are placed in the femoral vessels and peritoneum to cool organs until consent can be obtained. Spain leads in the use of uncontrolled DCD transplants.

Kidney Donor Risk Index and Kidney Donor Profile Index

The Kidney Donor Risk Index (KDRI) and the Kidney Donor Profile Index (KDPI) were developed by the US Organ Procurement and Transplantation Network (OPTN) and can affect the decision about accepting or rejecting a donor kidney.

The KDRI estimates the relative risk of post-transplant graft failure and is calculated from the donor age, ethnicity, creatinine, history of hypertension or diabetes, cause of death, height, weight, hepatitis C virus status, and whether the kidney was donated after circulatory death. The KDPI is derived from the KDRI score and is the percentage of donors in a reference population that have a KDRI score less than or equal to the donor's KDRI score.

For both living and deceased donors, consideration of donor suitability includes assessing donor kidney function (ensuring the donated kidney will provide adequate graft function for the recipient), the risk of transmission of infection or malignancy (to prevent harm to the recipient) and donor–recipient

immunology (see later). Donor assessment therefore involves measuring kidney function and examining the urine, screening for transmissible infections (hepatitis B, hepatitis C, and HIV) and screening for cancer. Potential donors with a history of cancer, apart from select cancers at very low risk of transmission (for example, early non-melanoma skin cancers and primary intracerebral tumours), are usually excluded from donation.

For living kidney donors additional considerations include:

- Ability of the donor to withstand the nephrectomy procedure
- Long-term renal and cardiovascular risks to the donor following nephrectomy
- Psychological state of the donor

The perioperative mortality of living kidney donation is 3.5 per 10 000 donors [7]. Long-term risk of end-stage renal disease (ESRD) in the donor is low, but probably higher than if the donor had not donated [8]. Long-term donor risk is an evolving field and informed consent is a crucial part of the donor workup.

Surgery

Surgical management of transplants begins with the retrieval of the kidney for transplantation from the donor. There are important differences in technique between deceased and living donors. In the setting of deceased donors, techniques vary depending on whether other organs are also being retrieved. Key elements include cooling of the organs, dissection of the vessels and perfusion of the kidneys with a solution which flushes out blood and cools the organ, providing a degree of protection against ischaemic and osmotic damage. Two important concepts with regard to the time period for which the donor kidney is deprived of blood supply are:

- *Warm ischaemia time*: the amount of time an organ remains at body temperature after its blood supply has been stopped or reduced. It basically refers to the period between circulatory arrest and commencement of cold storage. With in situ perfusion techniques, the warm ischaemia time is essentially zero in DBD donors. In the case of DCD donors, a kidney may function after 60 minutes of warm ischaemia time, but the rates of delayed function and non-function increase markedly after 20 minutes.

- *Cold ischaemia time*: the amount of time an organ is chilled or cold and not receiving any blood supply.

Minimization of the length of warm ischaemia time is key to reducing the risk of DGF, as is gentle handling. Once perfused and cooled, kidneys are either placed in an ice slurry or in a mechanical perfusion device for transportation to the location of recipient transplantation surgery. In general, cold ischaemic times of 24 hours or occasionally longer are well tolerated, although the risks of DGF increase with longer cold ischaemic times.

For living donors, various techniques of laparoscopic donor nephrectomy have largely replaced the traditional open nephrectomy that was the practice in the past. This has substantial advantages for the recipient in reducing postoperative pain and length of hospital stay, with no apparent disadvantage to the recipient [9]. In general, the left kidney is preferred because of the longer renal vein and easier approach laparoscopically, unless there are local anatomical factors for medical reasons (such as discrepant kidney size) which would require use of the right kidney.

Apart from the kidney, anatomical structures that are transplanted during a deceased donor kidney transplant usually consist of the following:

- Renal artery(ies), usually with a cuff of the donor aorta
- Renal vein(s), usually with a cuff of the inferior vena cava for the left kidney or the entire inferior vena cava for the right kidney (because of the shorter right renal vein)
- Ureter, with a generous amount of periureteral tissue

In laparoscopically recovered living donor kidneys, the donor artery and vein will be inevitably shorter than with a deceased donor kidney, as the living donor vena cava and aorta are obviously not available.

Kidney allografts (whether from living or deceased donors) are usually implanted in the right or left iliac fossa in adults, in an extraperitoneal position. In that location, arterial and venous anastomoses can be performed to the recipient's iliac vessels, together with implantation of the transplant ureter into the recipient bladder. The donor renal artery is anastomosed either to the internal or external iliac artery, and the renal vein is anastomosed to the external iliac vein. The ureter is then implanted into the bladder, usually with an extravesical technique. Many surgeons prefer to stent the ureteroneocystostomy to minimize the risk of leak or stenosis and remove the stent four to six weeks later cystoscopically. The recipient's (original) kidneys are left in situ, unless there is a medical reason for nephrectomy prior to transplantation, such as symptomatic massive kidneys in a patient with autosomal-dominant polycystic kidney disease.

Anaesthetic and perioperative management of kidney transplant recipients involve a number of important challenges. Patients are generally dialysis dependent and may present to surgery in varying states of volume overload. They often have background cardiac or vascular disease as a complication of their underlying renal disease. Avoidance of hypotension and tight control of blood pressure in the operative and immediate postoperative period is crucial, as the transplanted kidney is unable to autoregulate renal blood flow.

Immunological Issues

Prior to transplantation, the immunological compatibility of donor and recipient are assessed by means of tissue typing and cross-matching. The three main tissue typing considerations are:

- *Blood group*: ABO-incompatible blood group transplantation is generally not possible for deceased donor transplantation. For living donor transplantation it may be possible depending on the level of antibody titres. This requires special pre-transplant desensitization measures such as plasmapheresis/immunoadsorption and/or intravenous immunoglobulin (IVIG) and the possible addition of adjunctive therapies (splenectomy/rituximab). Rhesus antigens are not expressed on renal grafts and are thus not relevant for kidney transplantation. Despite the initial observation of higher rates of acute antibody-mediated rejection (AMR) in desensitized ABO-incompatible transplantation, long-term graft and patient survival are comparable with those of ABO-compatible transplantation.
- *HLA match*: the degree of matching at HLA-A, -B, and -DR predicts rejection and long-term graft outcomes. However, it is now common to perform transplants with 6/6 HLA mismatches and still have generally good outcomes.
- *Presence of donor-specific antibodies (DSAs)*: these are anti-HLA antibodies generated by the recipient, acquired via pregnancy, transfusion or

prior transplant. The presence of DSAs, especially at high titres, is a strong predictor of AMR and early graft loss. Approximately 16% of patients currently on the deceased donor allograft waiting list are highly pre-sensitized to HLA, defined as ≥80% panel-reactive antibody. Either high-dose IVIG or low-dose IVIG and plasmapheresis is used to desensitize potential recipients with pre-formed HLA antibodies to ensure a successful transplant.

In addition, donors and recipients are typically cross-matched using both complement-dependent cytotoxicity and flow cytometry methods. These methods test the recipient's serum against the donor's T or B cells (thus testing whether the donor's lympho-cytes serve as a target for the recipient's serum). The presence of positive anti-donor IgG HLA antibodies in the recipient's serum is a contraindication to transplantation.

Immunosuppression is required to prevent alloim-mune rejection of the renal graft. Immunosuppression is initially intense (induction) and then reduced grad-ually to a lower, stable dose (maintenance). Induction immunosuppression typically consists of intravenous methylprednisolone and, in most cases, monoclonal or polyclonal antibodies directed at depleting T cells or interfering with their proliferation. At the same time, patients are commenced on an antimetabolite agent (typically mycophenolate, but occasionally aza-thioprine or an mTOR inhibitor) and a CNI (tacroli-mus or cyclosporin).

Maintenance therapy usually consists of oral steroids, an antimetabolite and a CNI or mTOR inhibitor; there is substantial variation in immu-nosuppressant regimens between patients and between centres. The total burden of immunosup-pression is tailored according to immune risk and the risks of infection and cancer, and the choice of drug may be affected by their different side-effect profiles (Table 20.3).

Outcomes: Graft and Patient Survival

Outcomes of transplantation are considered at many levels. The most widespread and unambiguous meas-ure is graft survival. This metric counts both loss of graft function (requiring a return to dialysis) and death of the recipient as an endpoint. The likelihood of graft survival has progressively improved over time,

with one-year graft survival now approaching 95% in many countries (Figure 20.3).

Whilst the improved early outcomes directly trans-lates to better long-term outcomes, there have been concerns that there has not been much change in the rate of graft loss after one year (illustrated in the Kaplan–Meier graph in Figure 20.4, where the lines are largely parallel after the first 12 months for more recent transplants).

There are a number of key determinants of graft sur-vival, which can be broadly divided into donor factors, recipient factors and transplant factors. Amongst donor factors, older age, and a medical (rather than traumatic) cause of death are associated with poor graft survival. Living donors (whether related or unrelated) are associ-ated with superior outcomes to deceased donor trans-plants. Of the recipient factors, older age, second or subsequent (rather than first) transplant and the pres-ence of comorbidities (especially vascular disease or diabetes) are associated with poorer graft function. The transplant factors include the degree of immunological matching. The role of ischaemic time and DGF on long-term outcomes is debated, but both are likely to have a detrimental effect.

For potential recipients, however, the key compari-son is the expectation of quantity (and quality) of life with a kidney transplant compared to that during dial-ysis therapy. Usually a comparison of two different medical therapies would be subjected to a randomized controlled trial, but this has not been practical in the setting of kidney transplantation. Simple comparisons of mortality rates (or other outcomes) between preva-lent transplant and dialysis groups are subject to strong selection bias in favour of the transplant group. Several studies have attempted to minimize this by comparing the outcomes of recipients of deceased donor trans-plants with those on the waiting list; the latter group are assumed to have met the same standards to be placed on the waiting list. Studies using this approach have consistently shown higher mortality in the trans-plant group in the first three months (corresponding to the perioperative risk), followed by a progressive fall to a longer-term mortality rate around one-quarter that of the comparators [10–12].

Importantly, the benefits of transplantation are not simply restricted to longer life. There is a substantial improvement in quality of life with release from the time and dietary restrictions arising from dialysis. Numerous studies with a variety of approaches have demonstrated improved well-being, increase in phys-ical activity and better mental health. At a functional level, this is often associated with increased rates of employment [13–15].

Table 20.3 Immunosuppressive drugs commonly used in kidney transplantation

Drug	Mechanism of action	Common side effects	Common interactions[a]
Prednis(ol)one	Multiple	Weight gain Hyperglycaemia Osteopenia Impaired wound healing	
Mycophenolate	Antimetabolite	Diarrhoea Myelosuppression	Levels increased by cyclosporine
Azathioprine	Antimetabolite	Myelosuppression Hepatotoxicity	Allopurinol dramatically increases levels and toxicity
Tacrolimus	Calcineurin inhibitor (CNI)	Nephrotoxicity Tremor Diabetes Hair loss Diarrhoea	Cytochrome (CYP) P450 interactions Levels reduced by CYP P450 inducers: • Rifampicin • Anticonvulsants (barbiturates, phenytoin, carbamazepine) Levels increased by CYP P450 inhibitors: • Non-dihydropyridine calcium channel blockers (diltiazem/verapamil) • Azole antifungals • Macrolides (except azithromycin)
Cyclosporine	CNI	Nephrotoxicity Tremor Gout Diabetes (less than tacrolimus) Hypertension Hirsutism Gum hypertrophy	As for tacrolimus
Sirolimus/everolimus	Mammalian target of rapamycin (mTOR) inhibitor	Mouth ulcers Oedema Proteinuria Myelosuppression Impaired wound healing Hyperlipidaemia Diabetes	Increase the nephrotoxicity of cyclosporine

[a]Drug interactions are common with immunosuppressive medications. Owing to the narrow therapeutic window of these drugs, the prescription of any new drug should prompt the explicit consideration of the potential for drug interactions, and therapeutic drug level monitoring is an essential practice.

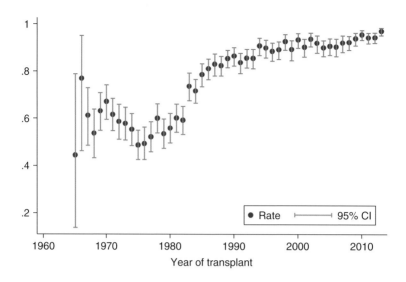

Figure 20.3 Graft survival at one year for kidney transplants performed in Australia. CI, confidence interval. ANZDATA Registry, personal communication.

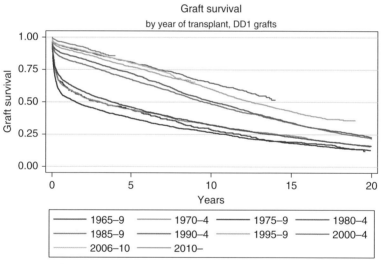

ANZDATA, all Australia & NZ deceased donor grafts, to 12/2013

Figure 20.4 Kaplan–Meier graph of graft survival for first deceased donor (DD1) kidney-only allografts in Australia, by era of transplantation (ANZDATA Registry, personal communication)

Complications

Surgical Complications

The rate of surgical complications after kidney transplantation is higher than with other procedures, as the concomitant doses of immunosuppression limit wound healing and increase the risks of infection. The clinical presentation of surgical and non-surgical complications of kidney transplantation may be similar (Table 20.4). For example, graft dysfunction may suggest rejection or a urine leak, whilst graft tenderness may suggest rejection or wound infection.

Acute vascular thrombotic events are a surgical emergency, as the viability of the kidney will be threatened by even a short period of warm ischaemia

Table 20.4 Early complications following kidney transplantation

Complication	Presentation	Investigation	Management
Transplant arterial thrombosis	Acute reduction in urine output, generally within the first 2–3 days post-transplantation, with minimal graft pain. Risk factors include hypotension, hypercoagulability, multiple-transplant renal arteries	Ultrasound (immediate) or laparotomy	Nephrectomy
Transplant venous thrombosis	Acute reduction in urine output, generally within the first week post-transplantation. Graft swelling and tenderness more prominent than in arterial thrombosis. May also be sub-acute presentation if thrombosis incomplete. Key risk factors include kinking of renal vein, hypotension, hypercoagulability, local compression (for example from a haematoma), and ipsilateral femoral deep vein thrombosis	Ultrasound (immediate) or laparotomy	Surgical exploration
Ureteric leak	Oligo-anuria; abdominal distension; increased volume of fluid through wound drain. Usually occurs during the first 2 weeks and may be due to distal ureteric ischaemia secondary to non-preservation of lower pole donor renal artery	Demonstration of collection on imaging – computed tomography (CT) or ultrasound – and on aspiration the fluid has a higher creatinine level compared with the serum creatinine	Usually surgical reimplantation
Obstructed ureter	Anuria (or oliguria from a partial obstruction). This can present as an early or late complication	Ultrasound or CT	Initially nephrostomy followed by stent placement for 4–6 weeks or surgical correction
Lymphocele	Typically occurs from 2 weeks to 6 months post-transplantation. Two types: • From donor lymphatics: collection immediately adjacent to the allograft and tendency to obstruct the proximal ureter and urine outflow to the bladder • From native lymphatics: collection distant from the transplant. May obstruct venous drainage from the leg, causing ipsilateral leg oedema	Ultrasound-guided aspiration of clear fluid with a creatinine level similar to the serum creatinine level is diagnostic (in contrast to fluid from ureteric leak or urinoma)	Depending on the size, observation, aspiration, sclerotherapy or laparoscopic creation of window into the peritoneal cavity is considered
Haemorrhage	External haemorrhage; hypotension and tachycardia; distension around transplant kidney	Haemoglobin; coagulation tests; CT/ultrasound	Depends on source and degree of haemorrhage
Wound breakdown	Wound dehiscence		Treatment of infection and control of hyperglycaemia

associated with arterial or venous thrombosis. If immediate imaging (usually ultrasound) is not available, then immediate operative exploration may be required to salvage the graft. Other diagnostic measures – increased lactate dehydrogenase (LDH), loss of perfusion on nuclear scanning – can diagnose renal infarction, but are not expeditious enough to permit graft salvation.

Infective complications of surgery are usually those of wound infection and urinary tract infection. Wound infections are particularly common after kidney transplantation, with an incidence of approximately 5%. Risk factors include obesity, diabetes, urine leak, retransplantation and use of more potent and high dose immunosuppression [16, 17].

Renal artery stenosis (RAS) is a potential complication of transplant surgery and is discussed later in the chapter.

Another late complication seen after kidney transplantation is incision hernia. The iliac fossa incision required for adequate surgical exposure is lengthy and divides multiple abdominal wall muscles. Risk factors for incisional hernia include obesity, diabetes, and postoperative wound infection [18].

Infections

Infections are more common in transplant recipients than the general population, reflecting the effects of therapeutic immunosuppression. Infections can be related to surgical complications, acquiring of healthcare-associated pathogens, reactivation of latent disease or augmented immunosuppression in graft dysfunction due to multiple episodes of acute or chronic rejection. Features of infections in the post-transplant patient include the following:

- Most infections occur in the first month and are related to technical complications of the surgery or invasive medical devices and commonly involve the genitourinary system.
- In between months one to six, infections with what are called 'immunomodulating viruses', cytomegalovirus (CMV), Epstein–Barr virus (EBV), human herpesvirus (HHV), hepatitis B virus (HBV), and hepatitis C virus (HCV), are very important. In addition to the clinical syndromes induced by these viruses, by altering the expression of cytokines and inflammatory mediators they lead to the creation of a permissive environment for opportunistic bacterial (e.g. *Listeria monocytogenes*, nocardia or toxoplasma), fungal (pneumocystis, aspergillus or *Cryptococcus*) or other viral infections.
- From six months onwards (late post-transplantation), most recipients are on minimal immunosuppressive therapy and infections in these patients are similar to those seen in the general population. However, 10–15% of these patients who are chronically infected with the immunomodulating viruses may now develop secondary clinical syndromes, such as colitis due to CMV, lymphoproliferative disorders due to EBV or chronic hepatitis from HBV or HCV.
- A minority of patients (5–15%) need higher levels of immunosuppression due to multiple acute rejections. These patients are more prone to develop opportunistic infections like pneumocystis, nocardiosis etc. (Table 20.5) associated with significant mortality and morbidity.

Table 20.5 Infections after kidney transplantation

Time	Infections
First 30 days	Typical perioperative bacterial infections: urinary tract infections, pneumonia, wound infections
1–6 months	Opportunistic bacterial infections (*Listeria monocytogenes*, *Nocardia*, *Toxoplasmosis*, and *Legionella*)
	Fungal infections (*Pneumocystis*, *Aspergillus*, and *Cryptococcus*)
	Viral infections (cytomegalovirus, Epstein–Barr virus, herpes simplex virus)
From 6 months (late post-transplantation)	Community-acquired pneumonia
	Bacterial urinary tract infections
	Opportunistic infections already mentioned (especially environmentally acquired)

- Peritoneal dialysis in the immediate pre-transplant setting is associated with higher risk of infectious complications after surgery.
- Antimicrobial prophylaxis with trimethoprim-sulfamethoxazole is given for the prevention of urinary tract infection, *Pneumocystis jirovecii* pneumonia and nocardiosis. CMV prophylaxis is indicated in most cases of renal transplant except when both donor and recipient are CMV negative.

Whilst the risks of all types of infections are increased at all stages, there is a typical pattern of risks which changes at various times (Table 20.5).

Urinary tract infections occur at a higher rate amongst kidney transplant recipients, particularly in the early postoperative period. Factors contributing to this include urethral catheterization, immunosuppression and the altered anatomy after transplantation. The transplant ureter is shorter compared to the native ureter, lacks innervation and does not have a functioning vesico-ureteric valve, leading to risk of vesico-ureteric reflux.

Infectious presentations amongst immunosuppressed recipients can often be atypical, with relatively non-specific symptoms. Given the higher rate of unusual pathogens, a low threshold is required for investigation and obtaining definitive diagnostic specimens (for example, a patient with fevers and chest infiltrates requires aspiration of the collections or bronchoscopy).

Recipients at the highest risk of viral infection are those who are seronegative at the time of transplantation and receive a seropositive graft. Acute primary EBV or CMV disease in the setting of immunosuppression can be disseminated and life threatening. Secondary disease (reactivation amongst those seropositive at the time of transplant) is generally less severe and occurs later. The risk is proportional to the degree of immunosuppression, with a particularly high rate amongst those who have received anti-CD3 antibodies.

Cytomegalovirus

CMV is a globally widespread virus and evidence of latent infection can be seen in 40–100% of the normal adult population, with higher rates in economically deprived communities. In renal transplant recipients, symptomatic disease due to CMV can be due to reactivation of latent disease or, less commonly, reinfection with a novel exogenous strain that typically occurs after the first month of transplantation.

Amongst the recipients of renal transplant patients in the USA, approximately 18% are CMV-seronegative recipients of kidneys from CMV-seropositive donors

(CMV D+/R-), 61% are CMV-seropositive recipient patients (CMV R+) and 21% are seronegative recipients of kidneys from seronegative donors (CMV D-/R-). Whilst both CMV D+/R- and CMV R+ patients are at increased risk of CMV reactivation, the higher risk is in the CMV D+/R- patients.

CMV can present in kidney transplant recipients as either CMV infection or CMV disease.

- *CMV infection*: laboratory evidence of CMV replication in blood regardless of whether signs or symptoms are present.
- *CMV disease*: defined as the presence of detectable CMV in a clinical specimen accompanied by other clinical manifestations. These clinical features are further classified as:
  - *CMV syndrome*: laboratory evidence of virus replication in blood accompanied by attributable symptoms and signs (e.g. fever, malaise, arthralgia, leukopenia, thrombocytopenia) in the absence of tissue-invasive disease.
  - *Tissue-invasive CMV disease*: demonstratation of clinical symptoms and signs of end organ disease, for example enteritis and/or colitis (commonest manifestation), hepatitis, nephritis, pneumonitis, meningitis, encephalitis, and rarely retinitis.

Serological tests are not of much use in the acute setting, as CMV-specific IgM antibodies can persist for up to six months after seroconversion, whilst CMV-specific IgG antibodies are often not detectable until two to three weeks following the onset of symptoms. Both conventional and shell viral culture techniques are limited by their low sensitivity.

CMV antigenaemia assays which detect CMV proteins (pp65) in peripheral blood leukocytes are more sensitive than cultures and have a rapid turnaround time of 24 hours. However, they have low sensitivity in patients with low neutrophil counts.

In suspected CMV amongst renal transplant patients, diagnosis is confirmed by polymerase chain reaction (PCR) for the detection of CMV DNA. Usually higher viral loads are seen in tissue-invasive CMV disease (mean baseline viral loads around 20 000 international units/ml) than in those with CMV syndrome (mean viral loads around 10 000 international units/ml).

Treatment is based on reduction of immunosuppression and antiviral therapy. Those with CMV infection (laboratory evidence of CMV) with no clinical signs and symptoms are treated with oral valganciclovir if reduction of immunosuppression does not lead to remission of viraemia within a week. Those with mild to moderate CMV disease are usually treated with oral valganciclovir. Intravenous ganciclovir is often required for those with severe CMV syndrome or tissue-invasive CMV disease. Treatment is continued until clinical signs and symptoms of CMV disease have completely resolved and there is absence of CMV viraemia in two blood PCRs performed at least one week apart. The typical duration of therapy is 21 days, but can range from 14 to 28 days or longer.

There are two approaches to the prevention of CMV infection: either routine prophylaxis (usually with oral valganciclovir or valacyclovir) or routine monitoring for evidence of viraemia with preemptive treatment. There is no definitive evidence favouring one strategy over another, however either of these strategies is superior to no treatment [19].

CMV prophylaxis is indicated in CMV D+/CMV R- pairings (highest risk), CMV D+/CMV R+ pairings, and CMV D-/CMV R+ pairings, with oral valganciclovir for periods ranging from three to six months. Essentially the only group of patients not offered CMV prophylaxis is when both donor and recipient are CMV negative.

Epstein–Barr Virus

From 90 to 95% of the adult population worldwide are seropositive for EBV. Whilst EBV is not believed to lead to acute problems with renal transplantation, an important long-term complication of EBV infection is the development of post-transplant lymphoproliferative disease (PTLD). Most cases of PTLD occur within the first post-transplant year. The more intense the immunosuppression used, the greater the risk of PTLD and the earlier it tends to occur. There is an increased risk of PTLD amongst EBV-negative recipients of EBV-positive donor organs. PTLD may present either early as a diffuse process infiltrating multiple organs, or late (5–10 years post-transplant) with more typical features of non-Hodgkin lymphoma [20].

Patients may present with non-specific symptoms or systemic signs such as fever, unexplained weight loss, fatigue, lymphadenopathy, gastrointestinal symptoms (including obstruction), hepatosplenomegaly, central nervous system symptoms or pulmonary symptoms that may otherwise not initially suggest a diagnosis of PTLD. A rising blood level of EBV viral load by quantitative PCR measurement in this clinical setting should raise concern for PTLD. Involvement of the allograft tissue can cause declining organ function, which is clinically and histologically difficult to distinguish from severe allograft rejection. Renal biopsy reveals diffuse lymphocytic infiltrate of such severity that it is difficult to visualize tubular architecture. Treatment consists of withdrawal or drastic reduction of immunosuppression. Standard chemotherapy and irradiation are of no use and the mortality rates are much higher than in standard lymphomas.

BK Virus

BK virus belongs to the polyomavirus group and prevalence rates in adults worldwide are up to 80%. It is a primary cause of tubulointerstitial nephritis; that is, BK virus nephropathy (BKVN) and the rarer ureteral stenosis [21] in renal transplant recipients and haemorrhagic cystitis in bone marrow transplant recipients. Although first described in 1971, BKVN emerged as a significant clinical problem in the mid-1990s with the advent of more potent immunosuppressive regimens [22].

BK virus normally has a predilection for renal and ureteric cells. BK-seronegative recipients who receive grafts from BK-seropositive donors seem to be at a higher risk for the development of BKVN compared to BK-seropositive recipients. Of note is that BKVN rarely occurs in the native kidneys of patients who undergo non-renal solid organ transplantation, despite similar immunosuppression.

Other risk factors for BK virus infection and disease include degree of immunosuppression, use of tacrolimus and/or mycophenolate, allograft rejection, older age, male sex, ureteral trauma, and diabetes mellitus (Table 20.6) [23].

BK viruria post-transplant is extremely common and is not necessarily associated with BKVN. It must be remembered that 20% of normal immunocompetent people have occasional viruria. In contrast, BK viraemia is a strong indicator of a risk of BKVN. Histologically, BKVN is characterized by tubulointerstitial inflammation and progressive fibrosis.

Table 20.6 Risk factors for BK virus nephropathy

BK virus-seropositive donor
Degree of immunosuppression
Use of tacrolimus and/or mycophenolate
Allograft rejection
Older age
Male sex
Ureteral trauma
Diabetes mellitus

BK virus infection progress through well-characterized stages, with initially BKV DNA detected in the urine, followed by detection in the plasma and, finally, in the kidney (i.e. BKVN). Viruria and viraemia may be detected weeks to months before there is a detectable increase in the serum creatinine, thus necessitating a need for screening and a preemptive strategy.

Patients usually present with an asymptomatic acute or semi-acute rise in serum creatinine or sometimes are diagnosed on surveillance biopsy. The onset of the disease occurs at a mean period of 10–13 months post-transplantation.

The presence of 'decoy' cells in the urine has been used as a screening tool for possible BKVN.

Transplant biopsy is required for a diagnosis of BKVN. However, because of the focal nature of early BKVN, the diagnosis may be missed on one-third of biopsies. At least two biopsies including medulla should be examined (BK has a predilection for the medulla).

A presumptive diagnosis of BKVN may be made in the absence of definitive findings on biopsy with sustained (more than two weeks' duration) urinary viral shedding and significant BK replication (plasma DNA PCR load >10 000 copies/ml) with or without kidney dysfunction.

There is no specific antiviral treatment for this condition. In the absence of strong evidence from randomized controlled trials, approaches to management are based on the reduction of immunosuppression. Other approaches (with varying levels of evidence) typically include:

- Change from tacrolimus to cyclosporine
- Introduction of mTOR inhibitor or leflunomide
- Cidofovir
- IVIG
- Fluoroquinolones

Pneumocystis Jiroveccii

Pneumocystis pneumonia (PCP) is a potentially life-threatening infection that occurs in immunocompromised individuals. Although the nomenclature for the species of pneumocystis has changed from *Pneumocystis carinii* to *P. jiroveccii*, as it was found that the former is seen in rats, the term PCP is still used because of widespread usage over the years.

The period of highest risk for PCP following solid organ transplantation is from one to six months post-operatively, particularly when prophylaxis is not given. It is also seen later in the setting of those who are maintained on higher doses of immunosuppression due to multiple episodes of acute rejection.

Acquisition of new PCP infections in humans is most likely by person-to-person spread. In the transplant patient, PCP typically presents as fulminant respiratory failure associated with fever and dry cough (in contrast to a more indolent presentation in HIV).

The typical radiographic features of PCP in HIV-uninfected patients are diffuse and bilateral interstitial infiltrates. PCP cannot be cultured and hence diagnosis depends on the microscopic demonstration of the organism in respiratory secretions. The most rapid and least invasive method of obtaining respiratory secretions is by sputum induction after inhalation of normal saline. However, the diagnostic yield of this procedure is not very high, and the patient might need bronchoscopy with bronchoalveolar lavage (BAL). PCR of BAL fluid or induced sputum can increase the diagnostic yield over conventional staining and microscopy alone.

PCP in immunosuppressed recipients can be life threatening. Treatment consists of trimethoprim/sulfamethoxazole orally in mild to moderate disease or intravenously in those with severe disease. In those with contraindication to trimethoprim/sulfamethoxazole, alternative drugs include clindamycin/primaquine, trimethoprim/dapsone, atovaquone and intravenous pentamidine.

Prophylaxis for *P. jirovecii* is routine, at least for the first six months and often indefinitely. The typical agent used is trimethoprim/sulfamethoxazole at low dose (for example three days per week [24]). Recent outbreaks in kidney transplant units have emphasized the benefit of longer-term prophylaxis [25–27].

Vaccination in Transplant Recipients

Vaccination amongst transplant recipients is an important area. In general, live vaccines should be avoided given the risk of uncontrolled proliferation in the setting of immunosuppression. These include varicella, smallpox, measles/mumps/rubella (MMR), bacillus Calmette–Guérin (BCG), and oral polio vaccines. When required, vaccination against varicella and measles should be administered prior to transplantation. Inactivated ('killed') vaccines are safe, and vaccination for influenza and pneumococcal disease should form part of the standard post-transplant care amongst immunosuppressed patients.

Diabetes Post-Transplant

Diabetes after transplantation is becoming an increasingly common management challenge. Broadly speaking, the challenge falls into two groups: the management of patients with known diabetes and the diagnosis and management of patients with new-onset diabetes after transplantation (NODAT). The latter has become increasingly common in the modern immunosuppressive era, with around 20% of non-diabetic patients developing diabetes in the post-transplant period [28]. The presence of NODAT is associated with an increased risk of graft loss, cardio-vascular disease and mortality.

The causes of deteriorating glycaemic control after transplantation are multifactorial, but the dominant one is immunosuppressive drugs, which in one analysis was estimated to account for three-quarters of the risk [29]. The key contributors are prednisolone and CNIs (tacrolimus has been shown to be a greater risk factor for NODAT than cyclosporine) [28]. The other major contributor is obesity. NODAT is associated with worsening cardiovascular risk amongst transplant recipients [30]. The average weight gain in the first 12 months after transplantation is around 4 kg. There is a 'U'-shaped relationship between weight change after transplantation and long-term outcomes. Evidence shows that excessive weight loss or weight gain is associated with poorer outcomes [31].

Blood sugar levels can often become unstable and elevated in the immediate postoperative phase due to perioperative physiological stress responses and administration of high-dose prednisolone. Management through this phase usually involves insulin infusion and supplemental intravenous fluids as required. There is some evidence that tight perioperative sugar control does have a beneficial effect on the risk of graft rejection [32], in addition to the more typical issues of wound healing and general health.

Management of diabetes in the longer-term post-transplantation (whether new onset or not) follows similar strategies to those of the general population. Minimization of immunosuppressive drug doses may be attempted where possible, but in general this approach has limited utility. The risk of catastrophic graft loss with reduction in immunosuppression outweighs the modest benefit of tight glycaemic control. There is little high-quality (i.e. randomized controlled trial) evidence to guide therapy in the post-transplant setting. All the usual oral agents can be used, following the usual modifications to account for kidney transplant function. This may limit the ability to use metformin in cases of impaired kidney function; many of the sulphonylureas have substantial renal clearance and will require dose modification. The half-life of insulin is also prolonged in people with reduced renal function.

Diet and lifestyle advice form part of standard management of diabetes amongst transplant recipients. There is clear beneficial effect of an intensive lifestyle modification programme (dietician referral, exercise programme and weight loss advice) rather than generalized lifestyle modification advice [33].

Hypertension after Renal Transplant

The following risk factors are believed to be associated with a higher incidence of post-transplant hypertension:

- Delayed and/or chronic allograft dysfunction
- Deceased donor allografts, especially from a donor with a family history of hypertension
- Presence of native kidneys
- Cyclosporine, tacrolimus and/or glucocorticoid therapy
- Increased body weight
- Renal artery stenosis (RAS)

The CNIs (cyclosporine and tacrolimus) are believed to cause hypertension by increasing both systemic and renal vascular resistance. Increased release of vasoconstrictors, particularly endothelin, has been thought to play an important role (as discussed in the section on CNI nephrotoxicity). Many physicians use a calcium channel blocker (dihydropyridine calcium channel blockers, e.g. amlodipine or nifedipine) in this setting, not only to treat the hypertension but also to potentially reverse CNI-induced vasoconstriction. One should be careful not to use the non-dihydropyridine calcium channel blockers (diltiazem and verapamil), as they are cytochrome inhibitors (CYP3A/4) and can lead to CNI toxicity by slowing down their metabolism.

It is important to identify post-transplant RAS because it is a potentially correctable form of hypertension. Although RAS can present at any time, it usually becomes evident between three months and two years post-transplant. The following are risk factors for post-transplant RAS:

- Operating techniques (such as improper suturing and trauma)
- Atherosclerotic disease
- CMV infection
- Delayed allograft function

Although direct arteriography is the gold standard investigation, Doppler ultrasonography by an experienced operator showing peak systolic velocity of ≥ 250 cm/s is diagnostic of more than 50% luminal stenosis. Both computed tomography angiography (CTA) and magnetic resonance angiography (MRA) can be useful if renal function is good. First-line treatment is usually percutaneous balloon angioplasty (with or without stenting). Whilst success rates are as high as 80%, almost 20% of patients will develop recurrent stenosis. Metallic stent placement is often helpful in those with recurrent stenosis. Surgical correction is difficult given the extensive fibrosis and scarring around the transplanted kidney. Surgery is usually considered only in patients with resistant hypertension or with proximal recipient arteriosclerotic disease. When RAS is detected in the first month post-transplant and scarring and fibrosis are less established, surgical correction is the treatment of choice.

Acute and Chronic Rejection

Rejection refers to alloimmune injury to the graft, and may be either cellular or antibody mediated, and acute or chronic. Rejection can only be definitely diagnosed by graft biopsy and histopathology. The occurrence of rejection, particularly that involving vessels – that is, vascular rejection – is associated with poorer long-term graft outcomes [34]. Over time, the frequency of acute rejection has dramatically reduced with the improvements in immunosuppression. Amongst the immunosuppressive agents, the most dramatic change was the introduction of cyclosporine, the first CNI, in the mid-1980s.

Acute rejection may occur any time after transplantation, but typically occurs within the first six months. After six months acute rejection is most often due to inadequate immunosuppression, either from non-compliance with medications or from excessive reduction in immunosuppression. Whilst very severe episodes may be marked by graft tenderness and fever, patients are mostly asymptomatic and acute rejection is detected by graft dysfunction (rise in serum creatinine) and histopathological evidence of immune-mediated injury.

Acute rejection should be suspected when patients have one or more of the following:

- New increase in serum creatinine of ≥25% from baseline *or* a serum creatinine that is higher than expected (such as in recently transplanted patients whose serum creatinine stops decreasing earlier than expected after transplantation)
- New-onset or worsening hypertension
- Proteinuria >1 g/day

Acute cellular rejection (Table 20.7) is characterized by interstitial infiltration with mononuclear cells and disruption of the tubules by the invading cells (tubulitis). Intimal or transmural arteritis can be seen in both acute cellular and antibody-mediated rejection, although it tends to be more severe in the latter. The major treatment options for acute cellular rejection include pulse corticosteroids, rabbit antithymocyte globulin (r-ATG; Thymoglobulin®), increasing baseline immunosuppression (e.g. increasing dose of tacrolimus) and, in severe or resistant cases, the use of T cell-depleting antibodies.

Acute antibody-mediated rejection is characterized by the presence of the complement split product C4d on biopsy and DSAs in serum. Biopsy features include neutrophil infiltrates of the arterial walls, mural thrombosis with intimal or transmural arteritis

Table 20.7 Differences between acute cellular rejection (ACR) and acute antibody-mediated rejection (AMR)

	ACR	**Acute AMR**
Donor-specific antibody in serum	Usually absent	Present
Tubulitis	Present	Absent
Vascular mural thrombosis and fibrinoid necrosis	Absent	Present
Neutrophil polymorphs in glomerular and peritubular capillaries	Absent	Present
C4d staining of peritubular capillaries	Absent	Present
Primary therapy	Pulse steroids, rabbit anti-thymocyte globulin, increase immunosuppression	Plasmapheresis, intravenous immunoglobulin, pulse steroids, rituximab

in severe cases. Typically, the tubulointerstitium is spared and there is no mononuclear infiltrate. The major treatment options include removal of antibodies by plasmapheresis, IVIG, pulse corticosteroids, increasing baseline immunosuppression, rituximab, and aggressive treatment of any concurrent cellular rejection. It must be remembered that cellular and antibody-mediated rejection may coexist.

Chronic rejection, also called transplant glomerulopathy or chronic renal allograft nephropathy, is the most common cause of graft failure after the first year. Under the new Banff classification, it is termed 'interstitial fibrosis and tubular atrophy' and graded mild, moderate, or severe depending upon the degree of interstitial fibrosis and tubular atrophy. Apart from the interstitial fibrosis and tubular atrophy, biopsy reveals thickened glomerular capillary walls with occasional double-contour appearance, resembling mesangiocapillary glomerulonephritis (MCGN), but without dense deposits). Peritubular capillary basement membrane splitting and lamination are seen in up to 60% of cases and are quite specific for this condition. Whilst chronic renal allograft nephropathy may also be observed in association with humoral anti-donor antibodies and the deposition of complement fragment C4d (suggesting an antibody-mediated chronic rejection), Banff 2013 recognized the entity of C4d negative antibody-mediated chronic rejection.

Prevention of chronic rejection consists of maintaining patients on triple therapy of prednisolone, CNI and an antimetabolite like mycophenolate. Treatment is difficult in established cases. The usual strategies consist of minimization/withdrawal of CNI, conversion of cyclosporine to tacrolimus and azathioprine to mycophenolate.

Calcineurin Inhibitor Nephrotoxicity

Whilst the CNIs cyclosporine and tacrolimus revolutionized the world of solid organ transplantation by prolonging graft survival, they are potentially nephrotoxic agents. CNIs can lead to both acute kidney injury (AKI), which is largely reversible with dose reduction, and chronic kidney disease (CKD), which is usually irreversible.

CNIs cause AKI by causing a dose-related and reversible vasoconstriction of the glomerular afferent arterioles, with a subsequent reduction in renal blood flow. The vasoconstriction is believed to be secondary to the following;

- Endothelial impairment, leading to reduced production of vasodilatory prostaglandins and nitric oxide (NO)

- Enhanced release of vasoconstrictors (endothelin and thromboxane)

Clinically it is often difficult to differentiate acute CNI nephrotoxicity from acute rejection. A high plasma level of CNI points to the former, but if creatinine does not trend downwards within 48 hours of ceasing the drug then an urgent renal biopsy should be performed.

CKD due to chronic calcineurin inhibitor nephrotoxicity (CIN) manifests histologically with patchy or striped interstitial fibrosis and tubular atrophy in the absence of inflammatory changes. Increased production of transforming growth factor-beta is postulated to lead to these scarring effects in the interstitium.

Whilst there has been some interest in the use of cold-water fish oil, thromboxane synthesis inhibitors, and pentoxifylline in patients with CIN, there is no known therapy to definitely reverse CKD attributed to CIN. Whilst the co-administration of calcium channel blockers has a role in minimizing CNI-induced renal vasoconstriction (as mentioned in the section on hypertension), they do not seem to have any beneficial effects on CNI-associated nephrotoxicity in the long term. The important preventive measure is to tailor the lowest possible dose of CNI for individual patients that will provide adequate immunosuppression.

CNIs are occasionally associated with thrombotic microangiopathy, which is an idiosyncratic complication and not dose related. CNIs can lead to hyperkalaemia with a mild acidosis due to type IV renal tubular acidosis. Hypophosphataemia and more commonly hypomagnesaemia from increased urinary losses may also be seen in patients on CNIs.

Delayed Graft Function

DGF refers to AKI in the immediate post-transplantation period and can be caused by donor events (either ante- or peri-mortem), warm ischaemia or traumatic handling at the time of organ retrieval, prolonged cold ischaemia or suboptimal perfusion or perioperative hypotension. Definitions vary, but the most common one is the need for dialysis within one week of transplantation. The incidence of DGF is higher in ECD allografts. The occurrence of DGF is associated with substantial short-term morbidity and prolongation of hospitalization, as well as poorer long-term outcomes [35].

Late Graft Loss

The function of a transplant kidney is closely related to its long-term outcomes, and deteriorating transplant function (defined as a progressive increase in serum creatinine concentration over time) is a strong marker for graft loss and increased mortality.

There are many causes of late graft loss, including:

- Recurrence of primary renal disease
- Chronic allograft nephropathy
- Repeated episodes of acute rejection
- Drug toxicity
- BKVN

In addition, the various causes of acute graft loss (including arterial, venous and ureteric problems) may also occur later, albeit less frequently.

Investigation in the setting of progressive graft loss would usually involve checking serum and urinary markers of kidney function, blood drug levels (for CNIs), as well as ultrasound imaging. A transplant biopsy may be required for a definitive diagnosis.

The risk of recurrence of primary renal disease depends on the nature of the original disease. Primary focal segmental glomerulosclerosis (FSGS), MCGN, and IgA nephropathy are the conditions which confer the highest risk for graft loss related to recurrence [36]. Some conditions (e.g. polycystic kidneys, Goodpasture's syndrome) do not recur in kidney transplants. Primary FSGS typically recurs in a florid fashion, often very early with pronounced proteinuria, and requires plasmapheresis. MCGN and IgA nephropathy tend to recur more progressively, with deterioration in graft function over a period of years marked by haematuria and proteinuria. Recurrence of IgA nephropathy is very common, with histological evidence in most grafts at five years [37]. There is some evidence that with maintenance steroids recurrence rates may be reduced [38]; however, there is no specific treatment for recurrent disease.

Chronic allograft nephropathy (discussed earlier) was in the past often attributed to chronic CNI toxicity [39]. However, it is increasingly recognized that chronic immune-mediated damage (in particular chronic antibody-mediated rejection) can also contribute to non-specific interstitial scarring, especially with more recent practice involving lower doses of CNI [40].

Cardiovascular Disease

Cardiovascular diseases are the commonest cause of death after transplantation. There are several risk factors, both classical ones (hypertension, dyslipidaemia, diabetes) and those related to transplantation (impaired kidney function and drug effects). Rates of cardiovascular mortality are however improving in transplant patients, both in absolute terms and relative to the general population [41].

Current clinical guidelines suggest using similar blood pressure and lipid targets as in the CKD population [42]. Whilst specific trials in the kidney transplant population are sparse, the prevalence of hypertension and dyslipidaemia is considerably higher amongst kidney transplant patients compared to the general population.

Cancer

Rates of cancer are increased after transplantation, with a threefold increase in overall incidence. Biologically this is related to suppression of the 'surveillance' role performed by the immune system. However, not all cancers are affected equally. Several common cancers (breast and prostate) do not have increased risk, whilst cancers associated with a virally driven aetiology (cervical carcinoma, Kaposi's sarcoma and non-Hodgkin lymphoma) have a substantially increased incidence rate [43]. Common cancers such as oesophageal, gastric, and colonic cancer are increased approximately threefold. The rates of lung cancer are also increased.

Recommendations and practice surrounding screening for cancer amongst transplant recipients vary [44]. There is some evidence that screening for colorectal cancer provides a reasonable cost–benefit ratio [45] and that conducting a screening colonoscopy in this group is safe practice [46].

Increased rates of non-melanoma skin cancer are substantial, with a predominance of squamous cell carcinomas over basal cell carcinomas (in contrast to the general population, in whom basal cell carcinomas are more common). In high-risk areas such as the state of Queensland (in Australia), half of transplant recipients develop a documented skin cancer within 20 years of transplantation. There is some evidence that this risk is affected by the type of immunosuppression, with lower rates associated with mTOR inhibitors. Unfortunately, this benefit is counterbalanced by higher rates of other complications [47].

Other Issues

Pregnancy

For women of childbearing age, one of the consequences of CKD and dialysis treatment is dramatically reduced fertility and increased rates of pregnancy-related complications. However, successful pregnancy is possible post-renal transplantation. In the absence of detailed information about the number of women attempting to conceive, reports comparing post-transplant women to the general population are subject to bias, but clearly suggest lower fertility rates [48]. Importantly, the risk of congenital malformations appears similar to the general population, although the rates of miscarriages and spontaneous abortions are increased. Similarly, the rates of preeclampsia and other pregnancy-related complications are also increased, with over half of women experiencing some form of medical complication during pregnancy [49].

Some of the relevant drugs contraindicated during pregnancy include mycophenolate, mTOR inhibitors and angiotensin-converting enzyme inhibitors or angiotensin receptor blockers [50]. Prior to pregnancy, immunosuppression regimens are usually modified to a combination of azathioprine, CNI (cyclosporine or tacrolimus), and prednisolone to minimize the risk of teratogenicity.

Kidney Transplantation in Disadvantaged Groups

The vast majority of the literature relating to kidney transplantation and outcome measures comes from the developed world. Kidney transplantation also serves an important role in the developing world. Further, dialysis therapy has only limited availability and can present a substantial economic burden on recipients. Costs associated with kidney transplantation relate to long-term immunosuppressive therapy, and are highly variable between countries depending upon local pharmaceutical pricing arrangements. In some situations, economic incentives are offered to pursue lower-cost options that result in inferior graft outcomes (for example, use of tacrolimus for the first year only, with azathioprine and prednisolone as dual therapy in the longer term).

Special issues which can arise in this context are ensuring adequate quality and safety of practice for both donors and recipients. In general, registries and standardized outcome reporting do not exist in many developing countries, hence accurate accounts of procedures performed or outcomes are not available to inform patient decisions.

Limited availability of kidney transplants in many areas has led to the practice of 'transplant tourism'. Condemned as unethical by the Transplantation Society [51], this involves patients travelling from one country (often a wealthy, developed country) to another solely for the purpose of transplantation. Ethical concerns arise in this situation about the source of transplants, including coercion and undue financial incentives for living donors, and the use of organs from executed prisoners as deceased donors. In addition to the obvious ethical and human rights concerns, there are also reports of an increased risk of infectious complications [52].

Other groups which experience substantially higher levels of disadvantage and poor health are the indigenous people of Canada, USA, Australia and New Zealand. Although there are important anthropological differences, there are similarities between these groups, with substantially higher rates of CKD (largely attributable to diabetes). For members of these groups, there is evidence of a relative underprovision of transplantation, together with poorer outcomes [53]. There are a variety of contributors to this, including an increased prevalence of comorbidities and reduced rates of living kidney donation as well as higher rates of CKD, diabetes, and other chronic diseases apart from occasional cultural and social issues.

Kidney Transplantation Combined with Other Organs

At times, kidneys are transplanted with other organs. The most common of these is a simultaneous kidney–pancreas transplant, for recipients with type I diabetes. This offers not just the benefits of kidney transplantation, but also the opportunity to prevent or limit the development of diabetic complications, particularly retinopathy and neuropathy. Acceptance criteria for kidney–pancreas transplants are generally more limited than for kidney-alone transplants, with most centres not accepting recipients over the age of 50 years. Pancreas transplantation is usually not offered to patients with type II diabetes.

The combination of kidney and liver is the other multiple-organ transplant performed on a routine basis. Candidates for this procedure have both severe chronic liver and kidney disease. A critical part of the evaluation is determining whether the kidney failure is irreversible.

The other scenario which arises occasionally is transplantation in a patient with a previous non-renal transplant whose kidney disease is caused by prolonged use of CNIs. Heart–kidney and lung–kidney transplant combinations are examples of this.

The Future

For people with ESRD, kidney transplantation is an established and viable treatment. Whilst outcomes have improved over time, there is still considerable mortality and morbidity, partly related to the need for long-term immunosuppression. The removal of the need for immunosuppression remains a long-term goal. Theoretically this can be achieved with the induction of a state of immunological 'tolerance'. Whilst there is active work going on in this direction, achievement of this goal and translation into clinical practice remain several years away.

References

1. Tilney, N.L. (2003). Transplant: From Myth to Reality. New Haven, CT: Yale University Press.
2. Vincenti, F. (2003). Immunosuppression minimization: current and future trends in transplant immunosuppression. *J. Am. Soc. Nephrol.* 14: 1940–1948.
3. Dilek, N., Poirier, N., Hulin, P. et al. (2013). Targeting CD28, CTLA-4 and PD-L1 costimulation differentially controls immune synapses and function of human regulatory and conventional T-cells. *PLoS One* 8: e83139.
4. Edozie, F.C., Nova-Lamperti, E.A., Povoleri, G.A. et al. (2014). Regulatory T-cell therapy in the induction of transplant tolerance: the issue of subpopulations. *Transplantation* 98: 370–379.
5. Touzot, M., Soulillou, J.P., and Dantal, J. (2012). Mechanistic target of rapamycin inhibitors in solid organ transplantation: from benchside to clinical use. *Curr. Opin. Organ Transplant.* 17: 626–633.
6. Summers, D.M., Johnson, R.J., Allen, J. et al. (2010). Analysis of factors that affect outcome after transplantation of kidneys donated after cardiac death in the UK: a cohort study. *Lancet* 376: 1303–1311.
7. Segev, D.L., Muzaale, A.D., Caffo, B.S. et al. (2010). Perioperative mortality and long-term survival following live kidney donation. *JAMA* 303: 959–966.
8. Muzaale, A.D., Massie, A.B., Wang, M. et al. (2014). Risk of end-stage renal disease following live kidney donation. *JAMA* 311: 579–586.
9. Brook, N.R., Gibbons, N., Nicol, D.L., and McDonald, S.P. (2010). Open and laparoscopic donor nephrectomy: activity and outcomes from all Australasian transplant centers. *Transplantation* 89: 1482–1488.
10. Wolfe, R.A., Ashby, V.B., Milford, E.L. et al. (1999). Comparison of mortality in all patients on dialysis, patients on dialysis awaiting transplantation, and recipients of a first cadaveric transplant. *N. Engl. J. Med.* 341: 1725–1730.
11. McDonald, S.P. and Russ, G.R. (2002). Survival of recipients of cadaveric kidney transplants compared with those receiving dialysis treatment in Australia and New Zealand, 1991-2001. *Nephrol. Dial. Transplant.* 17: 2212–2219.
12. Rabbat, C.G., Thorpe, K.E., Russell, J.D., and Churchill, D.N. (2000). Comparison of mortality risk for dialysis patients and cadaveric first renal transplant recipients in Ontario, Canada. *J. Am. Soc. Nephrol.* 11: 917–922.
13. Evans, R.W., Manninen, D.L., Garrison, L.P. Jr. et al. (1985). The quality of life of patients with end-stage renal disease. *N. Engl. J. Med.* 312: 553–559.
14. Laupacis, A., Keown, P., Pus, N. et al. (1996). A study of the quality of life and cost-utility of renal transplantation. *Kidney Int.* 50: 235–242.
15. Valderrabano, F., Jofre, R., and Lopez-Gomez, J.M. (2001). Quality of life in end-stage renal disease patients. *Am. J. Kidney Dis.* 38: 443–464.
16. Humar, A., Ramcharan, T., Denny, R. et al. (2001). Are wound complications after a kidney transplant more common with modern immunosuppression? *Transplantation* 72: 1920–1923.
17. Kuo, J.H., Wong, M.S., Perez, R.V. et al. (2012). Renal transplant wound complications in the modern era of obesity. *J. Surg. Res.* 173: 216–223.
18. Smith, C.T., Katz, M.G., Foley, D. et al. (2015). Incidence and risk factors of incisional hernia formation following abdominal organ transplantation. *Surg. Endosc.* 29: 398–404.
19. Fehr, T., Cippa, P.E., and Mueller, N.J. (2015). Cytomegalovirus post kidney transplantation: prophylaxis versus pre-emptive therapy? *Transpl. Int.* 28: 1351–1356.
20. Faull, R.J., Hollett, P., and McDonald, S.P. (2005). Lymphoproliferative disease following renal transplantation in Australia and New Zealand. *Transplantation* 80: 193–197.
21. Gardner, S.D., Field, A.M., Coleman, D.V., and Hulme, B. (1971). New human papovavirus (B.K.) isolated from urine after renal transplantation. *Lancet* 1: 1253–1257.
22. Barraclough, K.A., Isbel, N.M., Staatz, C.E., and Johnson, D.W. (2011). BK virus in kidney transplant recipients: the influence of immunosuppression. *J. Transplant.* 2011: 750836.

23. Jamboti, J.S. (2016). BK virus nephropathy in renal transplant recipients. *Nephrology* 21 (8): 647–654.

24. Zmarlicka, M., Martin, S.T., Cardwell, S.M., and Nailor, M.D. (2015). Tolerability of low-dose sulfamethoxazole/trimethoprim for *Pneumocystis jirovecii* pneumonia prophylaxis in kidney transplant recipients. *Prog. Transplant.* 25: 210–216.

25. Chandola, P., Lall, M., Sen, S., and Bharadwaj, R. (2014). Outbreak of *Pneumocystis jirovecii* pneumonia in renal transplant recipients on prophylaxis: our observation and experience. *Indian J. Med. Microbiol.* 32: 333–336.

26. Mulpuru, S., Knoll, G., Weir, C. et al. (2016). *Pneumocystis* pneumonia outbreak among renal transplant recipients at a North American transplant center: risk factors and implications for infection control. *Am. J. Infect. Control* 44: 425–431.

27. Chapman, J.R., Marriott, D.J., Chen, S.C., and Macdonald, P.S. (2013). Post-transplant *Pneumocystis jirovecii* pneumonia-a re-emerged public health problem? *Kidney Int.* 84 (2): 240–243.

28. Vincenti, F., Friman, S., Scheuermann, E. et al. (2007). Results of an international, randomized trial comparing glucose metabolism disorders and outcome with cyclosporine versus tacrolimus. *Am. J. Transplant.* 7: 1506–1514.

29. Montori, V.M., Basu, A., Erwin, P.J. et al. (2002). Posttransplantation diabetes: a systematic review of the literature. *Diabetes Care* 25: 583–592.

30. Armstrong, K.A., Campbell, S.B., Hawley, C.M. et al. (2005). Obesity is associated with worsening cardiovascular risk factor profiles and proteinuria progression in renal transplant recipients. *Am. J. Transplant.* 5: 2710–2718.

31. Chang, S.H. and McDonald, S.P. (2008). Post-kidney transplant weight change as marker of poor survival outcomes. *Transplantation* 85: 1443–1448.

32. Thomas, M.C., Mathew, T.H., Russ, G.R. et al. (2001). Early peri-operative glycaemic control and allograft rejection in patients with diabetes mellitus: a pilot study. *Transplantation* 72: 1321–1324.

33. Sharif, A., Moore, R., and Baboolal, K. (2008). Influence of lifestyle modification in renal transplant recipients with postprandial hyperglycemia. *Transplantation* 85: 353–358.

34. McDonald, S.P., Russ, G.R., Campbell, S.B., and Chadban, S. (2007). Kidney transplant rejection in Australia and New Zealand: relationships between rejection and graft outcome. *Am. J. Transplant.* 7: 1201–1206.

35. Butala, N.M., Reese, P.P., Doshi, M.D., and Parikh, C.R. (2013). Is delayed graft function causally associated with long-term outcomes after kidney transplantation? Instrumental variable analysis. *Transplantation* 95: 1008–1014.

36. Briganti, E.M., Russ, G.R., McNeil, J.J. et al. (2002). Risk of renal allograft loss from recurrent glomerulonephritis. *N. Engl. J. Med.* 347: 103–109.

37. Odum, J., Peh, C.A., Clarkson, A.R. et al. (1994). Recurrent mesangial IgA nephritis following renal transplantation. *Nephrol. Dial. Transplant.* 9: 309–312.

38. Clayton, P., McDonald, S., and Chadban, S. (2011). Steroids and recurrent IgA nephropathy after kidney transplantation. *Am. J. Transplant.* 11: 1645–1649.

39. Nankivell, B.J., Borrows, R.J., Fung, C.L.-S. et al. (2003). The natural history of chronic allograft nephropathy. *N. Engl. J. Med.* 349: 2326–2333.

40. Remport, A., Ivanyi, B., Mathe, Z. et al. (2015). Better understanding of transplant glomerulopathy secondary to chronic antibody-mediated rejection. *Nephrol. Dial. Transplant.* 30: 1825–1833.

41. Pilmore, H., Dent, H., Chang, S. et al. (2010). Reduction in cardiovascular death after kidney transplantation. *Transplantation* 89: 851–857.

42. (2009). (KDIGO) KDIGO, transplant work group special issue: KDIGO clinical practice guideline for the care of kidney transplant recipients. *Am. J. Transplant.* 9: S1–S155.

43. Vajdic, C.M., McDonald, S.P., McCredie, M.R.E. et al. (2006). Cancer incidence before and after kidney transplantation. *JAMA* 296: 2823–2831.

44. Wong, G., Webster, A.C., Chapman, J.R., and Craig, J.C. (2009). Reported cancer screening practices of nephrologists: results from a national survey. *Nephrol. Dial. Transplant.* 24: 2136–2143.

45. Wong, G., Li, M.W., Howard, K. et al. (2013). Health benefits and costs of screening for colorectal cancer in people on dialysis or who have received a kidney transplant. *Nephrol. Dial. Transplant.* 28: 917–926.

46. Collins, M.G., Teo, E., Cole, S.R. et al. (2012). Screening for colorectal cancer and advanced colorectal neoplasia in kidney transplant recipients: cross sectional prevalence and diagnostic accuracy study of faecal immunochemical testing for haemoglobin and colonoscopy. *BMJ* 345: e4657.

47. Knoll, G.A., Kokolo, M.B., Mallick, R. et al. (2014). Effect of sirolimus on malignancy and survival after kidney transplantation: systematic review and meta-analysis of individual patient data. *BMJ* 349: g6679.

48. Levidiotis, V., Chang, S., and McDonald, S. (2009). Pregnancy and maternal outcomes among kidney transplant recipients. *J. Am. Soc. Nephrol.* 20: 2433–2440.

49. Hebral, A.L., Cointault, O., Connan, L. et al. (2014). Pregnancy after kidney transplantation: outcome and anti-human leucocyte antigen alloimmunization risk. *Nephrol. Dial. Transplant.* 29 (9): 1786–1793.

50. Coscia, L.A., Constantinescu, S., Moritz, M.J. et al. Report from the National Transplantation Pregnancy Registry (NTPR): outcomes of pregnancy after transplantation. *Clin. Transpl.* 2010: 65–85.

51. 2008 PitISoTTOTCbTTSISoNiITAtM (2008). The declaration of Istanbul on organ trafficking and transplant tourism. *Clin. J. Am. Soc. Nephrol.* 3: 1227–1231.

52. Babik, J.M. and Chin-Hong, P. (2015). Transplant tourism: understanding the risks. *Curr. Infect. Dis. Rep.* 17: 473.

53. Yeates, K.E., Cass, A., Sequist, T.D. et al. (2009). Indigenous people in Australia, Canada, New Zealand and the United States are less likely to receive renal transplantation. *Kidney Int.* 76: 659–664.

Questions and Answers

Questions

1. Which of the following statements regarding C4d deposition is NOT correct?
   a. C4d is a fragment of C4 produced during the classic complement activation pathway
   b. C4d deposition is known to cause antibody mediated graft rejection in renal transplantation
   c. C4d deposition is known to cause cell mediated graft rejection in renal transplantation
   d. C4d deposition is often associated with donor specific antibodies in serum

2. Which of the following drugs interacts adversely with azathioprine?
   a. Ketoconazole
   b. Diltiazem
   c. Erythromycin
   d. Allopurinol

3. Which of the following diseases recurs least commonly after kidney transplantation?

   a. Primary FSGS
   b. IgA nephropathy
   c. Goodpasture's syndrome
   d. Mesangiocapillary GN

4. Which of the following is the current definition of an expanded criteria donor?
   a. Donor over the age of 70
   b. Donor over the age of 50
   c. Donor over the age of 50 with history of hypertension
   d. Donor over the age of 50 with two of the following – history of hypertension, serum creatinine greater than or equal to 1.5 of normal value, or death resulting from a stroke

5. CMV prophylaxis postrenal transplant is not indicated in:
   a. CMV-positive donor/CMV-negative recipient
   b. CMV-positive donor/CMV-positive recipient
   c. CMV-negative donor/CMV-negative recipient
   d. CMV-negative donor/CMV-positive recipient

Answers

1. c. C4d is characteristically absent in acute cell-mediated rejection
2. d. After oral administration and absorption, approximately 90% of azathioprine is converted to 6-mercaptopurine (6-MP). 6-MP in turn undergoes further metabolism by three different pathways – two of these convert 6-MP into inactive products while the third pathway results in the production of active metabolites. The two inactivating pathways are carried out separately by the enzymes thiopurine methyltransferase (TPMT) and xanthine oxidase (XO). Allopurinol is an XO inhibitor and hence leads to increased levels of 6-MP. The other three choices are all cytochrome P450 inhibitors. Azathioprine is not a substrate for the cytochrome P450.
3. c. Primary FSGS typically recurs in a florid fashion, often very early with pronounced proteinuria and is treated with plasmapheresis. MCGN and IGA nephropathy tend to recur in a more progressive fashion, with deterioration in graft function over a period of years. Goodpasture's syndrome typically does not recur post transplantation.
4. d. The standard criteria donor (SCD) is a donor who is under 50 years of age and suffered brain death from any number of causes. This would include donors under the age of 50 who suffered from traumatic injuries or other medical problems such as a stroke. The expanded criteria donor (ECD) is any donor over the age of 60, or a donor over the age of 50 with two of the following: a history of hypertension, a creatinine greater than or equal to 1.5 of normal value, or death resulting from a stroke.
5. c. *CMV* prophylaxis is indicated in CMV-positive donor/CMV-negative recipient pairings (highest risk), *CMV*-positive donor/CMV-positive recipient pairings, and CMV-negative donor/CMV-positive recipient pairings (essentially the only group of patients not offered CMV prophylaxis is where both donor and recipient are CMV negative) with oral valganciclovir for periods ranging from three to six months.

Index

Lecture Notes Nephrology: A Comprehensive Guide to Renal Medicine, First Edition. Edited by Surjit Tarafdar.
© 2020 John Wiley & Sons Ltd. Published 2020 by John Wiley & Sons Ltd.